Hartvig Dahl Horst Kächele
Helmut Thomä (Eds.)

Psychoanalytic Process Research Strategies

With 34 Figures and 36 Tables

Springer-Verlag
Berlin Heidelberg New York London Paris Tokyo

Professor Dr. Hartvig Dahl
Department of Psychiatry, State University New York
Health Science Center, Brooklyn, N.Y., USA

Professor Dr. Horst Kächele
Professor Dr. Helmut Thomä
Universität Ulm, Abteilung Psychotherapie
Am Hochsträß 8, 7900 Ulm
Federal Republic of Germany

Printed with the support of the Breuninger-Stiftung, Stuttgart

ISBN 3-540-50521-0 Springer-Verlag Berlin Heidelberg New York
ISBN 0-387-50521-0 Springer-Verlag New York Berlin Heidelberg

Printing: Weihert-Druck GmbH, Darmstadt
Binding: J. Schäffer, Grünstadt
2119/3140-543210 - Printed on acid-free paper

Table of Contents

Part I. Towards the Objective Analysis of Psychodynamic Structures

Part II. The Evolution of Single Case Study Methods

Introduction

Hartvig Dahl

This is a book about the future that we hope will arouse the curiosity of clinicians and point a direction for researchers. It marks the surprisingly rapid evolution of psychodynamic psychotherapy research from an applied toward a basic science, and, as its title implies, describes strategies to follow rather than results to live by. It was not always thus. A quarter of a century ago the editors of two volumes of psychotherapy research reports summarized the state of the field then:

> Although there has been a great accumulation of clinical observations and experimental findings, the field has made relatively little progress. There has been little creative building on the work of others (Parloff and Rubinstein 1962).

> Psychological research generally has tended to be insufficiently additive. Research people often find it hard to keep informed of related work done on the same site and elsewhere, and therefore do not build upon each other's foundation (Luborsky and Strupp 1962).

Twenty-five years later the state has significantly changed, as we hope will be adequately illustrated (though of course not proven) by the research strategies reported here. But for many of the intervening years psychodynamic psychotherapy research has served as handmaiden to other masters, employed both in attempts to demonstrate its efficacy over untreated controls, and to show its superiority over other treatment techniques including "placebos" (see Smith, Glass and Miller 1980). The first task is widely believed to have finally been settled in favor of the good effects of any psychotherapy, but the supposed superiority of psychodynamic therapies over others has not been proven.

Given this state of affairs a significant minority of psychodynamic researchers (including most of those represented in this volume) have subtly changed their agendas and commitments. They have come to regard their true goal as not simply to ask, "Does psychotherapy do *any* good?" but rather to ask fundamental questions about the nature of psychopathology, how psychotherapy addresses the pathology, and what the effects of the treatment interventions are on the pathology. Such questions are part of the strategies of a basic science in its own right, one with its own agendas, its own coherent problems, and its own methods for solving them. Its overall strategy is aimed at three things: (1) the detailed description of an individual patient's maladaptation, (2) the identification of the nature of interventions that succeed in changing those maladaptations, and (3) the development of mini-theories to explain the relationship between (1) and (2). In the process these researchers have rediscovered some very old basic categories, namely wishes and beliefs, and they have begun to study them divorced from the polemics and politics of past applied necessity.

Most remarkable of all, given the diverse backgrounds of the researchers, during the past decade there has been a demonstrable, and, we believe, quite unplanned convergence of both strategies and tactics. Within the more limited domain of the psychodynamic tradition (read loosely, Freudian) the convergence of strategies has been ever more apparent, as is the manifest concentration on *repetitive maladaptive structures* where each of these words is becoming increasingly well defined. Moreover, as should become clear to a careful reader, there is surprising overlap in the early findings.

We hope that one unanticipated but happy result of this convergence and shift toward a basic science strategy will be that psychoanalysts and psychodynamic therapists more generally might accommodate to this fledgling science and to both the new research insights and the mini-theories designed to explain them. Ultimately (say in another quarter century) we might hope that research findings will share equal billing with published clinical reports. Researchers are not longer mainly trying to demonstrate that psychotherapy products are safe and effective. Rather, they have begun to investigate *psychic structures under conflict* in their own right – an entirely different and more fundamental goal.

****

All of the contributors to this book were among those invited to participate in July 1985 in the 8th Workshop on Empirical Research in

Psychoanalysis prior to the International Psychoanalytic Congress in Hamburg. The workshop was organized by the Department of Psychotherapy (Prof. Dr. H. Thomä, Chair), the collaborative research program # 129, "Psychotherapeutic Processes" (Prof. Dr. H. Kächele, Director) of the University of Ulm and the Psychoanalytic Institute of Ulm, and was generously supported by the Breuninger Foundation of Stuttgart.[1] Originally our plan was to produce a simple Proceedings of the Workshop. But because of other commitments and the wishes of a number of participants to expand on or revise their contributions we decided on a simple collaborative volume. And curiously, our final classification of the chapters into two Parts, (I) Towards the Objective Analysis of Psychodynamic Structures and (II) The Evolution of Single Case Study Methods, also classified the contributors into Americans and West Germans! In fact, these categories seem to reflect quite different, though complementary, research strategies in the two countries, as will become evident to the reader.

In the spirit of our postulated paradigm change we emphasize the commitment to systematic *empirical* research by including, as Chapter 2, a complete transcript of a Specimen Hour which is a source of common data (to different degrees) for six of the Chapters (3-7 and 11). In the same spirit we have given pride of place in Chapter 1 to Strupp, Schacht and Henry's discussion of a principle whose time has come, not by design, but as an implicit consequence of the paradigm shift. This principle is that the description and representation, theoretically *and* operationally, of a *patient's conflicts*, of the *patient's treatment*, and of the *assessment of the outcome*, must be congruent, which is to say, must be represented in comparable, if not identical terms. Schacht, Strupp and Henry put it this way:

> The principle of the P-T-O Congruence proposes that the intelligibility of psychotherapy research is a function of the similarity, isomorphism, or congruence among how we conceptualize and measure the clinical problem (P), the process of therapeutic (T) change, and the clinical outcome (O) (p. 7).

Their claim is that the requirement for PTO congruence differs sharply from the procedures of a traditional psychotherapy treatment study in which, for example, the *problem* is evaluated by a set of diagnostic criteria (e.g. DSM-III, SCL-90, Beck Depression Inventory, etc), the

---

[1]Not all participants in the Workshop chose to contribute chapters to this volume.

treatment is evaluated by the "therapists' adherence to specified protocols" of a particular school of psychotherapy, and the *outcome* is assessed by a composite index of the repeated initial measures, an index which often has perverse measurement properties. By contrast, when there is PTO congruence, the representation of the psychopathology explicitly focuses on what the candidates for change are and thus explicitly points to what has to change if change is to occur; then the treatment measures can be explicitly examined for their specific effects on these candidates; finally, the outcome is measured in terms of explicit changes in the original psychopathology. Thus, this is tantamount to a theory of change independent of any particular brand of psychotherapy because the problem, its treatment, and the outcome are all intrinsically defined by the assessment of the pathology.

Although Strupp et al. explicitly formulated this principle, its true origins go back to Luborsky's (1977) first representation of a patient's problem as the Core Conflictual Relationship Theme (CCRT). This theme consists of three categories of events found in the patient's "relationship episodes" told to the therapist during treatment: a Wish (W), a Response from an Other (RO), and a Response from the Self (RS); the goal was to represent one or more of the most repetitive and important CCRT's for each patient. In Chapter 6 Luborsky and Crits-Christoph illustrate this method with two CCRT's that they found in the Specimen Hour. Then in Chapter 8 Crits-Christoph and Luborsky demonstrate the natural extension of this approach with the development of a measure to assess the degree to which the therapist's interventions accurately address the CCRT and by their assessment of the patient's degree of self-understanding of his own CCRT wishes and responses. And obviously the next step (already underway) is the assessment of the fate of the CCRT itself. Thus in just over a decade one particular mini-theory of pathology has led to a complete instantiation of the principle of PTO Congruence.

This implicit strategy is well represented in Part I of this volume. It includes Strupp et al.'s *Dynamic Focus* (Ch 1), Bucci's *Frames* (Ch 3), Dahl's *Frames* (Ch 4), Hoffman and Gill's *Patient's Experience of the Relationship with the Therapist* (Ch 5), Silberschatz et al.'s *Plan Compatibility* (Ch 9), and Teller's *Frames* (Ch 11). Each of these approaches depicts the central roles of *repetition*, *structure*, and knowledge *re*-presentation, including the careful, systematic description of a patient's manifest wishes and beliefs. For example, it is clear that the logic of Strupp et al.'s Dynamic Focus is exactly comparable to

Luborsky's although the former use four predetermined categories, having differentiated RO's into Expected and Actual RO's.

On the other hand Dahl's and Teller's and Bucci's Frames differ significantly in that for them the clinical events are specific for each patient and are simply and directly classified into the everyday common-sense categories (anticipating Edelson's (1985) later advice) that make up the Frame structures. They do not use a small set of predetermined categories that are assumed to be regularly arranged in a fixed sequential structure (e.g. W, RO, RS). Instead they permit each individual structure to be determined by the repetition of particular sequences of each patient's specific events as they emerge in the narratives of the free association itself. Nonetheless it is worth noting that thus far all the events that make up these Frame structures are easily categorized as special cases of wishes and beliefs, i.e., emotions and defenses. And clearly, interventions can be judged for the degree to which they address the Frame events and structures and outcomes can be judged by the fate of the Frames themselves.

Of course it seems likely that clinicians who are used to thinking in terms of unconscious libidinal and aggressive drives and hidden defenses will not only resist the strategy of using manifest content to represent pathology, but will believe it to be deeply implausible. Such persons might well find Hoffman and Gill's focus on different categories of transference manifestations a more fitting way to represent a patient's pathology. Nonetheless it is important to note that they too have consistently and firmly rooted their scoring in the manifest data of transcripts. One does not have to agree with all of their judgments about the Specimen Hour (e.g. the basis for the analyst's intervention in paragraph 51 and/or the overall rating of 3.0 which they assign to the analyst's conduct of the hour) to applaud their efforts to systematize the description of transference phenomena. Certainly the description of the problem in terms of the transference can lead to a systematic assessment of the degree to which the analyst's interventions accurately address transference manifestations. And presumably the outcome could be evaluated by changes in the transference manifestations.

On the other hand clinicians and researchers who are hungry for new and different psychoanalytic theories might be attracted by Weiss's (1986) hypotheses of "Higher Mental Functioning" and "Unconscious Pathogenic Beliefs." Weiss has postulated that the dynamic function of the therapist's neutrality lies in its effect on the patient's ability to express warded-off and unacceptable wishes and beliefs. Thus in treatment a patient repeatedly tests a therapist to find out what it is safe to express and the degree to which the therapist's response both contradicts the patient's pathogenic beliefs and fits the patient's "unconscious plan" to change. In Chapter 9 Silberschatz, Curtis, Fretter and Kelly report on their efforts to empirically compare predictions from Weiss's theory with those derived from standard analytic theory, using both psychoanalytic and short-term psychotherapy data. Ultimately Weiss's theory requires the formulation of a patient's "unconscious plan," but Silberschatz et al. do not deal here with the complex issues involved in formulating this plan; Caston (1986) has written about the procedure and the reliabilities of formulating this plan.

To the degree to which Koenigsberg et al.'s development of a method for describing therapist's techniques with Borderline patients is based on an implicit or explicit theory of the pathology of these patients, then their approach also implies at least PT congruence. Teller's concluding chapter of Part I will be considered along with the final chapter of Part II.

In sum, there has been an impressive convergence among a group of American dynamic psychotherapy researchers in the past decade. These approaches have *all* been characterized by: (1) *Mini*, *local*, *modest* theories about the *essential* characteristics of *typical* (meaning, *recurrent*) *maladaptive structures* of *behaviors* that are reliably definable and describable. Among these are CCRT's, DF's, FRAMES, and PERT'S.

For the first time, we have *converging research definitions of psychopathology* that have been translated into relatively narrow, formalized, structural descriptions. And the power of these descriptions is that they in turn can serve as guides for clinicians to likely *specific therapeutic targets*. In other words, the research categories, derived from many different sources, may ultimately, we hope, offer practical clinical foci, instead of the traditional situation in which clinical problems have defined research foci.

****

Beginning Part II, Kächele, Thomä, Ruberg and Grünzig state that "the tape-recording of psychoanalytic sessions should by now be standard procedure for those who are prepared to undertake serious empirical research on the psychoanalytic process" (p. 179). But of course they are not blind to the fact that "the number of those who expose themselves to this procedure is still small, nearly as small as the number of those willing to engage in the careful scrutinizing of what they do when practicing psychoanalysis" (p. 179). Later they directly confront one of the central issues involved:

> When a psychoanalyst asks a patient for informed consent to make audio recordings of the analysis he explicitly or implicitly informs the patient that the boundaries of the privacy of the consulting room are extended to involve other people, known or unknown to the patient.
>
> . . . In contrast, patients undergoing supervised analyses are rarely if ever informed of the fact and the implicit extension of the boundaries of privacy that it entails. It is curious that analysts who might be very uncomfortable with the first extension, which the patient knows about, are likely to be quite comfortable with the other extension of which the patient is typically ignorant. (p. 192)

This contrast also captures a major difference of the Ulm Psychoanalytic Institute form most other Psychoanalytic Institutes, American and European, namely its extraordinary commitment to empirical research. Its members, as part of the Department of Psychotherapy of the University of Ulm, have participated in establishing a large and significant database of recorded psychoanalyses and psychotherapies, successful and unsuccessful, as well as initial interviews, etc. As Mergenthaler and Kächele document in Chapter 13, many years ago they anticipated this need and the result now is the Ulm Textbank, far and away the largest accumulation of transcribed sessions. These are all stored in a protected computer system together with sophisticated classification and retrieval programs which make them a prized resource for interested and qualified researchers throughout Europe and America. There is little question but that the Textbank is now the true prototype for others to emulate. And its usefulness to English speaking researchers will increase as transcripts in English continue to be added.

Just as a significant portion of Part I has been organized around the Specimen Hour, five chapters of Part II deal with Case B from the Ulm Textbank: Kächele et al. (Ch 12), Grünzig (Ch 14), Neudert and Hohage (Ch 15) Hohage and Kübler (Ch 16), and Leuzinger-Bohleber and Kächele (Ch 19). These innovative approaches are nowhere better illustrated than by Grünzig's use of time-series analyses to study problems of sampling in Case B. His results speak for themselves. On the one hand he shows that several computer content-analysis measures applied to four quite different samples of the psychoanalysis all gave essentially similar results when they "spanned the whole treatment." On the other hand samples of the first and second halves of the analysis gave quite different results, as one would expect if significant changes in the patient had indeed occurred.

Few psychotherapy researchers haves used sophisticated time-series-analysis techniques. This is a shame because, as Grünzig's analyses show, despite using what might appear to the uninitiated as vastly over-simplified measures, when applied to testing carefully chosen clinical hypotheses, these methods have demonstrated their ability to empirically support one hypothesis over rivals. In principle these techniques are even powerful enough to allow one to answer questions about the *causal* nature of interactions between patient and therapist. As Grünzig puts it, "Who mainly influences or follows whom? Does the patient adapt to the therapist or vice versa or neither?" These are questions we all want to answer and we owe it to ourselves and to our field to master and use these methods.

Hohage and Kübler, in developing their measure of Emotional Insight, also anticipated Edelson's (1985) advice to use commonsense categories derived from manifest contents. Indeed common sense supports their claim that "raters do not have to be clinically trained because the judgments are based on the language characteristics and not on clinical inferences" (p. 244). Using sessions from Case B they applied five scales which, taken together, are meant to capture the concept of Insight. It is worth noting that their categories of Emotional Insight and Cognitive Access strongly remind one of Bucci's Referential Activity (Ch 3), which indexes the degree to which the verbal system accesses and represents nonverbal (read *emotional* in this context) contents. They support their claim of superiority for Emotional Insight over previous scales such as Meaningfulness, Productivity, or Experiencing by showing details of the interactions between the patient and analyst in hours 1, 2, and 7, including the interactions which correspond to plots of the course of four of their scales. Clearly this is another promising tool for assessing the effects of analyst/therapist interventions.

Researchers whose results are based on transcripts of audio recordings of therapy sessions regularly expect and receive pointed questions from analysts and therapists who are skeptical of their ignoring nonverbal and other information in the treatment setting. Such clinicians may take real comfort from Krause and Lütolf's research on facial expressions during treatment. What their meticulously planned and executed study shows is that a patient's facial expressions may indeed reveal both his central conflicts and his defensive expressions, such as masking anger and disgust by smiling. Moreover, their finding that the therapist smiled at the patient almost exclusively when the patient was *not* masking anger, raises the question of the curative function of such interaction. This is surely a salutary corrective to the omissions of most of the other contributors to this book and it speaks to the importance of encouraging further similar research.

At the same time, those who are skeptical of the value of using measures of manifest contents and scaling etc. should carefully read Neudert and Hohage's study on different types and sources of suffering during psychoanalysis. Indeed their interest in this question derived from the current theoretical controversies over the function of the analyst's abstinence in psychoanalysis (cf. Silberschatz et al., this volume). And their ingenious method of analysis permitted them to discover the answer in one block of hours in which the patient manifestly complained about the analyst more than at any other time in the treatment. This was demonstrably the result of the patient having learned from the analyst's abstinence (in this instance, refraining from being defensive) that it was safe to fully experience her fears of being observed and her fears of physical closeness to men, thus supporting Weiss's (1986) Control-Mastery hypothesis over the prediction of standard psychoanalytic doctrine.

Since Meyer is clearly addressing a fundamental (and nearly totally unresearched) question about the role of a clinician's "Mini-models" in the conduct of therapy it is important to distinguish his concept from the "mini-theories" described earlier in this introduction. Indeed the differences are apparent in Meyer's labels such as: "sadomasochism," "castration anxiety," "anal assault," and "inhibition of exhibitionistic wishes." Such terms, common in clinical papers and discussions, are conspicuously rare in the research literature. Why so? We believe that a substantial part of the answer lies in our Coda at the end of his chapter in which we note analysts' pervasive tendency to seek confirmatory evidence for their prior theories and the related tendency to use theoretical categories as initial classificatory schemes instead of following Edelson's (aforecited) advice to use commonsense categories first. Our emphasis on the fundamental role of starting at the surface, with manifest content, and theorizing at later stages, as illustrated elsewhere throughout this volume, is our basic response to Meyer and the large number of clinicians who will surely be sympathetic to his approach. Nonetheless, it must also be said that studies about "What

Makes Psychoanalysts Tick?" are conspicuously rare and fraught with difficult methodological problems.

Finally we are left with the last chapters of Parts I and II, which have to do with Artificial Intelligence (AI). What on earth are they doing here? What can AI possibly have to do with psychoanalytic and psychotherapy research? And what chutzpa enables Teller to propose AI as a basic science for psychoanalysis? In fact she goes so far as to suggest that if the disciplines that make up current Cognitive Science had been available to Freud he might well have created an AI model of the mind instead of the seventh chapter of *The Interpretation of Dreams*. Those who are curious for answers will have to review her arguments and decide for themselves whether her proposal for a Pattern-Directed Inference System (PDIS) is too much pie in the sky. Its conception is simple: it should do what analysts and researchers have demonstrated they *can* do, namely detect the many different repetitive maladaptive patterns of behavior that are illustrated in this book. Whether a computer program will be able to do the same is simply unknown at this time.

Leuzinger-Bohleber and Kächele have taken a different approach. They started with a psychoanalytic model of the mind that Clippinger (1977) incorporated in ERMA, a computer program that actually produced a convincing example of text from a patient in conflict. One of ERMA's central postulates is that the mind is composed of a number of independent, but interacting modules such as Freud (roughly, ego) and Calvin (superego). Then, turning matters on their head, they asked human judges to examine psychoanalytic transcripts of one "unsuccessful," two "moderately successful," and two "very successful" patients, to play computer, so to speak, and see if changes in the functions of the modules correspond to what one might predict clinically. The fact that the judges' ratings (and computer content analyses) discriminated the three outcome categories is itself warrant for pursuing further such approaches. But it is well to keep in mind that, although an AI model was used in this essentially clinical research, more direct contributions of AI methods and technology to psychoanalytic process research still await us.

Finally, let us say once more that our intent has been to outline strategies, not to proclaim conclusive findings. Nonetheless we believe that strategies such as these will indeed make it possible for some reviewers a quarter of a century from now to look back on what we have done as crude and elementary compared with what they will have achieved by then.

Author Index

Appelbaum, Ann, M.D., The New York Hospital, Cornell Medical Center, Westchester Division, White Plains, NY
Bucci, Wilma, Ph.D., Derner Institute of Advanced Psychological Studies, Adelphi University, Garden City, NY
Carr, Arthur, Ph.D., The New York Hospital, Cornell Medical Center, Westchester Division, White Plains, NY
Crits-Christoph, Paul, Ph.D., Department of Psychiatry, School of Medicine, University of Pennsylvania, Philadelphia, PA
Curtis, John T., Ph.D., Department of Psychiatry, Mount Zion Hospital, San Francisco, CA
Dahl, Hartvig, M.D., Department of Psychiatry, State University of New York, Health Science Center, Brooklyn, NY
Fretter, Polly, Ed.D., Department of Psychiatry, Mount Zion Hospital, San Francisco, CA
Gill, Merton M., M.D., Department of Psychiatry, College of Medicine, University of Illinois, Chicago, IL.
Grünzig, Hans-Joachim, Ph.D., Department of Psychotherapy, University of Ulm, Ulm
Henry, William P., Ph.D., Center for Psychotherapy Research, Vanderbilt University, Nashville, TN
Hoffman, Irwin Z., Ph. D., Department of Psychiatry and Behavioral Sciences, Northwestern Memorial Hospital, Chicago, IL.
Hohage, Roderich, M.D., Department of Psychotherapy, University of Ulm, Ulm
Kächele, Horst, M.D., Department of Psychotherapy, University of Ulm, Ulm
Kelly, Thomas J., M.A., Department of Psychiatry, Mount Zion Hospital, San Francisco, CA
Kernberg, Otto F., M.D., The New York Hospital, Cornell Medical Center, Westchester Division, White Plains, NY

Kernberg, Paulina, M.D., The New York Hospital, Cornell Medical Center, Westchester Division, White Plains, NY

Koenigsberg, Harold W., M.D, The New York Hospital, Cornell Medical Center, Westchester Division, White Plains, NY

Krause, Rainer, Ph.D., Department of Psychology, University of Saarland, Saarbrücken

Kübler, J. Christopher, Dipl.Psych., Department of Psychotherapy, University of Ulm, Ulm

Leuzinger-Bohleber, Marianne, Ph.D., Gesamthochschule Kassel, Universität, Fachbereich 1, Kassel

Luborsky, Lester, Ph.D., Department of Psychiatry, School of Medicine, University of Pennsylvania, Philadelphia, PA

Lütolf, Peter, Ph.D., Department of Clinical Psychology, University of Zürich, Zürich

Mergenthaler Erhard, Ph.D., Department of Psychotherapy, University of Ulm, Ulm

Meyer, Adolf-Ernst, M.D., Ph.D., Universitätskrankenhaus Eppendorf, II. Medizinische Klinik, Hamburg 20

Neudert, Lisbeth, M.D., Department of Psychotherapy, University of Ulm, Ulm

Rockland, Lawrence, M.D., The New York Hospital, Cornell Medical Center, Westchester Division, White Plains, NY

Ruberg Wolfgang, Ph.D., Department of Psychotherapy, University of Ulm, Ulm

Schacht, Thomas E., Psy.D., Department of Psychiatry, Quillen-Dishner College of Medicine, East Tennessee State University, Johnson City, TN, USA

Silberschatz, George, Ph.D., Department of Psychiatry, Mount Zion Hospital, San Francisco, CA

Strupp, Hans H., Ph.D., Department of Psychology, Vanderbilt University, Nashville, TN

Teller, Virginia, Ph.D., Hunter College and the Graduate School, The City University of New York, New York NY

Thomä, Helmut, M.D., Department of Psychotherapy, University of Ulm, Ulm

Part I.

Towards the Objective Analysis of Psychodynamic Structures

Problem-Treatment-Outcome Congruence: A Principle Whose Time Has Come

Hans H. Strupp, Thomas E. Schacht, and William P. Henry

1. Introduction

There is clearly no need to preach to readers of this book about the importance of process research; however, in keeping with the views of many colleagues we firmly believe that process research must be closely tied to research on therapeutic outcomes. The reasons are obvious: for one thing, outcome, in our view, is a more or less arbitrary way station; secondly, process research will remain in limbo unless concerted efforts are made to link process to outcome.

Our research group at Vanderbilt University has endeavored for a number of years to combine research on process and outcome. We have done it in a particular way: beginning with the Vanderbilt I study (Strupp and Hadley 1979), we have systematically employed various process measures (notably the Vanderbilt Psychotherapy Process Scale and the Vanderbilt Negative Indicators Scale) and studied various indices in relation to outcome measures (Gomes-Schwartz 1978; Sachs 1983). We have found it particularly useful – and recommend the approach to others – to proceed with process research in the context of a reasonably controlled outcome study. In the Vanderbilt I study, for example, we used two experimental groups and two control groups. Having defined a patient population and followed out an experimental design, we learned a great deal by studying intensively individual patient-therapist dyads. Specifically, we focused attention on "high" and "low" changers treated by the same professional therapist (Strupp 1980a, 1980b, 1980d). We remain firmly convinced that scientific understanding of the variables instrumental in therapeutic change will be best advanced through intensive study of individual dyads. Traditional group comparisons, in our view, can be invaluable because they help to define and demarcate a controlled context; however, to bring greater magnification to bear on the patient-therapist transactions which are, after all, the place where therapeutic change ultimately is located, we must turn to process research. As we said, we have a predilection for the kind of process research we have briefly sketched.

2. Why Time-limited Dynamic Psychotherapy?

There are several reasons for our research group's interest in time-limited dynamic psychotherapy:

1. From the standpoint of the researcher, short-term therapy provides practical and realistic opportunities for intensive study of the therapeutic process and outcome under reasonably controlled conditions, and with the hope that a particular research project can be completed in a tolerable period of time. As we know, adequate experimental controls are extremely difficult to implement in open-ended forms of psychoanalytic psychotherapy, especially in analyses that may last for many years. The researcher concerned with time-limited forms of therapy must, of course, assume that the basic dynamics of long-term therapy are observable in the shorter forms as well, and that contemporary time-limited psychotherapy is not the kind of inferior therapy it was once considered to be. The salient point is that the study of time-limited therapy affords research economies not otherwise obtainable.

2. From a clinical standpoint, there are great potential advantages that accrue to both patient and therapist when therapeutic progress is monitored at specific periods of time, say every six months. This procedure begins to question the practice of patient and therapist embarking on a journey without direction or goals. Thus, periodic assessment can aid in keeping patient and therapist "on course" (Strupp and Binder 1984).

3. It has long been known that most psychotherapies are, in fact, time-limited. Indeed the average patient seems to stay in therapy only for a few sessions (Garfield 1978). Apart from these considerations, modern clinical practice, notably in the United States, is being profoundly influenced by considerations of cost-effectiveness and accountability (Strupp 1986). Increasingly, psychotherapy is being compared to other treatment modalities (particularly drugs). Rightly or not, long-term therapy has come to be regarded as a costly and often risky investment of time, effort, and manpower. These developments are linked to the continuing dearth of hard empirical evidence supporting the traditional

claims of radical personality reorganization in psychoanalysis. Although I, for one, continue to believe that under propitious circumstances long-term psychoanalytic psychotherapy can produce changes obtainable in no other way, the research literature does not provide very convincing evidence in support of this position.

3. The Dynamic Focus

At the 1984 SPR meeting, Schacht, Strupp and Henry (1984)[1] presented an overview of a method for assessing interpersonal problems and dynamic conflicts. We have since begun to use it in our new process and outcome study (known as Vanderbilt II). A brief description of this project follows:

The Vanderbilt II Project, currently underway, is an intensive five-year NIMH-funded study of the process and outcome of a particular form of time-limited dynamic psychotherapy (TLDP) (Strupp and Binder 1984).

The TLDP approach was developed from principles and techniques of modern psychodynamic, interpersonal, and communications theories, and from results of previous research. The elements of TLDP are conceptually integrated around core interpersonal principles, such as understanding and using the therapeutic relationship as a technical parameter rather than simply as a nonspecific or common factor. TLDP addresses therapeutic problems in terms of the concept of self-sustaining interpersonal systems. These are patterns of repetitive interpersonal transaction and experience organized in a self-sustaining "vicious circle" (cf. Wachtel 1982) or, in cybernetic terms, a positive feedback cycle. This way of characterizing problems may be contrasted with alternate approaches that define problems in term of symptoms (such as anxiety, depression, obsessions, fears) or in terms of behavioral excesses or deficits (of assertiveness, aggression, social ability, self-regulation skills, etc.).

The treatment process in TLDP is articulated to the foregoing model of psychological problems. That is, therapeutic work in TLDP focuses on the recurrence of problematic patterns of interpersonal transaction within the patient-therapist relationship. According to

---

[1] The follow g section is based on this paper.

TLDP's working hypotheses, change occurs when this reenactment is uncovered and examined, and when the patient explores behavioral and experiential alternatives that disrupt self-sustaining vicious circles.

Although we have gained a good deal of experience with the approach we call "Dynamic Focus", we are still at an early stage of development. In the following we shall describe major concepts underlying our work on the Dynamic Focus and provide a brief example. We have also published a detailed description to which interested persons are referred: "The Dynamic Focus," Chapter 5 (Schacht, Binder, and Strupp 1984).

The Dynamic Focus[2] is an individualized process and outcome measure. It addresses the problem of gathering and organizing therapeutically relevant information. Of even greater importance, we seek to incorporate this information systematically into our form of time-limited dynamic psychotherapy (TLDP) which is central to the Vanderbilt II study (Strupp and Binder 1984). In other words, the Dynamic Focus is designed to (1) identify the patient's central "problem"; (2) guide the therapist's interventions; and (3) facilitate the study of the therapeutic process.

The TLDP Focus is grounded in two principles:

1. For the kinds of problems treated by TLDP, the primary arena for construing life experience is *interpersonal*. Consonant with the thinking of Harry Stack Sullivan and more recent exponents of the interpersonal schools, we hold that issues become evident in therapy primarily through the role they play in patient's transactions with significant others and, more immediately, with the therapist. The latter emphasis we share with such authors as Gill (1982) who point to the analysis of the transference in the here-and-now as the most fruitful focus for psychotherapy.

2. The primary psychological mode of construing life experience, for the therapeutic operations central to TLDP, is *narration* the telling of a story to oneself and others. Because patients are typically unaware of the underlying scripts, they live them out as if they represented absolute

[2] We have recently come to prefer the term Cyclical Maladaptive Pattern (CMP). Other researchers who are currently using similar concepts include Luborsky (1984) "Core Conflictual Relationship Theme"; Malan (1976a) "Dynamic Focus"; Mann (1973) "Central Issue"; Teller and Dahl (1981a, 1986; Dahl, this volume) "Frames."

truths rather than being simply versions of reality. Knowledge of a life story is acquired in the course of attempting to tell it (narration). Narration is thus a process of discovery, a kind of investigation. By retelling or renarrating one's life story in therapy, one gains a new understanding of its meaning and significance. This process, of course, is greatly aided by the therapist's gradual understanding and interpretations addressed to the emerging script or scenario.

The Dynamic Focus contains four structural elements which express, in schematized fashion, the following fundamental categories of action:

1. *Acts of self.* These may include all domains of human action, such as affects and motive (e.g. "I feel affectionate towards my mother" or "I wish my wife would pay more attention to me"); perceiving situations (e.g. "I sensed we were in a competition together"); cognitions (e.g. "I can't stop thinking about how ugly and inferior I am when I meet someone attractive"); or overt behaviors (e.g. "I can't refrain from avoiding eye-contact with my boss when I'm angry with him"). Acts of self include both private actions and public actions (e.g. feeling affectionate as well as displaying affection), and may vary in the degree to which they are accessible to awareness.

2. *Expectations about others' reactions.* These are imagined reactions of others to one's own actions and may be conscious, preconscious, or unconscious. To achieve a transactional understanding, these should be articulated in specific relation to some acts of self. Statements in this category should emphasize imagined anticipation of others' behavior. Expectations about others' reaction often take a form such as: "If I speak up, I imagine that she will disapprove of me" or "If I ask her out she will just laugh at me."

3. *Acts of others toward self.* These are observed acts of others that are viewed as occurring in specific relation to the acts of self. That is, these actions of others are performed in the patient's presence and appear (or are assumed) to be evoked by the patient's own actions. As above, "acts" may include all domains of human action, including both public and private actions. Acts of others are typically expressed in a form such as: "When I asked for the money he ignored me."

4. *Acts of self toward self (introject).* This category of actions refers to how one treats oneself (e.g. self-controlling, self-punishing, self-congratulating, self-destroying). These actions should be articulated

in specific relation to the acts of self, expectations of others' reactions, and acts of others which comprise the remainder of the format. An introject prototypically takes this form: "When my husband praises me I feel guilty and remind myself of my shortcomings" or "When I get angry I just try to slow myself down and think things through. I give myself all the time I need."

The following example outlines a problematic interpersonal transaction pattern that was observed first in the patient's current relationship with her therapist, and later was narratively integrated with her childhood history and her current marriage.

> *Presenting problem.* The patient complains of depression and marital difficulties.
>
> *Acts of self.* Frances assumes a passive interpersonal position in which she refrains from disclosing her inner self, avoids social contact by withdrawal or procrastination, defers and submits to other's wishes, and spends much time in private thinking and wondering rather than in active communication.
>
> *Expectation of others' reactions.* Frances expects that other people will ignore or reject her. She validates this expectation with recollections of being ignored or rejected by her mother and by various significant others.
>
> *Observed reactions of others.* Others find Frances' passivity unappealing and do not spontaneously recognize her distress and come to her aid. However, Frances does not see this as an understandable reaction to her passivity, but instead interprets this as evidence that others are actively rejecting and ignoring her.
>
> *Introject (how patient treats herself).* Frances views herself as helpless in a hopeless situation and neglects opportunities for change. Rather than endure the imagined negative reactions of others, she inhibits and controls herself and refrains from asserting her desires or complaints (hoping that this interpersonal passivity will make her mere presence more palatable to others).

4. The Dynamic Focus in Therapy and Research

The treatment process in TLDP is articulated to the foregoing model for understanding psychological problems. That is, therapeutic work in TLDP focuses on the recurrence of problematic patterns of interperworking hypothesis, change occurs when this reenactment is uncovered and examined, and when the patient explores behavioral and experiential alternatives that disrupt self-sustaining vicious cycles.

As this cursory discussion illustrates, the Dynamic Focus in our usage deals with patterns of interpersonal transaction which are a common unit of analysis for:

(1) defining problems,

(2) conceptualizing the treatment process, and

(3) evaluating outcome.

There are, however, further implications for process and outcome research which we will examine now in somewhat greater detail.

5. Principle of P-T-O-Congruence

Schacht, Strupp and Henry (1984)[3] proposed a fundamental integrative principle which may aid in the design of intelligible studies of complex psychotherapeutic phenomena. This principle – which is perhaps so obvious that it has been too easily ignored – is called the Principle of Problem-Treatment-Outcome congruence ("P-T-O congruence", for short). *The principle of P-T-O Congruence proposes that the intelligibility of psychotherapy research is a function of the similarity, isomorphism, or congruence among how we conceptualize and measure the clinical problem (P), the processes of therapeutic change (T), and the clinical outcome (O).*

By this principle, measures of the problem, the change process, and the outcome should ideally be fully congruent. That is, therapeutic outcome should be characterized in the same form and units of analysis as the clinical problem; and, the language used to describe both the problem and the outcome should lend itself to formulation of cogent theoretical links among the problem, the intervention process, and the therapeutic outcome. It is proposed that psychotherapy research can accommodate eclecticism – whether in the therapies studied or in the research methods – in direct proportion to the achievement of P-T-O congruence.

Illustration. P-T-O congruence may be most clearly visible when its absence induces a sense that a train of reasoning or a research method

---

[3] The following section is based on this paper.

Illustration. P-T-O congruence may be most clearly visible when its absence induces a sense that a train of reasoning or a research method has some logical or inferential weakness. A prototypic highly incongruent psychotherapy research design might appear as follows:

The example is of a comparative process and outcome study, in which Rational Emotive Therapy (Ellis 1970) and Interpersonal Therapy (Klerman, Weissman, Rounsaville, and Chevron 1984) are evaluated in the treatment of depression.

1. First, patients are selected for inclusion in the study (a group comparison) via various "therapy-neutral" characteristics, such as DSM-III diagnosis, MMPI or SCL-90 elevation, or scores on instruments such as the Beck Depression Inventory. A patient's scores on these various selection criteria essentially define the "problem" to which psychotherapy is to be addressed. The ostensible advantage of using a therapy-neutral common language for describing clinical problems is that such a language facilitates communication with colleagues. However, such neutral language also may insure that the problem is not defined in terms derived from the theories of behavior and change underlying the therapies being studied.

2. Second, consistent with the foregoing selection process, patients are treated for the problem of "depression," rather than for problems bearing a closer conceptual relationship to each treatment's underlying theoretical rationale. Thus, problems are not defined in terms of irrational beliefs or interpersonal deficits. Indeed, it is implicitly assumed that irrational beliefs or interpersonal deficits are important primarily as mediating variables which contribute to the etiology of the "real problem" of depression.

3. Third, evaluation of treatment process is primarily concerned with therapists' adherence to specified protocols, rather than with specifying how change occurs. "General" measures of treatment process may be employed (especially those emphasizing so-called "common factors" such as warmth and positive relationship). These general measures are conceptually distant from the way the problem and the treatment are characterized.

4. Finally, the battery of initial measures is repeated to characterize the therapy outcomes. Because the various individual measures have moved in different directions, (a common research finding) the investigator combines them statistically (factor analysis, effect-size calcu-

lations, etc.) to yield a composite outcome index. This composite index bears an uncertain conceptual relationship to anything that is directly observable or to any variables of specific theoretical importance. Little or no effort is made in the analyses to interpret the data from individual cases.

Further implications. The principle of P-T-O congruence implies that simply administering the same instrument pre- and post-treatment is not satisfactory, *unless* the instrument also articulates with the core dimension of the hypothesized therapeutic process. Frequently used pre- and post-measures such as MMPI elevations or SCL-90 symptom profiles typically provide only a pseudo-congruence. Such measures certainly have psychometric utility, especially for making comparisons to normative groups, but they lack heuristic value for the fundamental research task of understanding the nature of therapeutic change and the relationships between process and outcome. Ideal pre-post problem measures, in contrast, should carry some prescriptive implications for therapeutic action and appropriate therapeutic process. Such ideal measures are unlike DSM-III categories, for example, which appear to have little prescriptive value for psychotherapy in most cases.

In line with the foregoing, the principle of P-T-O congruence also implies that psychotherapy researchers should work toward refining representations of psychological problems so that so-called patient-dispositional variables or patient-selection criteria are incorporated into the original problem statement, rather than treated as extraneous mediating influences requiring separate analyses. We should assign patients to treatments using selection measures that are congruent with how we characterize the problem, the outcome, and the corresponding intervention and change processes. We ought not ask how patient dispositional characteristics influence the relationship of process to outcome; rather, we should seek to incorporate important patient characteristics into the initial definition of the problem, and hence into the definition of the appropriate process and eventual outcome. In this view dispositional variables should become an integral part of how the problem is characterized, and diagnostic concepts should be periodically revised to include these criteria.

In our view, all other measurement considerations are dependent on the principle of P-T-O congruence. Whether a measurement approach is individualized, standardized, or even reliable becomes a secondary consideration, since with P-T-O congruence the value of these other measurement properties is severely diminished. Use of psychometrically inferior measures, even with P-T-O congruence, illustrates the principle of "garbage in/garbage out." Using a psychometrically superior measure *without* P-T-O congruence is equally undesirable – an instance of "gold in/garbage out."

To readers familiar with both literatures it should be apparent that, on the whole, researchers studying behavioral therapies have often been more successful than their psychodynamically oriented counterparts in approximating the requirements of P-T-O congruence. However, the principle itself militates against overzealous attempts to export this limited success from its natural theoretical context.

For example, psychodynamic researchers are sometimes criticized for failing to include behavioral measures, such as role-playing or in-vivo observations of target behaviors. These complaints ignore the fact that definitions of the form and content of problems vary across theories, and that a measure which enhances P-T-O congruence for a behavioral therapy may fail to adequately represent events of crucial interest to researchers working form an alternate theoretical base. P-T-O congruence is not a property of specific measures taken in isolation (although certain measures are undoubtedly more theory-relevant than others). Rather, P-T-O congruence is context-dependent; it is a property of the logical inter-articulation of measures across the domains of problems, treatment processes, and outcomes.

The research challenge in studying TLDP involves translating the conceptual integration (around principles of interpersonal dynamics) into a research method that, via P-T-O congruence, preserves an opportunity to map the conceptual integration onto subsequent empirical observations. In applying the principle of P-T-O congruence to the design of the Vanderbilt II project, the study clearly could not be limited to traditional measures of symptoms, traits, target complaints, goals, and so forth, since these are not "problems" in a form that TLDP purports to treat. Therefore, the traditional battery of measures is being supplemented by efforts to develop additional procedures more conceptually consistent with the problems TLDP is designed to address. With respect to this more general end of enhancing P-T-O congruence, the following considerations emerge:

1. First, to articulate with TLDP's underlying theoretical premises, the measure should characterize a self-sustaining pattern of action and interaction, and it should reflect TLDP's emphasis on the interpersonal domain. To characterize patterns may require a measure

on a different order from, say, a Likert scale or a frequency count of target-behaviors. The idea of measuring a pattern alters assumptions that characterize linear and numerically incremental models of change, as reflected in attempts to measure "more" or "less" of a trait, symptom, behavior, etc. Linear or incremental models typically assume that all change may be reduced to either positive or negative, and that outcome judgments may be arrayed correspondingly. In contrast, outcome in TLDP may also involve transforming a self-sustaining pattern of maladaptive action into a self-limiting or self-extinguishing pattern. This kind of transformation reflects a qualitative change in the organization of behavior that is difficult to express in terms of numerical increments with fixed relationships to judgments of "good" or "bad." More traditionally, a change in a transactional pattern might be characterized quantitatively as an altered conditional probability that, given certain precipitating events, the entire vicious cycle would be enacted. Again, however, judgment of whether this represents a positive or negative outcome cannot be reduced to a simple context-free numerical indicator without risk of conceptual distortion.

2. Second, because a transaction pattern unfolds over time, and because at any one time the pattern exists both as present behavior and as future potential, dynamic assessment is preferable to static assessment. A static assessment is made in cross-sectional fashion by simply "freezing the action" and applying a measure. Static assessment is commonly used to measure "levels" of various symptoms, traits, dispositions, etc. Most self-report questionnaires and observer ratings in current use involve static assessments. Dynamic assessments, in contrast, involve a dialectical interaction between assessment, trial intervention, and reassessment. The clinical wisdom of this approach to assessment is reflected in the various forms of trial therapies advocated as part of the patient-assessment process in most brief psychodynamic treatments. Dynamic assessment is most useful when we wish to identify a person's *potential* to learn or adapt, or when we wish to see how a complex transaction pattern unfolds over time. Cross-sectional measures cannot adequately describe the nature of problems that are conceived in this essentially longitudinal manner.

3. Third, because of the potential for idiosyncratic or highly patient-specific problems, measures should permit individualized assessment. However, while patients should be able to serve as their own standard for comparison it is also desirable to be able to make some group comparison.

6. Structural Analysis of Social Behavior

In applying the principle of P-T-O congruence to TLDP, it is immediately apparent that patterns of interpersonal transaction are a common unit of analysis for defining problems, conceptualizing the treatment process, and evaluating outcome. Hence, any model of interpersonal behavior that is capable of representing interpersonal transactions has the potential, in theory, to enhance the P-T-O congruence of research on TLDP. While other general models of interpersonal behavior might be applied to this task, we have elected to incorporate Lorna Benjamin's (1974) model for the Structural Analysis of Social Behavior (SASB). The SASB model is a detailed, conceptually rigorous, and psychometrically advanced descendant of Leary's (1957) original circumplex model. The SASB permits interpersonal behaviors or their intrapsychic analogues to be represented mathematically as points on one of three interrelated two-dimensional coordinate planes or "surfaces." Any interpersonal process or content may be described mathematically by locating it in one or more points on the SASB surfaces, according to highly reliable coding procedures developed by Benjamin, Giat, and Estroff (1981). Similarity, difference, and change may then be quantified by reference to the well-known mathematical properties of the interpersonal circumplex.

SASB and P-T-O Congruence. SASB coded formulations of the focus can be applied to numerous research questions. Using the SASB as a common, theoretically cogent metric, it becomes possible to search meaningfully for relationships among *any* aspects of psychotherapy expressible in interpersonal terms – problem definition, treatment process, or outcome. Two closing examples will illustrate:

1. Congruence between problem definition and outcome measures can be enhanced by using the TLDP focus as an individualized measure of treatment outcome. A working hypothesis is that a successful therapy should be accompanied by changes in the patient's transaction patterns. Such changes may be characterized, quantified, and tracked with the dynamic focus/SASB combination. It is also possible, as Luborsky (1977) and Levine and Luborsky (1981) have suggested, that in a successful therapy a main transaction pattern does not always change. Rather, what may change is the patient's sense of mastery or control over the problematic transactional events. This latter possibility is addressed in two ways: first, via follow-up interviews, and second, via an experimental measure of interpersonal locus of control that is integrated with the SASB model, thereby permitting evaluation of the mastery

dimension in relation to the specific interpersonal areas targeted by the focus formulation (Schacht and Henry 1983).

2. Congruence between the problem definition and the treatment process will be enhanced by using the focal narrative as a benchmark for raters of therapeutic process. The extent to which patient and therapist reenact the focal interpersonal pattern, as opposed to understanding it while resisting reenactment, may be estimated from direct SASB coding of the interpersonal process and content of critical sessions. Along a related line, since maintenance and effective pursuit of a focus are hypothesized to be a central aspect of TLDP technique, the focal formulation will be used as the reference point for anchoring assessments of therapists' adherence to this technical guideline. By using the focus as a rating benchmark it thus becomes possible to evaluate an individualized aspect of the therapeutic process as well as the outcome. In contrast to homogeneous process "dimensions" like warmth, empathy, and so on, a therapist's adherence to a focus is a highly individualized aspect of the therapeutic process, and, consistent with the principle of P-T-O congruence, one that is closely articulated to the initial understanding of the problem.

7. Concluding Comments

Only modest progress has been made in the search for a common metric for evaluating psychotherapy outcomes. Unfortunately, there are no universally shared definitions of "mental health," and different psychotherapies disagree on conceptualizations of a patient's "problem" and preferred therapeutic interventions. We do great conceptual violence to psychotherapy research when we insist that, say, two different therapies, each based on very different ideas about the nature of psychological problems, be compared in terms of their effects on yet a third kind of problem that is defined in a way not consistent with a given form of therapy but rather in terms of descriptive diagnostic taxonomy such as DSM-III. Thus, researchers continue to employ measures that are derived from descriptive traditions but are unrelated to a theory of change. In short, current outcome measures often fail to capture unique and complex but also essential "clinical realities." To remedy these problems, there has been a widespread call for the development of change criteria specific to the individual patient. However, specificity and individualization are not panaceas, and they cannot compensate for the more fundamental problems we have mentioned. The Dynamic Focus approach is one attempt to come to grips with the basic issue of problem-treatment-outcome congruence and to facilitate study of the therapeutic process.

In the Vanderbilt II study we have begun to apply this approach. First, we are using a so-called Interpersonal Assessment Interview (IAI) which is designed to elicit, in a semi-structured form, the patient's narrative of his or her interpersonal difficulties. The assessment clinician seeks to obtain the pertinent information by focusing on the four action categories we have discussed (acts of self; expectations about others' reactions; acts of others toward self; and acts of self toward self (introject)). The next step is to construct a Dynamic Focus. To this end, two members of the research team study videotapes of the assessment interviews. We have found that in many cases it is relatively easy to distill a Dynamic Focus; however, there are other instances when the task is difficult if not impossible. It is our impression that the more difficult it is to identify a focus, the more difficult it is for the patient to form a viable therapeutic alliance. At the moment we are beginning quantitative analyses of the therapeutic process by means of SASB. We consider this a promising venture and also are encouraged by the work of colleagues represented in this volume. These approaches, we believe, hold considerable promise for the future of psychotherapy process research.

The Specimen Hour

Anonymous

Transcript of Hour 5

This is the verbatim transcript of the fifth hour of the tape-recorded psychoanalysis of a 28-year old married woman. The transcript was carefully prepared and punctuated to reflect the disfluencies and fragmentation that are characteristic of much of spoken language. In this session the analysand spoke 5244 words and the analyst 247. Substitute proper names have been used, e.g. David is the woman's husband.

The complete set of rules used for transcribing can be found in: Dahl, H. (1979a, pp x-xii). Among these are the following: The analyst's speech is enclosed within a pair of slashes; the transcriber's descriptive comments are enclosed within parentheses; all the rest is the analysand's speech. A letter followed by an underline (w_) or hyphen (w–) indicates a stammer or false start. A pause is a period from 15 seconds to 1 minute; a silence is greater than 1 but less than 2 minutes; longer silences are timed to the nearest minute. In this hour the patient's chuckles are always slightly nervous chuckles.

The paragraphs are numbered with a # sign: references in several chapters use this # sign to identify paragraphs in this transcript.

(3-minute silence, occasional stomach rumbles)

#1

Something that's been on my mind today is the relationship I have with the girl who is my assistant this year and was last year. And (sigh) well, it took me quite a while to get used to her last year and I imagine it was a variety of reasons. But at the beginning of this year things were going quite nicely and I was quite pleased with the kind of things she can do and not feeling at all annoyed by her, which was part of the trouble I had last year, although at times she's a, a type of person that I don't feel completely sympathetic with, I guess. And uhm, because of the other assistant having left, she's having to fulfill both of the functions to an extent and, and both of the teachers, myself and the other teacher, are to make adjustments too, so that she can help us both out.

#2

And today was the first day when she was really officially working for both of us. And I, I found all over again I was beginning to react to her the way I had last year which upset me very much because I know that some of it's, is the way she is and, and maybe I am annoyed by that kind of a person, but some of it's got nothing to do with her. And I think it had something to do with just sharing her and, and the fear that she might prefer working with the other girl or being in the other room. And, I think it also, when I'm faced with the aspect of sharing her, I, I also have to face that perhaps sometimes I'm not treating her quite the way I should be. And, and this is another reason why I become almost jealous of who she works with. (Sniff) And then I think well, I will try to be fairer to her since it is something within me. It has nothing to do with her, but I still can't seem to maintain that. I still seem to treat her the same way I used to. And, I think I'm, well, I don't really know how she sees it. I don't know whether she thinks there's anything wrong with the way I treat her at all.

#3

I think what I do to control her is to uhm, through controlling what she does with the children in the classroom. And I know I want to be the, the definite one in control in the classroom. And, and I know that I want to have a response from the boys that, as long as I have it, then it's all right for her to have it too. But I, I know I respond very much to any time that she has a very warm response and, and I don't – (pause)

#4

But she's also a type of person that bothers me and, and I don't know quite why it is. She's very boisterous and kind of (sniff), well, coarse is too strong a word, but, well, just loud and, I think in a way unfeeling, although she can be very kind and with the boys she's quite sensitive to them and, and I think has a real sense of them as individuals and, and people and, and I think she has a sense of people in general as being worthwhile. But, on the other hand, somehow there is something insensitive about her.

#5

For instance, she never really thought about this other girl at all. Now, I can't, I can't pretend that I had any idea at all that this girl had anything as serious in her problems in her life as she did, but I reacted to her as a person and thought some things were strange about it, but Betty, the girl who's my assistant, didn't even have any reaction to her as anything being strange about her. Or, I don't know, it just, it could have been anybody there at that time and she'd relate to them all exactly the same way. And I guess this bothers me that, uhm – Gee I don't know exactly what about it bothers me (chuckle), but it does. And uh, in being kind of noisy and loud she's the kind of person that just sort of – she will enter a room or a conversation or anything and just throw herself right in without kind of feeling her way or listening to what's happened before or feeling the atmosphere or any of these things. And again, this annoys me. And I don't know exactly why it is. I think perhaps part of it is because then, if I'm involved, she'll kind of jump right in and take over and, and she doesn't sort of defer to me, which I'm sure is part of why it annoys me.

#6

But even beyond that I think that kind of a person bothers me because uhm, even before I began to work with her when she applied, sh–, I was overwhelmed with all her enthusiasm and, and pleasure in everything. It just seems like it was practically everything. Now she's beginning to react. Some things are good and some things she doesn't enjoy which, you know, is only normal, but at first it just seemed like she just loved everything, and, and that also would make me feel (chuckle) as if I just wanted her to be quiet. (Sniff)

#7

And I don't, I don't really know how to handle it, both within myself how I feel, and, and how I should handle it in terms of our relationship in the job we have. Last year, uhm, this whole, the whole loudness of her personality bothered me anyway, just from the aspect of what we were trying to do within the room, because we have to keep a very quiet tone at this school. And uhm, I was trying to tone her down in the room without just telling her that she h_ had to just completely change herself, because that's not fair either.

#8

And at one point my supervisor blamed me for her conduct, conduct within the whole school. And I became very defensive (chuckle) I think, at the time, partly because the condact (sic), conduct she had was just the kind that I didn't like anyway. And I, I, I don't know, I guess I just didn't feel it was totally my responsibility. I mean, this other woman had hired her knowing she was that kind of a person. (Sniff, clears throat)

#9

And I think if – I think a lot of it's – my wanting to subdue her – is just so I'll be dominant. But some of it too, is for what's happening to the other boys who will become easily overexcited and out of control, for this school. I don't think for some schools they would, it would seem out of control. But for Lakehurst, uhm, very little will already become out of control. And so I have to watch that. And I just don't know, I, I don't know how to be honest with myself, and how much I want to subdue her for that good, and how much of it's just to control her, and then how much I have a right to even do anything. I mean, this is the kind of person she is. (Pause)

#10

I suppose it's also just wondering what the function of friendly advice is anyway. If you're a good friend of somebody, not that I'm saying this is the situation I'm in, but just makes me wonder, when you're a good friend of somebody, how much, from your point of view, you should advise your friend and how much you should keep quiet, because the person is what they are and, and your point of view is going to be different from theirs in any case. (Sniff, stomach rumble, pause)

#11

(Sniff) That's another funny thing too, because with all my problems in controlling my own life, feeling control over myself in the areas that I'd really want to, which I suppose is just knowing what I am and what I want to do and being happy about what I am doing and what I am being, but still I am very free with advice to other people when they ask me, and I feel as if I really know the answer. And sometimes I think my advice is pretty good (chuckle) but I can't seem to apply any of it to myself. (Clears throat, sniff, pause)

#12

In fact, regarding myself, I find decisions extremely hard. And, if I do make one, even if it's just a minor thing, like, for instance with my husband, what we're going to do for an evening if we want to go out, then I, if I do make that decision, then I have, then it has to be that way and it can't be any other way. And, I c–, I can't seem to adjust it if something makes a change in plans necessary. (Sniff) Or something that he used to do an lot, Dave used to do a lot, would be to, in talking about whether we'd go away for a weekend or not, he'd say, "Well, I can't be sure I can get away." And then we'd decide, well, we won't be going. And then on Thursday he'd say, "OK, we're going." And I would just find I – there was no reason I couldn't go – but I would just find that I practically could not get myself together and go away for a weekend, which involved little more than just packing a few clothes.

#13

Oh, it involved a lot more I guess, because it usually, when we made that kind of a s– decision, it would be to go to the house my parents have in Northwood, so it would mean calling them up on the telephone and I just couldn't bring myself to do that. So he'd always have to do that. (Pause)

#14

But even then, it, we'd have to go through a – he'd have to say, "Well, why don't you think you can go?" And then I'd give one reason. "All right, but can't you do this?" "OK," or "I can do that," and then, "Why else can't you go?" And then we'd go through a whole list of things that I would think up on why I couldn't go. And I'd have to have him help me answer every single one of them before I could make up my mind I could go. And then we'd usually have a fight too before I could decide that I could go. And my decision would be based more on the fact that I realized then I'd been unreasonable in fighting with him about it. (Sniff, clears throat, silence, occasional stomach rumbles)

#15

It's funny about the telephone too, because (sniff) I have a very funny reaction to it. I, I never like to make telephone calls, and I'll do anything to put off making them if I can. But then once I get on the telephone (chuckle) I find it very hard to terminate a conversation. (Sniff, pause, sniff) I don't know why I have this feeling. I can't believe it's from just something I saw my parents do in itself, but my father used to always hate to make telephone calls too and there – if he was supposed to call some friend of theirs about something, he would go through all sorts of excuses why he couldn't or he'd argue with my mother about who should call and try to get her to call. And it was almost like she were treating a little boy, making him call this time. (Sniff, pause)

#16

In fact, unless it's business he's still fairly strange on the phone. It's only occasionally, when there's been some real topic that he can talk about that's right there on his mind, that he isn't ill-at-ease on the phone. And usually if I get him when I'm calling he'll practically gasp, "Well, here's your mother," or "I'll get your mother." And then, and then, once he's called her, if he's waiting for her to come, he'll talk to me, and then he can be fine. And, and (stomach rumble) it's just somehow he has to know that she's coming, so he's not stuck talking to me. (Sniff) But I also panic if I know sh–, when I call if suddenly I find out she's not there and I'm going to just have to talk to him. It seems a mutual kind of reaction at this point. (Sniff, pause, stomach rumble)

#17

Because that sort of typifies our whole relationship. I think we're always (chuckle) panic stricken when we find we're going to be alone together with each other. (Sniff) And I don't, I can't quite figure out why it is, except he has one characteristic which I think I must find annoying, (sniff) or I don't find I'm equal to it, because he's constantly, on anything that he's talking about, asking for reassurance that he's right or th_ that I agree. (Sniff) And if, if you don't agree, it just doesn't get you anywhere to say it, unless you can sort of have a general discussion about something but so often they don't stay on a general level. (Tch) And, I don't know, I just find I can't respond after a while to being asked constantly to support him. (Pause, stomach rumble) I suppose now I'm thinking consciously, when he asks me things either that I don't agree and I can't answer, "Yes, I agree," or "I don't think it's that important so why do you keep on asking me if I don't think the same thing?" I mean, it doesn't matter if I think the same thing or not. (Sniff)

#18

Because I, I (chuckle) was just thinking I probably do the same thing with David. Last night in particular, I was talking with him about – I don't know, I just seemed to be in a funny mood by the time he got home. He got home sort of late, and it wasn't that he was late, because I knew he would be. But I guess he didn't immediately respond to me in the way I wanted him to or – I don't know what it was, because I imagine that somehow I was already in some kind of a mood. And (sniff) at one point I was talking to him, and I know I was talking to him wanting either confirmation that I'd done the right thing or a suggestion on what would be a right thing because I wasn't sure. I was upset about something I'd done and I didn't want him just to listen to me say it. I wanted him to actually react to it, and either suggest another course of action or, or approval that well, I guess that in the circumstances that wasn't that bad a thing to do. And, and he just didn't say anything, except sort of mutter under his breath. And so I got furious at him and (sniff) I imagine in a way it's the same kind of thing that my father always is doing. (Pause, stomach rumble)

#19

Because the thing I did that – it wasn't that important a thing I did that I was upset about, but it was indicative of something I'm doing all the time – was, uhm, the particular incident was, I have two boys in school who are constantly together. They were friends before. And it's disruptive to the class now because they're, whenever we're doing some kind of a group activity, they're so busy moving around inside the group, staying together and then changing places in the – if we're sitting on the f_ floor up in the front they'll be changing places where they're sitting – and so they sort of tunnel through the whole group and they're talking together and everything. And it really isn't good for them anyway, just in their cutting out other people so that they are only together within themselves. And I'm trying to encourage them to separate themselves from each other as much as possible. And once in a while if I'm really tired and worn-out and there they are disrupting the group again, I get a little annoyed at them on – again, though I know I shouldn't.

#20

And yesterday – I had been thinking about calling the parents – and yesterday – just to let them know that, if the children were kind of upset at what I was doing, the reason for it would be this, and that they, if they wanted to support it, they could by explaining that there were lots of boys to be friends with at the school and that type of thing. And – but I hadn't called them and I saw one of the mothers at the dismissal when she came to pick up her boy. And I never like talking to parents then because it was just too confusing. But of course I just said something to her that was, you know, chatty. And then, and then I suddenly found myself starting to talk about this problem, which I hadn't intended to at all. And I, I was kind of surprised at myself when I was talking and, then I just couldn't keep quiet (chuckle). I couldn't stop it, or say well, we better talk about this another time or anything. And I just seemed to get in deeper and deeper and I'm always doing this.

#21

I always seem to talk before I think and say things I don't mean or give them a connotation I don't mean to give them or bring them up at a time that they just shouldn't be brought up at all. And I, I consciously try to do, to control this now, because it's terrible when you're dealing with mothers who are putting a great deal of pressure on their children anyway. They misconstrue everything you can say and, and there I went again.

#22

And I think I was upset too because it, it's almost like immediately hitting the parent with something negative rather than first indicating to them that on the whole things are very good, because they are. And, and again this is something I do and, and I had a lot of trouble with my student reports last year because I do this. I seem to kind of assume the positive and then put all my energies into pointing out the negative things.

#23

/ This happened yesterday then? /

#24

Yes.

#25

/ Before you left school? /

#26

Yes.

#27

/ You mentioned yesterday o_ or the day before that uh things would occur to you during the day – /

#28

Mm.

#29

/ – that you had looked forward, as a matter of fact, before you started the analysis to be able to come in and talk about them. What strikes me as you tell me this is that you went home after you left here and talked to David about it – /

#30

Mm.

#31

/ – wanting reassurance, but not here. /

#32

You mean not seeking reassurance here?

#33

/ I mean, yeah, it's one of the things that apparently didn't occur to you (chuckle) to mention here. (Stomach rumble) I don't know what to make of it, except to just – I, I, I take note of these (chuckle) – /

#34

Mm.

#35

/ – different things that you've said that you, ahead of time, wanted to be able to have a place to talk about, things like that, for example, that trouble you. /

#36

Mm. Now, well, I don't think I, well, that's not true. I do seek reassur_surance wherever I talk, (chuckle) even here, but I don't think that – I think if, if I bring something up here I, I already know that –

#37

/ You won't get it. /

#38

Uh, that's not the point. Yeah, and so even though I would like to get it –

#39

/ Could that be in – one of the reasons it didn't come up? (Chuckle) That's really what I'm getting – /

#40

(Interrupting) I can't remember whether it even, you know, did come into my mind yesterday. It may have, but uhm, you know, sometimes I, especially when I first come in, I find I am here and I just have a flood of things, but nothing's really, but yet there's nothing. I d–, it's hard to explain. You know, there are – perhaps I'm selecting now, I don't want to talk about that, no I can't about that, and you know, then I'm selecting what I can (chuckle) talk about or feel I can, but uhm, I don't, I don't even remember that – I'm, I'm not sure how, how long after I spoke to the mother I even began to think I shouldn't have done it too. You know, how long it took me to react to what I'd said. Oh, I must have reacted right away, but perhaps that was one of the things that I pushed away from my mind and wouldn't face that I'd made a mistake on, because I will do that too.

#41

/ B_ but uh if it did occur to you and you mentioned it here, you would not expect reassurance now, from me? /

#42

I think not. I think now I –

#43

/ From David you want it and you're angry if you don't get it. /

#44

Yeah.

#45

/ Hmm. /

#46

Well, I thought – I can't say not here, although I think I'm becoming less apt to seek it here. I think I want to be reassured that (chuckle) you're listening, but uhm, because I feel very funny (chuckle) just talking aloud. But I don't know whether I seek reassurance beyond that. But with David I do beyond that. No, well, that's not true, because one thing I was, I did talk to him, and it does come to my mind now, uhm – and this affects things that I sometimes find I can't even bring up yet – is your reaction to some things I might say. So I suppose there again, it's your approving or disapproving. (Pause) And of course, what it boils down to is I'm sure you're going to (chuckle) disapprove, so I'm afraid of saying them. (Pause, stomach rumble)

#47

It's funny how we – I asked David about it too – and, and, I don't know, we, we've been debating how much we should talk about our experiences anyway, and I imagine that we really don't s_ speak much about it. In fact, I don't really talk to David about it at all now, except when a question comes up in regard to (sniff) his reaction to being analyzed. And uhm, I did ask him if he, when he's thinking about things, does think in terms of how his analyst would react and, and he used the word "shock." He's, I think at one point he said something to his – that he was afraid he might shock him and this was what was keeping him – and I was just thinking it was interesting, the different way we use our reactions because I don't care whether I (chuckle) shock you or not. It's whether you disapprove. (Pause)

#48

And this makes me think of uhm, (stomach rumble) friendships I've had with other people and, something that I don't like to admit, because I don't approve of it (chuckle), so I can't imagine anybody else would, but I seem to have to find fault with just about everybody that I'm friendly with to some degree whether it's just a small degree or a larger degree. And, even though in a way I might feel inferior to them, and I imagine I feel inferior to a lot of people, I still have to find fault with them and maybe criticize them to David, I don't know. I always have to openly criticize them, but in any case I have to kind've done that and then I can go on to a re–, a, some kind of friendly relationship with them. And until I've done that I can't really accept them as somebody that I want to be at all close to in any way at all. And, and if I can't, if I find I can't be critical of them in some aspect, then I just can't seem to be around them at all. I, I, I don't know, it's more than sort of being, well, it's not being in awe of them. It's just feeling very uncomfortable, I guess, with them.

#49

/ So your thoughts turned from thinking about whether I would approve or disapprove of things you say to what you've just been talking about. /

#50

Mm.

#51

/ There any connection? Does it follow perhaps that uh you (stomach rumble) have some criticisms of me that have occurred to you? /

#52

(Pause) I think if I had, I would have (chuckle) suppressed them too much to admit them. (Clears throat, sniff, pause) Uh, perhaps one – I'm starting with one that's less (chuckle) personal, one that I'm sure still is occurring to me at times, although I don't think it functions as much in my thinking now as it might have – is uhm, sometimes wondering if all this really does get anywhere, and (sniff), you know, if it isn't some sort of a hoax. But that's partly because I was brought up to think of it as being something that really didn't do any good for anybody and just costs a lot of money. I don't think that occurs to me as much now.

#53

I found it, I think I found it hard to come in here and lie down on the couch, with just you, being a man, in the room. But then that's, that could be any man, I suppose. (Pause)

#54

I do suppose though, if, if uh, something occurred to me about you, even if it weren't a criticism, I don't know that I feel, I think I, I feel I can't talk about it, because it seems like kind of an intimate type of thing and, and I just am not, I don't know, I just never made personal remarks to anybody (chuckle) before I knew them for a long time.

#55

In fact, I was kind of horrified last night at myself. I had a course a_ after I left here and uhm, (sniff) it uhm, it's an art course for teachers (sniff) and we were working on rubbing things for texture. And at one point I noticed the professor's tie, which was a very nubby coarse woven one, and although it would have been too soft to rub, I just (chuckle) reached out and held it out and said, "Well, this has a wonderful texture," which it did. But I was horrified at myself, because I've just never done anything like that before. And then I was sure his reaction was horror too, that I had been so forward. I don't know what it was actually, but at the time I was sure it was just horror. (Pause)

#56

Because several things have occurred to me while I've just been talking, shall I get off the other subject (chuckle)? (Sniff) I can't decide whether to – well, maybe I'll come back to it. Uhm, well, one thing is just a variation on my talking too much. When, at this same course last night, uhm – I'm, I'm usually very quiet when I'm, am new in a course and, and I don't like to say anything. But once I stop feeling that, once I've said something, whatever it is, then I just go the opposite way completely, and I get extremely aggressive. And at the time I don't realize I'm taking over, but then afterwards, if I think about it, I can see that I really did kind of take over or ins–, keep pushing myself into the conversation to the point where others might just say, "Oh well, I'm not going to bother trying to talk." And I do this, I've noticed, sometimes in conversations too, that I'll either try to anticipate what somebody's going to say and then continue on with what I'm thinking, or keep talking when I should stop because they're about to say something and then they won't, then they'll never say it. And that way I control the conversation. But the conversation might not get anywhere, or certainly nowhere near where it could have if I had stopped talking when it was time to. (Sniff)

#57

And the other thing I was thinking of when I was speaking of my reaction to psychoanalysis being, well, a questionable thing for all the money that it costs, is, uhm, just my reaction to money and handling it and saving it and all, which again has come up recently, because, uhm, the other day David and I were talking about, or I was talking (chuckle) about, having a budget, because this year is going to have a lot more expenses than we're (sic) ever had before. And, and I just don't feel I handle money very well anyway. I'll spend what's there and (sniff) if it's in the bank, I'll, and I can get my hands on it, I, it just sudden–, it just seems to disappear and I'm not really consciously spending it, or, I, in fact, I'm usually consciously being very miserly and, and ungenerous with my money (chuckle). But (sniff) somehow it seems to disappear – that I have no sense on where I can save and where it's stupid to save.

#58

And we had a, I guess a little bit of a fight (chuckle) about that too, because I, I have no reason to insist that somehow we make some savings if we can, but I was insisting that we should be able to make some savings and that no matter what, we should have some savings. And he would say, "Well, what are we saving for?" And I wouldn't know, except that I'd been brought up that you always made savings if you could, so somehow I just felt I had to have savings. But then when it came down to it, he said, "All right, well, you can put the savings aside with your money." And of course that wasn't (chuckle) what I had in mind. (Laughing) I guess what I really wanted was to have all the hardship with him and then I'd still be free to let money slip through my fingers. (Chuckle)

#59

(Sniff) But I do feel guilty sometimes too, if, uhm, for instance, if we use some money for our entertainment and then don't have very much for gifts or something like that, then I feel kind of guilty. (Stomach rumble) Well, I guess I look upon gifts as being more (sniff) – I'm not, well, I think I'm not too good at thinking of what somebody would want, and I'll try really hard and then, when I fail there, I think well, if you spend a lot of money it makes up for the fact that you couldn't think of anything (chuckle). (Sniff) Or else things I can think of always seem to cost a lot of (chuckle) money. I don't know which way it works.

#60

(Sniff) But then I'll have no sense about something like buying clothes. I'll absolutely buy nothing for a long time and then I'll suddenly go out on a big splurge, not meaning to. I'll just go looking and then I'll start finding things and then I justify it, well, I don't look very often so when I do find something I should just get it. But then I, I'm getting better at this now, because I'm getting better at knowing what I want and don't want and controlling my choices, but even then I might spend quite a bit of money suddenly. And I used to be terrible about shoes. I just, I wouldn't know what I wanted so then I'd end up buying all sorts of things. Well, I suppose it's all part of making decisions and making choices. (Pause)

#61

Because that (chuckle) is, well even this I find hard to say, and it's, it's silly, but just in thinking about clothes and wearing what you want, uhm, just in, in noticing what you've worn since I've started coming and the, the variety and the freedom that you seem to have and, and I think I've been sort of envious of that. (Sniff) I feel very embarrassed (chuckle) saying that.

#62

(Sniff) In fact I – just in thinking about people at school now who are very clothes conscious and they're always, if you come in with something they like, they'll compliment you on it. And even then I'm beginning to do this now and it's partly almost consciously because it's the way you have to do things at this school. But it's not just that, it's really sort of a gesture of friendship, I guess, to anybody, that if you like something somebody has on, acknowledging it. And I'm just, I, I just still find that hard. And it's almost like I notice it (sniff) but it doesn't register on my mind as something important to say to the person, even though I'm pleased if somebody will say it to me. I guess I'm just still so concerned with, with myself and what I'm thinking that I might register I like what they have, but I can't keep it as an important thing and, and feel it's important to tell them. (Sniff, stomach rumble) And I used to always justify this that, well, I'm not going to be one of these girls that just thinks about clothes all the time and that's all they talk about. But if I'm honest with myself I guess I think (chuckle) a lot about clothes. (Pause, stomach rumble)

#63

/ Our time's up. /

Converging Evidence for Emotional Structures: Theory and Method

Wilma Bucci

1. Introduction

The task of the psychoanalytic researcher is in part to verify what the clinician already knows. For much of what the researcher finds the response of the clinician must be, "I knew that all along." But the goal of research must also be to discover what we have previously had no access to, and what we seem to know, but wrongly. You can see that the work of the researcher is in some respects like that of the patient as well as the therapist. All participants in the psychoanalytic enterprise are attempting to detect psychic structures that have previously been unrecognized. At all levels, the achievement of new knowledge, the "surprise", depends on the articulation of connections and associations so that gaps can be uncovered and ambiguities resolved.

Psychoanalysis is essentially a theory of mental representation or in Freud's terms, of psychic structure. In contrast to behaviorist theories, which are concerned with regularities of external and observable events, theories of mental representation deal with internal and private phenomena that can be known directly only by their experiences, and are sometimes unconscious and inaccessible even to them. The necessity for research, and the difficulty of doing such research, both arise from this epistemological focus.

The observation of structure requires a Structure Detecting (SD) device. The only adequate SD device for detection of psychic structure in oneself or others is the human mind. However, the mind is also the quintessential Structure Constructing (SC) device. In clinical intuition the detection and construction processes are intertwined. The problem of suggestibility – the patient's vulnerability to the analyst's interpretations – is a special case of this general epistemological issue. The responsibility of the researcher is to find the level of meaning at which the detection of structures may be distinguished from the construction of them. For this purpose, consensual validation is not sufficient; consensus is itself subject to the problem of suggestibility. A system of propositions with well-defined, *testable* implications, which may be evaluated by independent observers, is required.

The psychoanalytic researcher can lead rather than follow the clinician by looking at clinical material in the context of a systematic theory that gives meaning to observation, and by providing an observer, a third "eye," on the psychoanalytic dialogue. The theory provides the context that defines the domain of "facts." Subjective experience and objective events alike derive their meaning, and their status as fact, from this theoretical network. Private experience can have the status of fact, existing prior to and distinct from its representation in some observable form such as language or behavior, but characterized in terms of a network of observables. The impact of the observer, and particular characteristics of the observer, can be included as variables in the network. Through a complex interaction of theory and monitored observation, it becomes possible to escape the pitfalls of both the hermeneutic and positivist positions.[1] The interlocking systems of propositions of the theory, their observable implications, and definitions based on these implications, are formalized in "manuals." In these terms, manuals go far beyond a static "cookbook" role, and constitute the core of this research approach, i.e., manuals determine the meaning and direct the identification of "facts."

This paper will present a brief outline of the dual code model of mental representation that provides the theoretical context of our approach, and will describe two types of systematic evaluation procedures, or "manuals" that permit us to develop converging evidence for nonverbal structures and for structural change. We will then briefly describe several preliminary studies that have been generated in the context of this research program.

---

[1]The position taken here, as to the espistemological status of the concept of psychic structure and the possibility of empirical testing of psychoanalytic theory, is at variance with the position of Schafer (1980), Spence (1982), Gill and Hoffman (1982b) and others. For a critical discussion of the positions of the former two authors see Bucci (1985). The spurious identification of positivism with science, and the implications of this for the hermeneutic argument have been discussed by Leeds, J. (1986).

2. Outline of the Dual Code Model

The dual code model of mental representation provides a theory of the mental apparatus that is compatible with psychoanalysis, but that is informed by the new perspectives on mental functioning brought in by the cognitive revolution of the late sixties. The model rests on an extensive body of experimental evidence developed by Paivio (1971, 1978) and others. The supporting evidence for dual coding over alternative theories of mental representation, and the application of dual coding to psychoanalytic theory have been discussed by Bucci (1985).

According to the dual code model, verbal and nonverbal representations are registered in symbolic form, in separate systems of schemata in the mind. The two codes have their own intrinsic and independent organization, but are connected by a complex body of referential links. There are both separate schemata within each system and interconnections between the systems, in development and throughout life. Both codes are capable of representing a wide range of information in symbolic, structured form.

Verbal Representations

The verbal system is the abstract code of language and logic, generally accepted as the optimal mature representational form by developmental psychologists such as Bruner (1967) and Piaget (1952). Theories of mental representation based on verbal mediation entirely dominated experimental psychology for half a century, from the advent of Watsonian behaviorism (1913) until the cognitive revolution of the middle sixties. In language, we attribute properties, assign entities to categories, and apply logical distinctions; we also develop systems of associations based on the sounds of speech. The elements of the verbal schemata are lexical items, which may be registered in the form of both phonological and semantic features. Examples of semantic schemata include hierarchical tree structures or other types of network structures, which represent the shared knowledge of the culture, as investigated by Collins and Quillian (1972) and others. In a very different domain, the systems of rings postulated by Lacan (1968) would constitute another format of the verbal system. Through such verbal structures the meaning of words *in terms of other words* is derived.

Nonverbal Schemata

In contrast to the verbal system, which is specialized for representing abstract properties and category membership, the nonverbal system is specialized for representing *concrete properties of things*. The nonverbal schemata are made up of representations of all manner of imagery and perceptual experience, including sights, sounds, tastes, and smells; somatic and visceral experiences, and motoric representations. Representations of somatic experience may include bodily states such as thirst and hunger, and feedback of functions such as heartbeat, muscle tension, and respiration. Representations of movements include facial expressions as well as other actions, and may be in the form of motor programs to direct action, kinaesthetic feedback from action, or more formal structures that are abstractions of operations on objects.

The schemata of the nonverbal systems are built on experience, reflecting shared perceptual properties of things, or sequence of events as they occurred. Many, but not all, of the nonverbal schemata are unique to an individual life. Representations of things are connected because they occur in the same place at the same time, because they play interacting roles in the same functions or events, or because they look or feel or taste alike; and one image will evoke another through such connections. Ice and glass are associated because they are perceptually similar – both shiny and clear. The sights and sounds of autumn leaves and the feel of cool air, may be connected in a schemata which also includes the return from vacation and the feelings associated with shortening days. The visual experiences of a tennis ball moving in particular direction at different speeds, the sight of the net, the lines of the court, and the movements of one's opponent are entered into complex computations which also include representations of movements of one's entire body, including eyes, hands, shoulders, feet and knees. Other memory schemata may include stored imagery, bodily experiences of pleasure or pain, and representations of characteristic behaviors, e.g. to approach or avoid certain persons (or categories of persons); these schemata may be associated with (or constitute) emotional states. The nonverbal schemata may play themselves out without the intervention of language, but may also interact with the verbal schemata in complex ways. The formation of schemata in the nonverbal system begins before language is acquired, and continues, with varying degrees of interaction with language, throughout life.

Emotional schemata are structures in the nonverbal system, made up of the elements of that modality, including imagery, representations of movement, and representations of bodily experience. This aspect of the model is derived from the psychoanalytic theory of the emotions developed by Dahl (1978), based on Chapter Seven of "The Interpretation of Dreams" (Freud 1900a). Thus, for example, the emotional schemata that characterize wishes are made up of images of the desired or feared or hated object; representations of consummatory acts; and bodily sensations – what we feel when we love or hate. The organization of the emotional structures are determined by the interactions of early life; these are the underlying structures that are activated in the transference.

Referential Connections

The two coding systems, based on different organizing principles, are joined and affect each other through the referential links. This must be so because we can name what we experience, and we can identify what has been named.

The referential connections are most direct for concrete and specific words and the entities to which they refer, and less direct for abstract concepts and words. Thus referential connections would be most direct for words like 'orange' or 'apple', less direct for supercategory terms such as 'fruit' or 'food' which do not have specific referents, and still less direct for words such as 'truth', 'beauty' or 'goodness'. Such words can be connected to imagery indirectly through other words, or may be interpreted entirely in the verbal networks without reaching the nonverbal system at all. Similarly, there may be representations on the nonverbal side that are difficult or impossible to put into words, e.g. perceptual, motoric or emotional representations that have never been verbalized. These would include representations laid down early in life before language has been acquired. Nonverbal schemata that do not themselves have referential connections to language may interact, via the associations within the nonverbal system, with those that do.

People differ in the strength of their referential connections as a matter of competence. An individual may also show fluctuation in activity of the referential process as a function of interpersonal context or somatic or emotional state. The fluctuation in activity of the referential process affects capacity to translate nonverbal experience into words, or to bring the words of others to bear on the nonverbal schemata. Where referential linkage is sparse or inactive, the two systems retain the modes of organization intrinsic to their own schemata.

Where referential linkage is active, the schemata of the two system will interact. Thus the schemata of language and logic and the experiential and episodic structures of the nonverbal system will each be reflected in and lead to reorganization of the other.

3. Application of the Dual Code Model to Psychoanalytic Theory

The psychoanalytic account of the mental apparatus is inherently a dual code approach. The basis for the division of the mental apparatus, and the characteristics associated with each part, have shifted with the evolution of the theory; however the premise of dual representation remains inherent throughout. On the one hand, the mental representation of material that has never been verbalized, or where the links to words have been lost, is a fundamental tenet of psychoanalytic theory, present in all its forms. The system of private nonverbal representations is associated with dreams and regressive mental functioning, and not with conscious thought. On the other hand, verbalization is viewed as a necessary condition for rational, productive thought. This view may be traced throughout Freud's writings, from its basic formulation in "The Interpretation of Dreams" (Freud 1900a), to the posthumous statement in "An Outline of Psychoanalysis" (Freud 1940a).

What the Freudian model lacks and the dual code theory contributes is the concept of nonverbal representation as a structured and organized system in normal, rational adult thought, existing alongside the verbal representational mode. Imagery is encoded and organized in its own special format in the mind. We may not be aware of our nonverbal structures, just as we may not be aware of many important facets of our verbal thought; nevertheless, we perform complicated mental operations by generating images and comparing them; by moving ourselves and the objects of our world in imagination through time and space.

Psychoanalytic treatment takes place primarily in words, but the structural change that is sought is in the nonverbal system, particularly the emotional schemata that determine what we perceive and how we feel and act. The nonverbal structures may be known through words, but exist independently of them. Given the system of dual coding of mental representations outlined here, the primary danger is not that the words spoken in the session will penetrate and rearrange the patient's memory schemata, as Spence (1982), Schafer (1980) and others have argued, but rather that the verbal communications will not reach the nonverbal schemata at all – will leave them untouched and unchanged. Where the psychoanalytic dialogue does bring about a change it is all too likely to be in the verbal schemata alone. It follows that the effectiveness of therapy depends on the operation of the referential connections, which link words that are spoken in the session to the nonverbal, particularly the emotional structures. Anything that facilitates the referential process will facilitate change in the nonverbal schemata; this is what we mean by structural change.

Within this theoretical framework, we have begun to develop two types of manuals that I will describe briefly here. One manual outlines procedures for detecting nonverbal, particularly emotional, structures that emerge as repetitive patterns in language and behavior. The other outlines linguistic measures that reflect the activity of the referential connections between verbal and nonverbal systems, and the degree to which nonverbal material is being retrieved and expressed.

4. Procedures for Detection of Emotional Structures

The detection of significant emotional structures has generally been seen as the domain of clinical intuition. This is a core challenge for research. Here we directly confront the question raised above, of whether the detection of structures (SD) can be distinguished from the construction of them (SC). This challenge has been addressed by Luborsky (1984) in the development of the concept of the "Core Conflictual Relationship Theme " (CCRT), and by Gill and Hoffman (1982b) in the concept of the "*Jxr*", i.e., the implicit manifestation of the transference relationship as inferred by judges in communications not manifestly about the relationship. Each of these concepts refers to underlying patterns represented in the manifest content; however these concepts involve a particular systematic organization; thus involve imposition of structure to that extent. In contrast, Teller and Dahl (1986) have sought to identify repetitive patterns in the free association of an analytic patient, without imposing structure in any sense. Their assumption is that significant emotional structures, schemata of the nonverbal system, are manifested repeatedly with many different objects and in many contexts. Such structures could be found in observations of behavior, i.e., by following individuals through the varied contexts of their lives. They can also be detected by a pattern matching procedure in the "free association" of an analytic patient. "Free" association is of course determined rather than free – determined by the structure of the nonverbal schemata, although the connections may not be reflected in the logical structures of the verbal system. Building on the approach of Teller and Dahl, two related pilot studies have been carried out: one to detect patterns in the free association of an analytic patient; the second to detect similar patterns in the behavior of young children at play.

Detection of Repetitive Patterns in Free Association

Leeds and Bucci have carried out an experiment to see if it is possible to detect repetitive structures in the text of an analytic session by following a system of rules specified in a manual (Leeds 1986). The method involves successive stages of simple judgments, made by different sets of judges. The multi-judge, multi-stage method precludes imposition of an interpretation on the sequence, thus disabling the SC device. The judgments involve stepwise increases in level of generalization, i.e., a process of categorization applied to the output of the preceding stage. Reliability is assessed at each judgment stage. The procedure is as follows:

1. One set of judges divides the text into idea units. The boundary of an idea unit is marked where the focus of the narrative shifts or a new idea is introduced. In some cases, the division into units follows the natural divisions of speech in a dialogue. In other cases long utterances may be subdivided or shorter ones combined; this is of course necessary for the long continuous narrative flow of free association in psychoanalysis.

2. The idea units are taken out of the context in which they appear in the hour and rearranged in random order, for presentation to the second set of judges.

3. The second set of judges translates the sentences in the idea units into propositional statements, each containing at least a subject and an action, with qualifiers and nonsubstantive words removed.

4. These judges also remove all references to specific actions, times, and people and replace them with coded category terms. These are general categories, e.g. "act," "object," numbered to distinguish between them, e.g. "act 1;" "act 2." This coding is not applied to experiential terms, i.e., those that refer to the patient's reactions and reflections, such as "I felt terrible," "I was confused," "I was surprised;" these are retained in their specific surface form.

5. A third set of judges then looks for repetitions of structures in the output of Stage 4, the generalized propositional sequences. A number of different types of analyses can then be carried out as part of the pattern matching procedure at this stage.

The method of step-wise generalization and categorization outlined here was applied to the text of the Specimen Hour (see page 15), the fifth hour of the psychoanalysis of a young married woman. Good reliability was achieved by the judges at each stage. The procedure may be illustrated by comparing the manifest content of the text with the coded output of Stage 4.

The following excerpt is an example of an idea unit, as segmented by the judges, in the format of the manifest content of the text. The patient is describing an experience as a teacher in an elementary school:

> (#20) ... And I never like talking to parents then because it was just too confusing. But of course I just said something to her that was, you know, chatty. And then, and then I suddenly found myself starting to talk about this problem, which I hadn't intended to at all. And I, I was kind of surprised at myself when I was talking and, then I just couldn't keep quiet (chuckle). I couldn't stop it, or say well, we better talk about this another time or anything. And I just seemed to get in deeper and deeper and I'm always doing this.

The following is the same unit in generalized propositional form, the output of judgment stage 4:

I never like doing (act 1) (time 1)

It was confusing.

I (act) to (object 1).

I start to (act 1).

I hadn't intended to.

I was surprised at myself.

I couldn't stop (act 1).

I couldn't say we'd better (act 1) (time 2).

I seemed to get in deeper and deeper.

I'm always doing this.

For purposes of this pilot study, the Stage 5 analysis, i.e., the search for repetitive structures, was then applied to a subset of the idea units from the session. We selected idea units that began with a reference to the patient's performing some action, or reflecting upon it, e.g. "I (act)," "I like to (act)" or the negation of such statements, as in the excerpt above. There were seven such units. We then looked for regularities in patterns associated with the general category of action. In 6 of the 7 cases, we found essentially the same general pattern: The patient begins with a negation of action or a negative reflection on action; then progresses from negation to starting to act, to acting, to an expectation of not being able to stop. This pattern is illustrated in the example above. In only one passage (#55, see page 26; lines 328 to 337 in Figure 1, page 44) was there an instance of an action taken without a preceding negation and the accompanying negative expectation. The patient's experience of this deviation was very clear: "I was horrified; I've never done anything like this before; I'm sure the other person was horrified too."

What we found then in this pilot study was a clear pattern of negative attitude or ambivalence over action, and an expectation of being unable to stop once an action is undertaken, repeated in different contexts, and with different objects. This study was very important in demonstrating that it is possible to identify significant repetitive patterns reliably in the text of a therapy transcript, while stringently precluding the operation of "intuition" and the imposition of structure on the text, i.e., disabling the SC device. Patterns detected by this approach are *there* to be found; not constructed by the observer in any sense. In future work, we will attempt to go deeper in plotting more intricate schemata of the nonverbal system by this means; here the numerical coding of specific subtypes within a given category becomes crucial. Different patterns can emerge based on specific constellations of actions, times or objects, i.e., the patient does this but not that, here but not there, with one person but not another.

Once these repetitive patterns have been identified, the next step is to demonstrate that they reflect structures in the nonverbal system, rather than verbal schemata. This position has been supported by several different kinds of converging evidence, including observation of emotional structures in the behavior of young children; and comparison of the incidence of emotional schemata to fluctuations in level of Referential Activity in the patient's speech.

Detection of Repetitive Patterns in Children's Behavior

It is a fundamental postulate of psychoanalysis that significant emotional structures can be laid down in early childhood long before full linguistic competence is acquired. We would expect these structures to be manifest repetitively in sequences of behavior of children seen in different interpersonal contexts, as well as in language.

In one pilot study, Davies and Bucci have explored the feasibility of detecting structures in the behavior of young children, which are similar to those detected in the free association of an analytic patient, using a similar method. The children were seen in two peer play situations, and in interactions with their mothers.[2] Procedures were developed for the coding and transcribing of behavioral sequences. The step-wise judgment and categorization procedures outlined above were then applied to the coded observations.

Repetitive patterns were first identified in the mother-child interaction. These patterns were then shown to be repeated or reflected in the peer play context, with the child assuming either corresponding or complementary roles in the two contexts. This study is of considerable interest in showing the emotional frame structures in formation, i.e., in the interaction of early life in which the schemata consisting of images, actions and somatic experience are formed. In principle, the repetitive patterns detected in the behavior of children would be expected to relate, in a complex but systematic manner, to the repetitive patterns detected in behavior in adulthood, and even to the structures detected in free association, if such continued observations were possible for an individual's life. The results of this study support the theory outlined here in showing emotional structures in pure culture, i.e., directly in behavior, rather than inferred to the nonverbal system from verbal representation. In these terms, the study provides evidence that emotional schemata of this sort are *there* to be found, i.e., present in the nonverbal system, not constructed in the psychoanalytic dialogue.

5. Linguistic Indicators of Emotional Structures

Another source of evidence for the presence of emotional schemata as representations in the speaker's mind lies in the nature of language itself.

---

[2]This study is based on data previously collected by J. Kagan, J. S. Reznick, J. Davies and J. Smith at Harvard University in 1982.

According to the dual code model, the degree to which the referential connections between the verbal and nonverbal systems are activated, and emotional structures are expressed is reflected in linguistic features and qualities of language style. In our basic experimental work during the past several years, we have discovered a number of measurable linguistic features and qualities that are likely to be used by individuals with active referential connections between language and imagery statements, i.e., individuals characterized as high in Referential Activity (Bucci and Freedman 1978; Bucci 1984). These include qualities of language style measured by rating scales, counts of specific content items, and other measurable and quantifiable features. The linguistic analysis serves as a verification procedure for the presence of nonverbal structures. The measures are defined in the manual for scoring Referential Activity (RA) language style,[3] and will be described briefly here:

Qualities of Verbal Expressions: the RA Scales

Scales reflecting the linguistic qualities of "Concreteness", "Specificity", and "Clarity" have been developed as measures of Referential Activity:

1. *Concreteness* is defined in terms of degree of perceptual or sensory quality – the degree to which a verbal expression refers to properties of actual things or events, in any sense modality, rather than to abstract concepts.

2. *Specificity* refers to amount of detailed description of persons, objects, places, or events.

3. *Clarity of Expressions* refers to quality of focus of the narrative. The outlines of the ideas or imagery as expressed in the speech are clean, not blurred of fuzzy. Clarity does *not* refer to logical or grammatical organization. Texts can be rated as high in clarity even if the speaker moves from idea to idea without the basis for the connections being evident, if each "shot" is well-focused.

The choice of these dimensions is based on both experimental research and literary criticism, as discussed in detail elsewhere (Bucci and Freedman 1978; Bucci 1984). The referential connections are more direct for concrete and specific entities and the words which refer to

[3] Bucci, W. *Instructions for scoring Referential Activity (RA) in transcripts of spoken narrative texts.* Manuscript, Derner Institute, Adelphi University, 1985.

them; less direct for abstract concepts and terms (Paivio 1971; 1978). Language that is high on these dimensions has a quality of immediacy, as if the speaker is reliving the experience in imagination; such language makes the experience come alive for the listener or reader as well (Strunk and White 1972).

The three dimensions are conceptually distinct but generally highly intercorrelated. They are interpreted as manifestations of the same underlying dimension, the closeness of the connections between language and the nonverbal representational system.

In addition, a measure of overall imagery level is used which provides a global rating of the degree to which the rater feels imagery (in any sense modality) is present in the speaker's mind, and the extent to which the text evokes corresponding imagery in the rater. This measure also correlates highly with the average of the three scales described above.

All dimensions are rated on a scale of 0 to 10. No clinical expertise is required of the judges, and good reliability is obtained after brief training.

Other Measurable Features of RA Language

In addition to the scales, a number of linguistic features have been identified that are associated with active referential connections and more direct access to imagery. These include: lesser use of first person singular pronouns, greater use of direct quotes, stylistic use of the present tense in describing past events, and use of figures of speech such as metaphor, in which concrete images represent complex ideas. The various RA language style indicators may be combined, in a weighted function, to yield an overall measure of activity of the referential connections in any segment of text.

RA as an Indicator of Clinical Process

The model implies that high RA language will be associated with greater ability to express emotional experience, and with more effective analytic work. This implication has been supported in several studies in which fluctuations in RA in patient speech were compared to independent assessments of the clinical process in psychotherapy and psychoanalysis.

1. Increase in patient RA level following "plan compatible" interventions

In one study, in collaboration with Fretter, Silberschatz, and Curtis at the Mt. Zion Hospital in San Francisco, RA level was rated for approximately 300 excerpts drawn from three completed short term psychotherapy cases conducted at Mt. Zion. Segments of patient text were selected that preceded and followed therapist interventions independently rated as to their "plan compatibility," i.e., their pertinence to a patient's problems, needs and goals (Sampson and Weiss 1986). The clinical evaluation of the therapist's interventions and the selection of text segments were carried out by the Mt. Zion group; scoring of the RA rating scales was carried out by us. All segments were presented in randomly rearranged form for RA scoring. Residualized gain scores were calculated representing the variance in post-intervention RA not predicted by the pre-intervention RA level. Significantly higher residualized gain scores on all RA scales were associated with plan compatible vs. non-compatible interpretations. That is, interventions that were plan compatible, in the terms of the Mt. Zion approach, facilitated access to nonverbal structures as measured by pre to post-intervention change in level of patient RA. In this sense, we would also argue that the change in patient RA level serves as a verification of the correspondence of the intervening interpretation to the patient's underlying nonverbal representations, and thus serves as verification of the validity of the "plan" itself.

2. Higher RA level in "work" over "resistance" sessions

In another study, RA level of language was found to be higher in analytic sessions characterized primarily as "work" than in those classified as "resistance" hours. This study was carried out jointly with Hartvig Dahl at Downstate Medical Center. In previous work, Dahl (1972, 1974) had selected ten *work* hours, ten *resistance* hours, and five *middle* hours from transcripts of 363 hours of a single analytic case. The classification was made on the basis of computer content-analysis techniques, and was confirmed by judgments of three experienced psychoanalysts with a reliability of .90. In this study, RA level was scored using a different computer-aided content analysis procedure. This involved matching words in the texts of the sessions with a list of words independently rated for semantic dimensions relevant to RA and generating a score on these dimensions for each session. For this study, we used a word list constructed by Toglia and Battig consisting of 2,854 words scaled along the dimensions of concreteness and imagery (as well as five other semantic dimensions that will not be discussed here). The results showed the use of both concreteness and imagery words to be highest in the work sessions, and lowest in the resistance sessions ($F=18.31$, $p<.001$ for concreteness; and $F=17.64$, $p<.001$ for imagery). In addition to its theoretical and clinical significance, this study is also important in demonstrating that linguistic qualities relevant to the RA dimension can be carried by individual lexical items independent of syntactic structure. Thus it supports the possibility of obtaining automatized or partially automatized counterparts of the RA measures, for future larger scale clinical applications.

6. Converging Evidence for Nonverbal Structures in the Specimen Hour

These two studies provide background for our application of this approach to the Specimen Hour, Hour 5 of a young woman's psychoanalysis. Fluctuations in RA level were compared to incidence of emotional structures in the course of the hour. The typed transcript was divided into idea units, following the procedure outlined in the Leeds and Bucci study above. Referential Activity level was scored for each unit. Graphs of this sequential variation were constructed for patient and therapist separately. An independent clinical evaluation was carried out to identify the incidence of emotional structures in the text.

Analysis of RA Level

The patient's speech in the course of this hour was segmented by the judges into 38 idea units. Referential Activity level for each unit, scored on a scale of 0 to 10, is shown in Figure 1, according to line number in the typed transcript of the hour.[4] The horizontal line, at 5, marks the midpoint of the RA language style Index.

The first result that emerges is a predominance of low RA utterances in this session; 24 of the idea units or 63% were scored as below the midpoint of 5 on the RA scale, and 14 above. We would expect that the relatively low RA level seen in this session relates to high resistance levels at this early stage of the analysis, and that RA level will increase with clinical progress in successful therapy. (We have verified this in another study which includes ratings of RA level in later sessions of this treatment.)

---

[4]The segmentation into idea units by the judges is a distinct process from the paragraphing of a text by a transcriber; numbering of the idea units and the text paragraphs do not necessarily correspond.

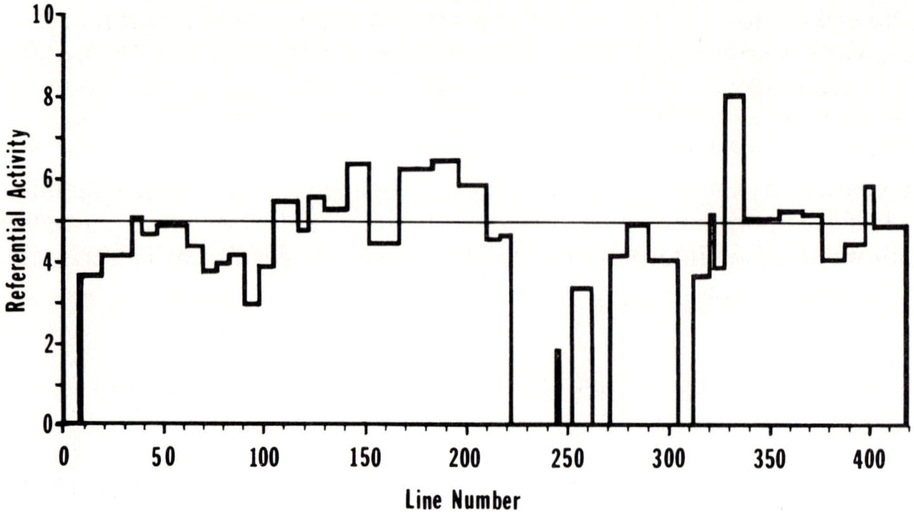

Figure 1

Excerpts from high and low RA utterances in this session may be used to illustrate the nature of the RA language style dimension. The following excerpt (lines 92 to 98 in Figure 1), represents the low RA point of this session:

> (#10) I suppose it's also just wondering what the function of friendly advice is anyway. If you're a good friend of somebody, not that I'm saying this is the situation I'm in, but just makes me wonder, when you're a good friend of somebody, how much, from your point of view, you should advise your friend and how much you should keep quiet, because the person is what they are and, and your point of view is going to be different from theirs in any case.

This paragraph is a characteristic low RA utterance. The language is abstract, general and vague, lacking in specific and concrete detail, and does not evoke imagery in the listener. (Later on in the treatment, this analyst will often respond to such utterances with interventions such as "You're being obscure," "Can you be more specific," "Can you be more concrete.")

In contrast, here are lines 328 to 337, the high RA point of the session:

> (#55) In fact, I was kind of horrified last night at myself. I had a course a_ after I left here and uhm, (sniff) it uhm, it's an art course for teachers (sniff) and we were working on rubbing things for texture. And at one point I noticed the professor's tie, which was a very nubby coarse woven one, and although it would have been too soft to rub, I just (chuckle) reached out and held it out and said, "Well, this has a wonderful texture," which it did. But I was horrified at myself, because I've never done anything like that before. And then I was sure his reaction was horror too, that I had been so forward. I don't know what it was actually, but at the time I was sure it was just horror.

This passage illustrates many features of high RA language style - a specific incident, rich in concrete sensory detail, and including stylistic features such as direct quotes. The passage gives the impression of immediacy of the experience in the speaker's mind, and evokes a corresponding experience for the listener.

Incidence of Emotional Structures

In this study, the identification of the emotional structures was done by one clinician[5] following the general definition of frame structures outlined by Teller and Dahl (1986), rather than by the rigorous multi-judge, multi-stage procedure used in the Leeds and Bucci study. The purpose of this preliminary analysis was to get a comprehensive picture of the underlying emotional patterns for the entire hour. The identification of the emotional frame structures was entirely independent of the language style assessment.

The major types of wishes identified in this session were, first, desires for *support and reassurance,* and second, a wish for *closeness and togetherness.* These are expressed in relation to several different subjects and objects. The patient and her father are both described as experiencing such wishes. The wishes are directed by the patient toward many objects, including her husband, the children in her classroom, and the analyst. The patient also repeatedly demonstrates an *expectation that the wishes will not be fulfilled,* and expects or fears that her action in seeking gratification is likely to be *uncontrolled.* Thus, she *delays* the action of seeking gratification of these wishes, and in some instances

---

[5]George Moroz, then at Downstate Medical Center.

controls the emergence of the experience of the wish – thereby insuring that gratification does *not* occur when she wants it. The identification of these wishes and expectations and their interaction in emotional frame structures are discussed in detail by Teller and Dahl (1986). We may note that this structure corresponds to the repetitive pattern found in the Leeds and Bucci study, although arrived at independently, using a different text analysis procedure.

Convergence of RA and Emotional Patterns

We can now look at the distribution of these emotional structures in the transcript of the session in relation to fluctuation in the RA level of the patient's speech as shown in Figure 2.

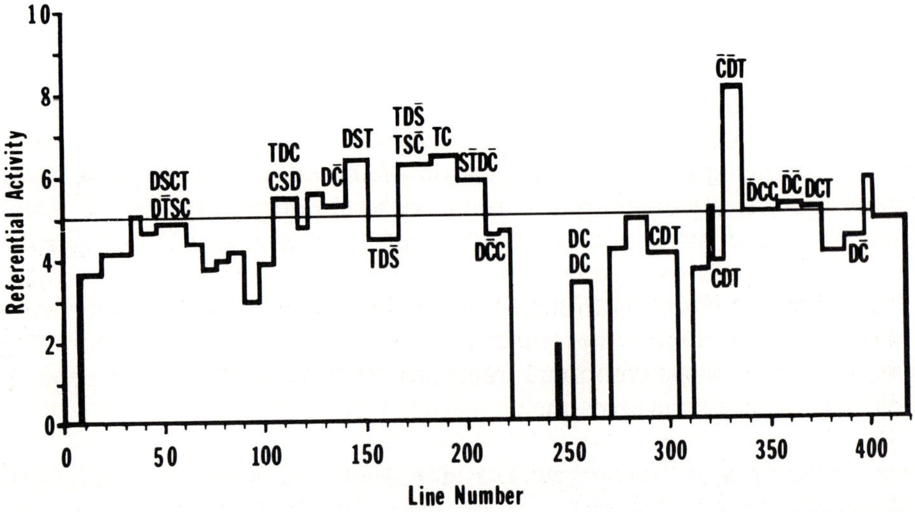

Figure 2

Each of the emotional frame structures and their negations are represented by a sequence of letters denoting the component themes; S = a wish for reassurance or support, T = a wish for togetherness, D = a defense of delay, C = a defense of control. (A negation of a theme in the narrative is represented by the standard notation of a bar over the theme letter.) For this session, which included 38 utterance units, a total of 21 emotional frame structures, each built upon two or more of the four basic themes were found; some utterance units had more than one emotional structure, some had none. The findings are summarized in Table 1:

Table 1 Emotional Frame Structures in High vs. Low RA Idea Units

		Emotional Frame Structures		
	Idea Units	EFS Total	Wish Structures	Defense Structures
High RA	14	14	11	3
Low RA	24	7	3	4
Total	38	21	14	7

Of the 21 emotional frame structures found in the hour, 14, or two-thirds of them, were in the 14 high RA utterances - an average of one per unit. In comparison, there were only seven theme structures in the 24 low RA utterances or about one for every three and one half units. It is striking that the only units in the first part of the session where the judges rated the language style as near or above the midpoint of five on the scale are also the only units in which emotional frame structures were identified by the clinician, i.e., lines 40 to 62. Here two complex instances of emotional frame structures emerged as the patient described a specific person, rather than talking in abstract and general terms. The next point at which the RA scoring emerges above the midpoint is in paragraph 12, lines 106 to 117, and this paragraph is immediately succeeded by a sequence of segments in which frame structures are identified and in which the language is consistently rated as above the RA midpoint. Here, in lines 167 to 210, is where we meet the three paragraphs discussed in detail by Teller and Dahl (1986). As the patient's language begins to drop below the RA midpoint, in paragraphs 21 and 22, lines 211 to 222, the therapist intervenes to ask a specific question, focusing the patient precisely on the core resistance of delay and its associated structures that emerged in this period. The analyst appears to be responding intuitively to the fluctuations in language style represented in this chart; we may note that the concepts presented here provide a systematic theoretical basis for interventions of this nature.

There were only two instances in the entire session of an expression of a wish without an accompanying non-negated defense structure; these were in paragraphs 19 and 55, the two highest RA points of the hour. The latter segment, highest in this session on the RA scales (#55 above), was in the clinician's scoring a clear expression of a wish for closeness or togetherness, with the two defense structures negated. This unit includes the passage that was referred to in the Leeds and Bucci study above as the only instance of a direct action without initial delay or control.

These data provide a strong demonstration of converging evidence for emotional structures in the free association of an analytic patient. The assessment of emotional structures and the evaluation of linguistic quality were carried out by applying distinct concepts and following independent procedures, but show striking correspondence. The findings are of considerable interest in demonstrating that significant fluctuations in RA can be reliably discerned within a session, and in providing evidence that these fluctuations have clinical significance. Passages marked as containing emotional frame structures were significantly higher in Referential Activity level than those not so marked, indicating more direct access to nonverbal experience in the associative process of the patient at those points. Furthermore, the passages highest in RA contained the only unmitigated expressions of wishes in the transcript.

These findings are interpreted directly in the context of a dual code model, and have significance as verification procedures in those theoretical terms. We may also suggest that the concept of the Core Conflictual Relationship Theme (CCRT) introduced by Luborsky (1977 and this volume); and the concept of implicit manifestation of the transference relationship *(Jxr)* studied by Gill and Hoffman (1982b and Hoffman and Gill this volume) might also be understood, in the terms of the dual code model, as reflecting basic emotional structures, analyzed in different terms and found by different means. On that basis, we would then expect RA level also to fluctuate in relation to incidence of either CCRT's or *Jxr's*. We would also expect some correspondence of the emotional frame structures to both of these other types of structures. These correspondences remain to be tested in future work.

7. Conclusion

The important point that we have tried to make here by presentation of this preliminary research is that in the context of a coherent and systematic model of the mental apparatus, the linguistic indicators provide a means of *external and shared* validation of the presence of *private and internal* emotional representations. Thus we are not confined within the hermeneutic circle, but can point to evidence for emotional structures that are present independent of their verbal report, and that are detected by observers rather than constructed by them.

There may be operational indicators other than language style, in other aspects of the patient's behavior, that show that nonverbal representations have been activated, as Freud (1937d) told us, and we're also interested in studying those. But language is the basic medium of the treatment, and the most available and useful data source. For the researcher language is important as an observable and shared indicator of the extent to which private nonverbal representations have been tapped, and of the nature of these underlying structures. For the clinician or the patient, words are the primary medium of communication – the means by which structures may be changed. Nevertheless, it is the nonverbal structures and not the words that are the object of treatment. Poets, like analysts, deal in words, but recognize that words are important because of the nonverbal experiences that are evoked. Heine makes this distinction quite concretely:

> Worte! Worte! keine Taten!
> Niemals Fleisch, geliebte Puppe,
> Immer Geist und keinen Braten,
> Keine Knödel in der Suppe! (Heine 1967, p. 245)[6]

I would argue that the "Knödel in der Suppe", the matters of physical and emotional substance that stand behind the words, are the appropriate subjects and objects of psychoanalytic research, and ultimately, of the treatment process.

---

[6] "Words! words! no deeds! Never flesh, beloved doll, always spirit, and no roast meat, no dumplings in the soup!" Heinrich Heine, *Selected Verse* prose translation by Peter Branscombe; Middlesex, England: Penguin Books, 1967.

Frames of Mind

Hartvig Dahl*

1. Introduction

In the past decade psychotherapy researchers' strategies have converged on a set of closely related methods for the systematic description of patient's conflicts, of the processes of change in treatment, and of their relationship to the outcomes. Hoffman and Gill's coding of the *Patient's Experience of the Relationship with the Therapist* (PERT), (this volume), Luborsky's *Core Conflictual Relationship Theme* (CCRT), (1977, 1984, this volume; Levine and Luborsky 1981), and Strupp et al.'s *Cyclical Maladaptive Patterns* (CMP), (this volume; Schacht, Binder and Strupp 1984) each adopt a slightly different version of an interpersonal focus on the patient-therapist dyad. Others such as Horowitz's (Horowitz et al. 1984) *Configurational Analysis* and Slap's *Schema* (1986; Slap and Slaykin 1983) emphasize systematic description of internally represented *States of Mind* (Horowitz 1979) in patients and of the role of these states in the processes of change.

These strategies are summarized in Table 1. All of them share two fundamentally important commitments. First and foremost they focus on *repetitive structures*. And second, the detailed nature of the structure is a central function of the particular descriptive method employed. This is most clearly illustrated in the case of Luborsky's CCRT. Luborsky is concerned with identifying one or two *content themes* that capture a patient's central conflicts, but in so doing he imposes a uniform *structure* on the way this conflict is represented by always specifying the same *three* components of a *relationship episode*. These are, (1) a wish about

---

*I first chose the title of this chapter for a presentation to an American Psychological Association Division 39 Research Panel (April 1985) entitled, *Templates of Mind: The Thematic Analysis of Psychoanalytic Data*, unaware that in 1983 H. Gardner had puplished his theory of multiple intelligences under the same title. As the reader will discover, my use of the expression is completely different from Gardner's.

an object, (2) a real or anticipated response from the object (RO), and (3) a response from oneself (RS). Similarly, Strupp et al.'s and Hoffman and Gill's methods yield structures that are direct reflections of their methods. After I have presented an alternative to these approaches I will return to make some comparisons.

Table 1

RUBRIC	FIRST PUBLICATION	REPRESENTATION
PHANTASY	Freud (1897)	Phantasies rather than actual events postulated as etiology of neuroses.
FANTASY	Arlow (1969a, 1969b, 1980)	Clinical summaries of recurrent manifestations of unconscious fantasies.
CCRT	Luborsky (1977) Levine and Luborsky (1981)	Sequential structures extracted from a patient's relationship with objects.
CA	Horowitz (1979)	Configurational Analysis: a systematic method of case formulation.
FRAME	Teller and Dahl (1981a)	Sequential event structures extracted from a patient's discrete narratives.
PERT	Gill and Hoffman (1982b)	Coded instances of a patient's experience of the relationship with the therapist.
SCHEMA	Slap and Slaykin (1983)	Clinical summaries of recurrent themes.
TLDP (CMP)	Schacht, Binder, and Strupp (1984)	Dynamic focus on a patient's cyclical maladaptive patterns of action.

I did not start out to look for repetitive structures in my work with my colleague Virginia Teller (see this volume). We made our discoveries after several years spent with Rubinstein (see Rubinstein 1978) studying the structure of the implicit reasoning processes of psychoanalytic clinicians. Our method was to examine specific clinical hypotheses about a patient paired with specific pieces of evidence from transcripts of the patient's sessions (Dahl 1983). We had clinicians rate the degree to which the evidence supported the hypotheses and then we studied the logical (and illogical) relationships between the pairs rated high and low. In short, unlike those researchers mentioned above, our agenda was something far removed from the structures that we eventually discovered.

2. Frames

In 1981 Teller and I first reported our discovery of repetitive structures in the free association of a patient in psychoanalysis (Teller and Dahl 1981a) and have published a detailed report of some of their characteristics (Teller and Dahl 1986). As a name for these structures we chose Frames, Marvin Minsky's (1975) term for stereotyped knowledge structures that have many desirable theoretical features. Here I will briefly summarize some of the features of three such frames (one of which is also examined for different purposes by Teller in this volume), all found in the transcript of the Specimen Hour (this volume), of a tape-recorded psychoanalysis. I will include some extravagant, and to some, I am sure, fanciful claims about them, claims that imply, or surely ought to imply, a program of empirical research.

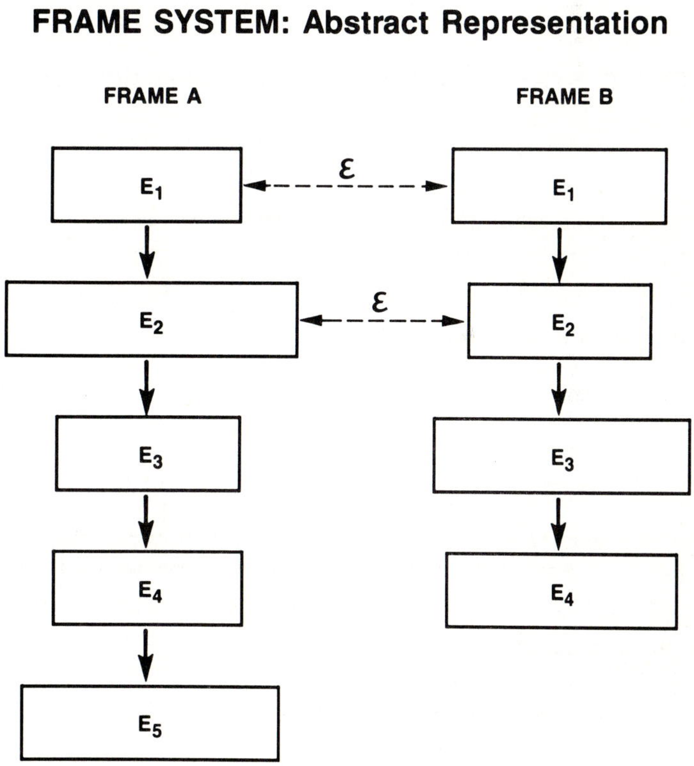

Figure 1

Figure 1 illustrates some of the basic properties of Frames. A frame is an Event Sequence Structure. Events are variables whose values may include mental and other events such as acting, perceiving, believing, knowing, wishing, feeling, being in certain states, etc. The relationship among the events is defined by their sequential order, indicated by the arrows. The dotted lines between the corresponding events in Frame A and in Frame B represent the fact that some events in two or more frames may be similar or may overlap in some way.

Figure 2 shows the values of each event for two specific frames that we labeled DELAY and SUPPORT. For each frame we distinguish between a Prototype in which the value of a specific event is completely justified by evidence from the manifest content of the transcript, and Instantiations, which are repetitions of a prototype. For example, *Having Conflicts* is a summary of specific patient statements taken from the transcript; and each of the values of the other events is also either the patient's literal statements, a close paraphrase, or a summary of several statements.

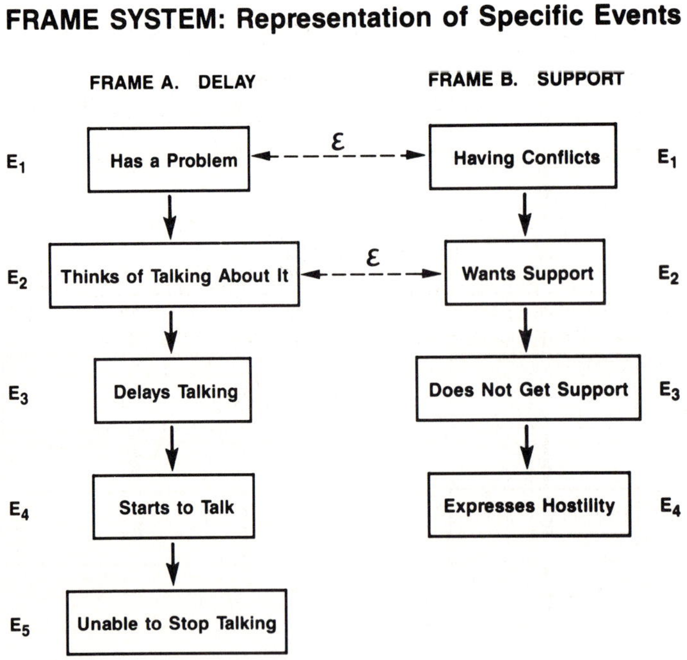

Figure 2

To illustrate, Table 2 is the text of paragraph 18, from which the prototype for the SUPPORT frame was constructed. Table 3 shows all of

Table 2

\# 18 Because I, I (chuckle) was just thinking I probably do the same thing with David. Last night in particular, I was talking with him about – I don't know, I just seemed to be in a funny mood by the time he got home. He got home sort of late, and it wasn't that he was late, because I knew he would be. But I guess he didn't immediately respond to me in the way I wanted him to or – I don't know what it was, because I imagine that somehow I was already in some kind of a mood. And (sniff) at one point I was talking to him, and I know I was talking to him wanting either confirmation that I'd done the right thing or a suggestion on what would be a right thing because I wasn't sure. I was upset about something I'd done and I didn't want him just to listen to me say it. I wanted him to actually react to it, and either suggest another course of action or, or approval that well, I guess that in the circumstances that wasn't that bad a thing to do. And, and he just didn't say anything, except sort of mutter under his breath. And so I got furious at him and (sniff) I imagine in a way it's the same kind of thing that my father always is doing. (Pause, stomach rumble)

Table 3 Support Frame

PROTOTYPE:
Talking to Husband

1. JUSTIFICATION for **HAVING CONFLICTS**
   Statements about "the thing I did":
   . . . either confirmation that I'd done the right thing or a suggestion on what would be a right thing because I wasn't sure. I was upset about something I'd done.

   . . . that wasn't that bad a thing to do.

2. JUSTIFICATION for **WANTS SUPPORT**
   I was talking to him wanting either confirmation that I'd done the right thing or a suggestion on what would be a right thing.

   I didn't want him just to listen to me say it. I wanted him to actually react to it, and either suggest another course of action, or, or approval that, well, I guess that in the circumstances that wasn't that bad a thing to do.

   ASSUMPTION: Spoken approval is one kind of support.

3. JUSTIFICATION for **DOES NOT GET SUPPORT**
   And, and he just didn't say anything, except sort of mutter under his breath.

4. JUSTIFICATION for **EXPRESSES HOSTILITY**
   And so I got furious at him.

WARRANTS FOR INDUCTIVE GENERALIZATION
I probably do the same thing with David.

Last night in particular, *I was talking with him. . .*

. . . and (sniff) I imagine in a way it's the same kind of thing that my father always is doing.

the evidence used to justify each of the four events in the SUPPORT frame. The data in this figure were taken from a single, succinct narrative that the patient told to the analyst about an episode with her husband. This is typical – a single narrative forms the basis for a prototype or a repetition. In three short paragraphs (18, 19 and 20) consisting of 612 words, we found one prototype and two instantiations for each of the DELAY and SUPPORT frames. In cases where there is no evidence for a particular event in an instantiation, the value in the corresponding prototype event becomes the predicted value in the instantiation.

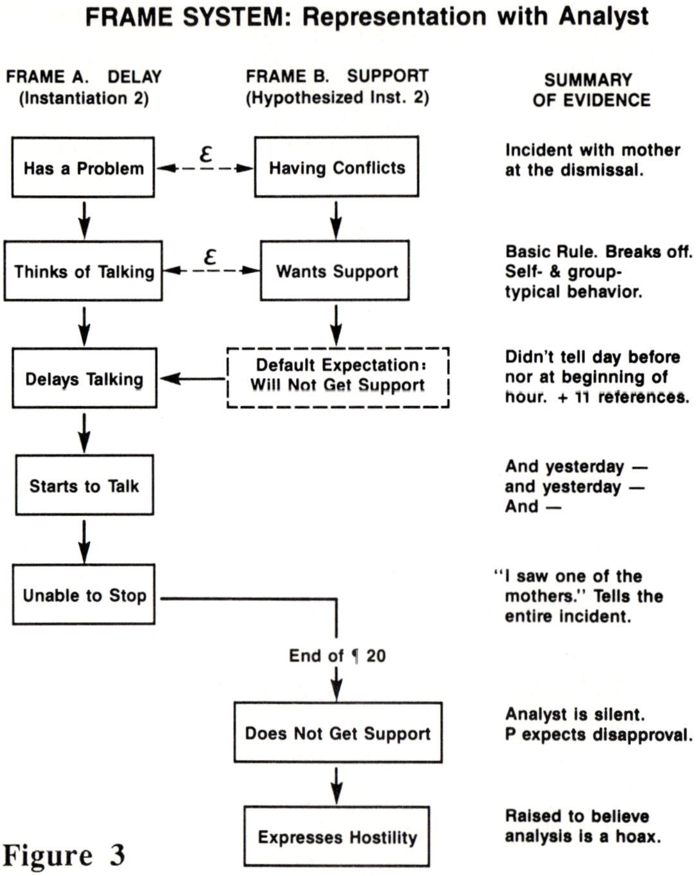

Figure 3

3. Frames of Mind

It does not stretch the imagination to think of the SUPPORT frame as a *wish* frame and DELAY as a *defense* frame. Our clinical knowledge would lead us to expect that these frames might interact with each other. Indeed much of the explanatory power (aside from predictive power) of these frames lies in their hypothesized interactions. Figure 3 allows us to explore such an interaction and to formulate a rather precise prediction about the patient's (P) interaction with the analyst (A).

On the day before this session P found herself in a conflict over an incident at her school, but she failed to tell A about it at her session later that afternoon. During the next hour (Hour 5) she started to relate the incident, but broke off and then made eleven abortive references before finally coming to the point. The steps in this are summarized in the right-hand column. Each event represents one of P's states and the arrows indicate transfer of control from one state to the next.

Thus P, in a state of conflict, wanted support for what she did, but she *believed* that she would not get it (default value from the prototype), which produced a "transference" expectation that A would not fulfill her wish. According to standard theory this is the occasion for a defense against the actual or anticipated unpleasure and the arrow shows a transfer to the *Delays Talking* event in the DELAY frame. Shortly afterward (#20) P finally told A about the incident. At this point there was no data to instantiate the last two events in the SUPPORT frame; we may therefore take the default values from the prototype as predictions and look to the rest of the session for evidence.

Indeed, direct confirmation was forthcoming. A little later, in response to a question by A, P said that not only did she not expect his approval, but was certain to get his active disapproval. Then toward the end of the session she confessed that she was raised to believe that analysis is a hoax, that it doesn't do any good and just costs a lot of money – possibly the only criticism she could think of at the time. It should be clear that these predictions need not necessarily have been confirmed; and, had they not been, that would have reduced the weight of evidence for the existence of this particular instantiation.

Figure 4 represents a different hypothesis about P's interaction with two boys in her school and their mothers. It is meant to illustrate the implicit side effects and/or the self-fulfilling intended consequences of two actions in the DELAY frame. The double-line arrows identify this particular type of interaction, one which we might hypothesize to be causal. P wanted the parents' support, but believed that she would not get it (default prototype value). As before, we hypothesize that this expectation aroused a defense and we think of control again being transferred to the *Delays Talking* event. By not calling the parents, P assured that she would not get the support she wanted. Later, she finally began talking to the mother at the dismissal even though she herself felt that complaining to the mother about her son in the presence of the other children and mothers was inappropriate. Common sense lets us understand that this was a covert expression of hostility.

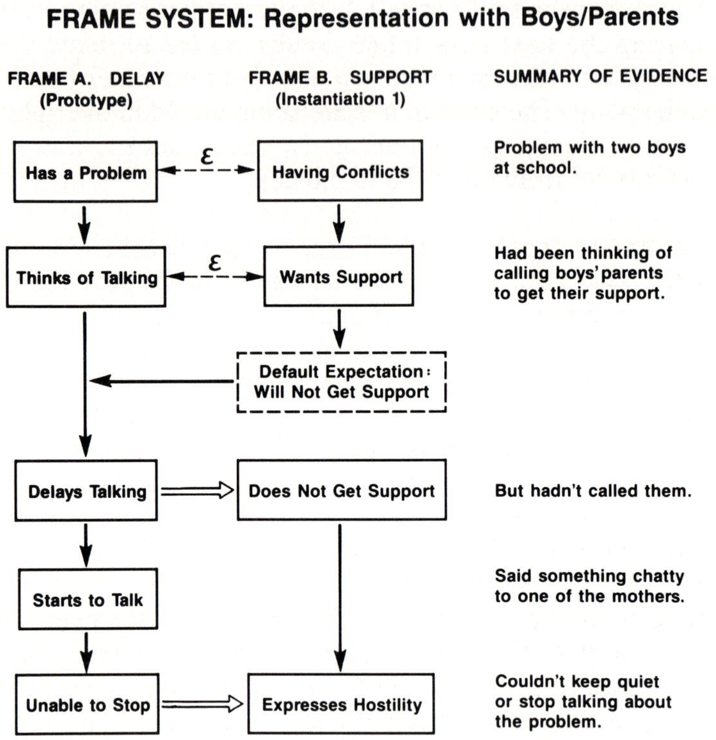

Figure 4

There are at least three other frames to be found in Hour 5. Two of them we have called TOGETHERNESS and CONTROL. Georges Moroz (1984)[1] has shown that these two, along with SUPPORT and DELAY, form a variety of clusters that are distributed throughout the hour. And Bucci (this volume) has demonstrated that Moroz's distribution is highly correlated with the distribution in Hour 5 of Bucci's (1984) measure of Referential Activity, a group of scales that assess how concrete, focused, and specific the language in the transcript is. Intuitively this fits both our common sense and our clinical belief that narrative episodes or Luborsky's "relationship episodes" give us direct, clear, coherent and significant information about a person's wish-defense organization.

---

[1] personal communication

One of the advantages of identifying and reasoning with and about frame structures, as compared with say, clinical themes, is that such reasoning is disciplined and constrained by three factors: (1) by the need for specifying the evidence explicitly and precisely, (2) by requiring that the sequence of events itself be repeated and, (3) by the ability to make and confirm or disconfirm specific clinically relevant predictions. These constraints constitute the heart of one answer to both Spence's (1982) worry about "soft pattern matches" and Grünbaum's (1984) concern about contamination and suggestion. On the one hand it is hard to see how frame structures can be suggested to a patient and on the other it is difficult to hide misclassifications given the requirements for literal or close paraphrases that we impose on what counts as evidence. Moreover the specific predictive powers allow us to systematically assess the degree of supporting evidence for any instantiation.

Most clinicians at least implicitly believe in the centrality of the recurrent manifestations and the influence of both conscious or unconscious fantasies in patients' lives. While they might quibble about the relatively mundane content of the two frames I have illustrated, they should not find the idea of frame structures and their interactions at all unfamiliar. Arlow (1969a, 1969b) for example, has provided convincing and informative accounts of the clinical manifestations of repetitive more or less unconscious fantasies. And in 1980, in a brilliant analysis of the movie *Blow-Up*, he described three different event structures, which had the essential characteristics of frames, as varieties of derivative representations of primal scenes. One of them recurred five, one four, and one three times in scenes of the movie. So we must assume that gifted artists such as Antonioni have their own ways of detecting and representing frame structures. Nonetheless the scientific problems associated both with clinical reports and with artistic creation are also recurrent and are the fundamental motivation for all the searches for structure to which I have already referred.

4. Comparison of Frames with other Repetitive Structures

Luborsky's (1977) CCRT's are recurrent structures, but their structure is at least partly imposed by the Wish/RO/RS sequence Luborsky defined. I say partly because intuitively this sequence makes a lot of sense as a candidate for a perfectly general structure that is built into all of us. We *do* wish about others, we *do* expect and observe their responses, and we *do* then respond ourselves. The uniformity of the structure is appealing as a way to eliminate a lot of individual variability that otherwise might obscure whatever patterns are to be found and as a way to make easy comparisons among patients. However the determination of a central theme by frequency or preponderance might sometimes lead one to overlook some less frequent themes that interact with the "central" theme.

Strupp et al.'s CMP's posit four "action categories" as basic elements of structure: (1) acts of self, (2) expectations about others' reactions, (3) acts of others toward self, and (4) acts of self toward self. Again, intuitively such categories are very appealing, but they carry with them limitations similar to those of the CCRT's.

Hoffman and Gill's codings of the PERT, like CCRT's and CMP's, begin with a set of predetermined categories, albeit quite different. Their categories of implicit and explicit transference references and experiences are obviously relevant to any therapy that employs the theoretical concept of transference. But this strength is also the PERT's central limitation, namely, its *exclusive* focus on the transference. Only empirical studies can ultimately decide the correctness of this view.

Horowitz's Configurational Analyses are much too complex to do justice here, but therein lies one of their limits. Their very richness and individuality as well as their imposition of many preexisting categories deprive them of the benefits of simplification that are the real strengths of CCRT's, CMP's, and PERT's.

Finally there remain the persistent hopes of clinicians, as embodied in Slap and Slaykin's resurrection of Bartlett's (1932) concept of the Schema, that they might yet contribute to our systematic knowledge. But schemas, with their structure, categories, and other properties nonsystematically described or defined, are subject to all the limitations of traditional clinical methods.

The most important way in which Frames differ from the preceding recurrent structures is in the fact that they are composed of categories of events that are explicitly represented in the discrete narratives told by a patient under instruction to free associate. Unlike structures using predetermined categories, Frames inevitably reflect the unique internal structure of a particular patient's memories, both conscious and unconscious, of a wide range of recurrent events such as wishes, beliefs, defenses, emotions, and actions. It is the belief in the causal role of these memories for the patient's adaptations that makes them important.

5. Frame Claims

Now for the extravagant, if not grandiose, claims, or more precisely for a mixed bag of hypotheses about the characteristics of Frames, loosely strung together. I propose them in full knowledge that we have little or no evidence for some of them, because I believe that we either now have, or will have in the next decade or so, the means to empirically investigate all of them. The claims then comprise an implicit program of research to which Bucci, Teller and myself all hope to contribute. Indeed we have already begun a variety of studies designed to reduce our ignorance and help clarify our hypotheses. We will be delighted if others join in. So here goes:

Frames

(1) are represented in the mind in *nonverbal* code in a dual code system of mental representations (see Bucci 1985),

(2) especially as *structured sequence of memories of emotions* (see Dahl 1978, 1979b)

(3) that are the *residues of early relationships with objects* (Gedo 1979);

(4) they *endure over time* and

(5) *across conflicts, objects, and situations*, and

(6) in principle *can account* for a wide spectrum of both *repetitive, neurotic, maladaptive behavior* and *normal, adaptive behavior*;

(7) they *permit specific predictions* of wishes and beliefs, and

(8) provide the *framework for a theory of change* independent of any particular theory of technique.

As part of the program of research, Leeds (1986) is applying a newly developed systematic method for objectively identifying repetitive frame structures in Hours 1 through 5 of the same case as Hour 5 in this volume. Davies (1988) is using the same method to try to identify in the behavior of 3-year-old children frame structures that recur in their interactions with their mothers and with two other 3-year-olds.

6. Final Frame

As Teller (this volume) describes in detail, the last frame that I will discuss was constructed differently from those I have just illustrated.

Instead of first finding a prototype and then looking for instantiations, Teller took seriously an inductive generalization that the patient reported about herself in Hour 5.

Figure 5 shows the simple, but nonetheless unusual structure of the CRITICAL/FRIENDLY (C/F) frame along with the evidence that

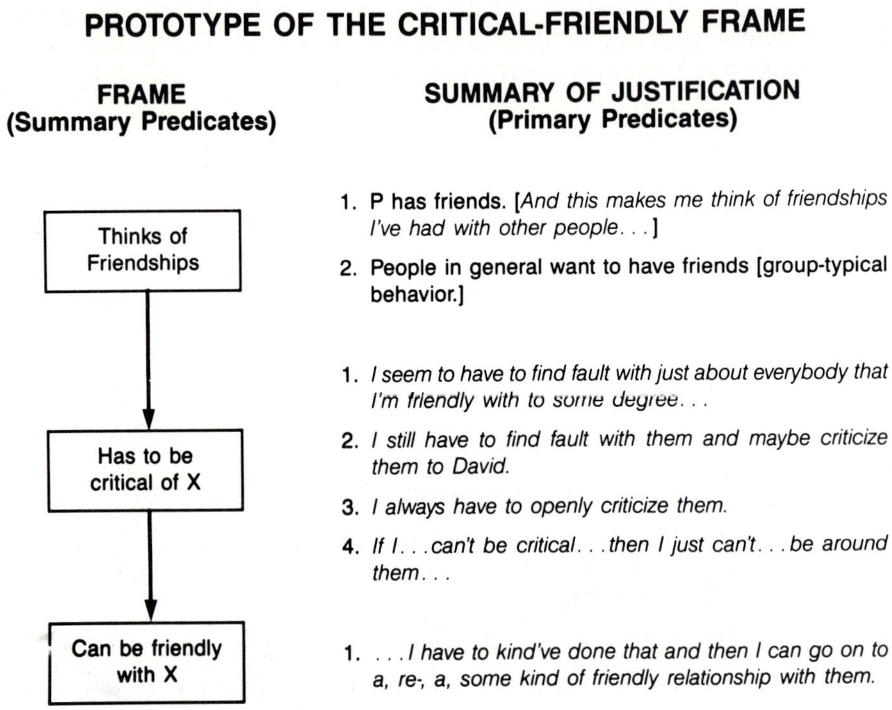

Figure 5

justifies each event. What makes this frame particularly interesting is that the logical status of the Critical event appears to be that of a necessary but not a sufficient condition for being able to be friendly. Thus C —> F but not vice versa. And, although the patient was obviously aware of this contingency, we found no evidence to indicate that she was in any way aware of the origins of her compulsion, nor of each instantiation, most importantly her enactment of the frame in the transference with the analyst (see Teller loc. cit.).

If we take the patient's self-description seriously we can then predict two empirical consequences: (1) critical behaviors are likely to outnumber friendly behaviors since friendly behavior does not automatically follow critical behavior, and (2) her critical behavior toward people should clearly precede friendly behavior. Very recently I rediscovered a study by L. Horowitz (1977), which, in retrospect, seems almost to have been designed to test these two hypotheses, although his rationale for doing the study rested on different grounds from our C/F Frame. His data consisted of the process notes of the first 100 hours from the same case as Hour 5. Horowitz investigated the change over time in two types of behavior: Friendly (F) behaviors, which he defined as those that bring persons closer together, and Critical (C) behaviors, defined as those that create distance between people.

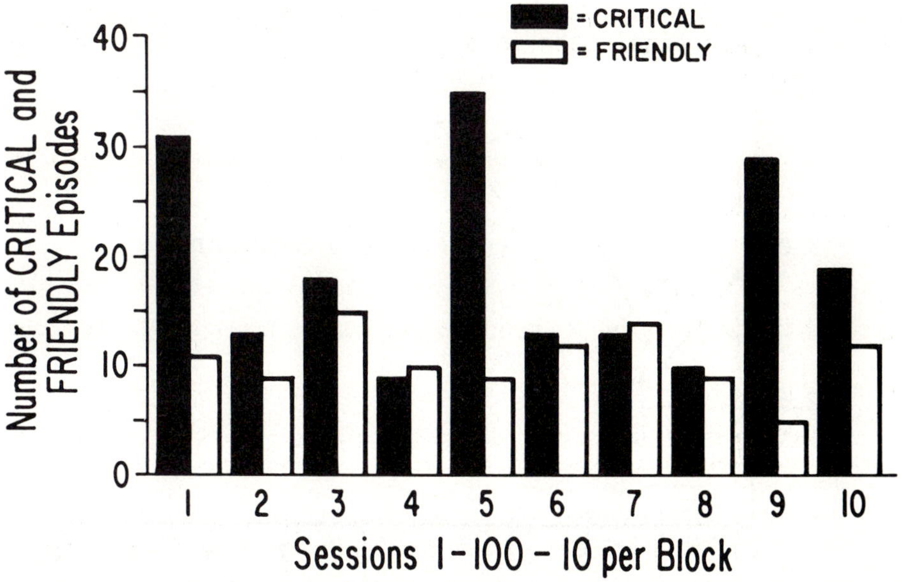

Figure 6

Three clinicians read through the entire 100 hours and identified all instances of both types of behaviors in 10 blocks of 10 hours each.[2] Figure 6 shows the distribution in each block of the total of 190 C behaviors and 106 F behaviors that were identified. A t-test of the difference in frequency between the C and the F behaviors in each of the

[2]Horowitz graciously provided me with the mean values on each scale for each of the ten blocks.

blocks ($t=2.49$, $df=9$, $p<.05$) supported the first hypothesis that the patient should exhibit more critical than friendly behaviors.

Next, four different clinical judges independently rated each behavior on a four-point scale designed to assess the directness of expression of the behavior. For C behaviors, a rating of 1 meant expressing a criticism indirectly to a third party and a rating of 4 implied a direct confrontation or criticism of a person, and similarly for F behaviors. The means of these ratings (no reliability measure was given) for each block of 10 hours are plotted in Figure 7.

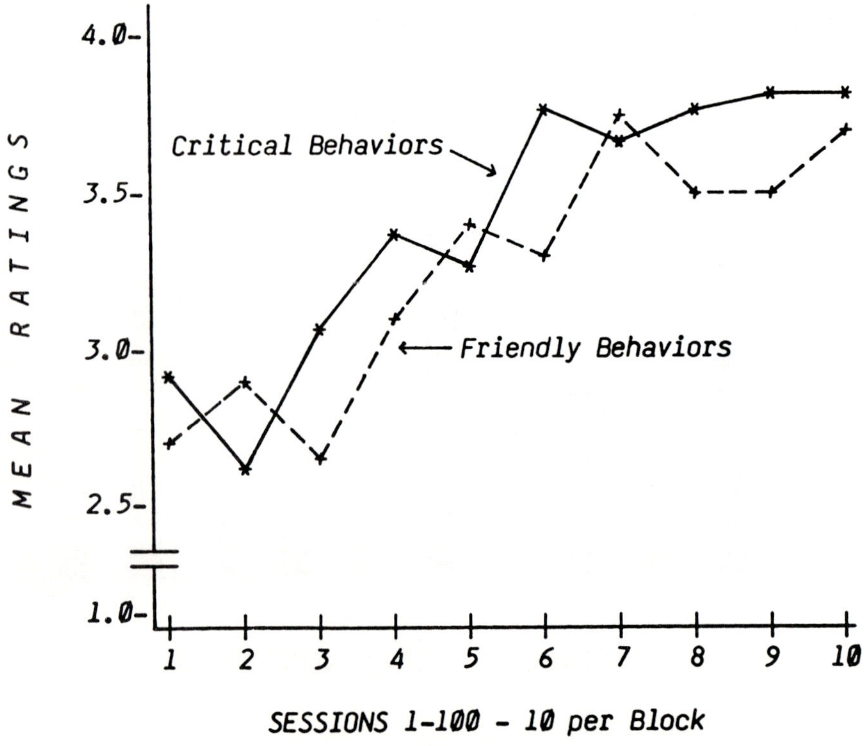

Figure 7

Note that the ratings of both behaviors increased over time: $r_{cf} = .83$. But the correlations of each behavior with time are even higher: $r_{ct} = .92$ and $r_{ft} = .90$. If time is partialled out there is no correlation between C and F: $r_{cf \cdot t} = .01$. Thus both C and F behaviors increased over time but were unrelated to each other in the same blocks of hours.

However, Figure 8 shows a dramatic change in the relationship when the C behaviors from block *n* are compared with the F behaviors from block *n+1*. Now the similarity of the curves is apparent and the first order lagged correlation, $r_{c(f+1)} = .97$. But here again, both C and F are highly correlated with time. Nonetheless, when time is partialled out of both, $r_{c(f+1)\cdot t} = .89$, df=6, p<.005. In a test of the logical possibility that if F were lagged one block (to see if F might precede C), $r_{f(c+1)\cdot t} = .26$, ns. Thus the empirical test supports the second prediction derived from the CRITICAL/FRIENDLY frame, namely, that critical behavior must precede friendly behavior.

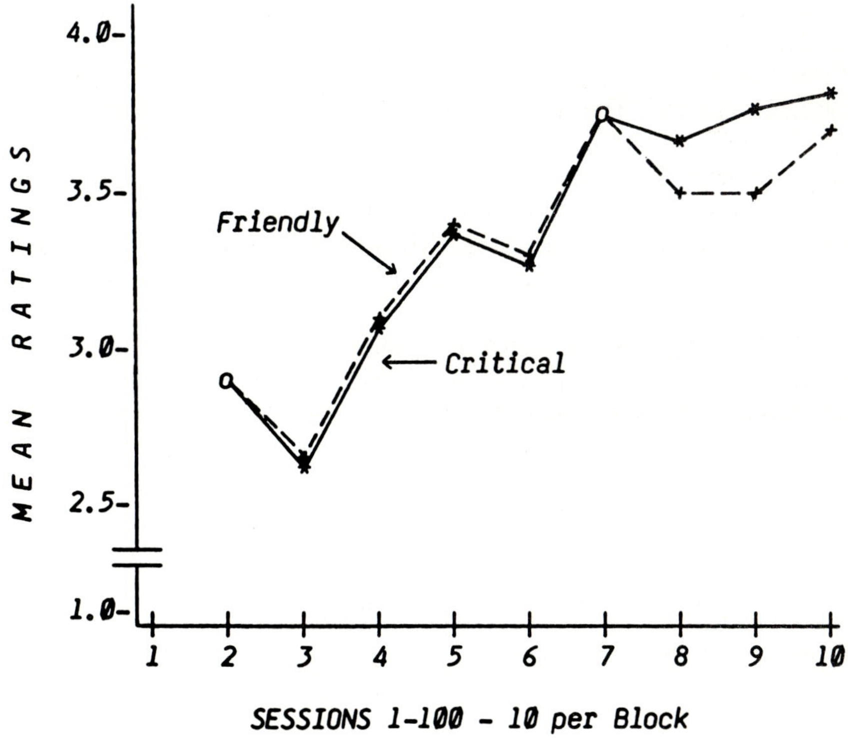

Figure 8

7. The Future of Frames

Research on Frame structures is proceeding in three essential directions. First, detailed descriptions of the general characteristics of and methods for finding Frames (Dahl and Bucci, In Preparation) are forthcoming. These will include illustrations of systematic applications to the first five hours of the Hour 5 psychoanalysis (Leeds 1988). Second, we are exploring the question of the *fate of the Frames* in the course of the same psychoanalysis, specifically the fate of the five Frames (with a total of 20 instantiations) that we have thus far identified in Hour 5. Scott Miller, a graduate student at Adelphi University, has traced their fate in the course of the analysis. During three hours at the height of the transference neurosis, as independently identified by Jones and Windholz (Submitted), four of the five Frames were still in evidence, but several instantiations of them had one significant event added at the end of their structures, an event Miller dubbed "Realization" because the patient indicated her beginning awareness of both the existence of the Frames and their roles in her transference struggles. As might be devoutly wished, in the last three hours of the analysis the five structures had either disappeared or radically altered. The SUPPORT Frame changed from a maladaptive to an adaptive structure; the third and fourth events, "Does Not Get Support" and "Expresses Hostility" were replaced by: "Insights" (which implied having felt support in the analysis) and "Wishes" (for the future). Similarly, these same two new events replaced the last two events in the one remaining instance of the TOGETHERNESS Frame.

And third, but perhaps most important, are questions of both the reliability of the identification of Frame structures (which Miller is pursuing) *and* their presence in the behavior of young children, as predicted by Frame Theory. In her doctoral dissertation Davies (1988) has found Frame structures in the behaviors of three-year-old children, structures that are unique to each child and, as the theory predicts, recur with different children as well as with the child's mother. Finally, it is clear that we will also need much work on the similarities and differences among the different repetitive structures that have been described in this volume.

A Scheme for Coding the Patient's Experience of the Relationship with the Therapist (PERT): Some Applications, Extensions, and Comparisons

Irwin Z. Hoffman and Merton M. Gill

1. Purpose

In this paper we will review the principal features of our scheme for coding transcripts of audio-recorded sessions of psychoanalysis and psychoanalytic psychotherapy (Gill and Hoffman 1982b). Throughout the paper the scheme will be referred to as the PERT, standing for the Patient's Experience of the Relationship with the Therapist. We will then illustrate the way the coding scheme works by applying it to the Specimen Hour. The Specimen Hour will also be utilized to introduce some extensions of the scheme that we feel are promising. We will conclude by comparing and contrasting our coding method to Luborsky's Core Conflictual Relationship Theme or CCRT (Luborsky 1977) and to Dahl's Frames (Dahl, this volume; Teller and Dahl 1981a, 1986).

2. Background

Theoretical Framework

There are several theoretical propositions from which the method derives and which it can also help to test. A fuller exposition of the theoretical underpinnings of the scheme can be found elsewhere (Gill 1979, 1982; Gill and Hoffman 1982b). The major propositions that inspired the development of the method can be represented briefly as follows:

1. That analysis of transference is an important aspect of the analytic process.

2. That, all else being equal, the analytic process itself and, ultimately, the outcome of an analysis is enhanced by good work on the

transference and, specifically, in terms of the contribution of the analyst, by good transference interpretations.

3. That collaborative exploration of the patient's experience of the relationship in the here-and-now is at least a very important aspect of the analysis of transference, the whole of which encompasses interpretation of genetics. At most, it seems to us that it is also possible that this aspect of the process has important potential, in itself, to promote insight at the same time that it creates the opportunity for a special kind of new interpersonal experience with the analyst; one which interrupts repetitive patterns of interaction and which can promote change. From our point of view, the extent to which interpretation of transference which is inclusive of genetic interpretation is decisive with regard to the therapeutic action of analysis as compared to the explication of the patient's experience of the relationship in the here-and-now is an open question and an empirical question.

4. That the transference involves a perspective on the interaction which has its origins in the past but which at the same time is relevant to the present ambiguous situation with the analyst. This perspective has a certain degree of plausibility. What adds to the plausibility of the patient's viewpoint is the fact that the patient himself does many things to promote the repetition with the analyst or therapist of old patterns of interaction.The patient attempts to elicit responses from the analyst which are consistent with the patient's transference-driven expectations (Hoffman 1983). Our position on transference is in keeping with the broad movement known as constructionism which is reflected in many fields including literary theory, philosophy of science, and psychology as well (Gergen 1985; Stern 1985; Protter 1985).

5. That much of what the patient experiences in the present in relation to the analyst is conflictual. The patient wants both to expose and to hide many aspects of his experience of the relationship with the analyst. The inclination to reveal and the resistance to revealing these conflictual aspects of the patient's experience result in communications which are, in effect, compromise formations, so that frequently the patient's experience of the relationship with the therapist is communicated in disguised form.

6. That the job of the analyst is, in part, to help to discern the latent meanings of such disguised communications and to encourage their

exploration through either active interpretation or simple encouragement to the patient to elaborate on an idea that he has merely hinted at. We see this as an interactional process in which reciprocal or shared resistances to direct communication are overcome by the participants. For his part, in the act of interpreting, the analyst lets the patient know that he has overcome whatever resistance he might have felt to hearing what the patient feels about the interaction. When the analyst invites the patient to communicate directly about a sensitive matter in the relationship, there is likely to ensue a reduction in the part of the patient's resistance which had been an accommodation to resistance attributed to the analyst.

These theoretical propositions influenced the choice of variables involved in the PERT and the manner in which the coding operation is carried out. They also have had continuing influence on our ideas for extending and developing the scheme.

The Immediate Purpose of the Scheme

With these background propositions in mind, the aim of the PERT is, first of all, to track the course of the patient's experience of the relationship with the therapist in a session of analysis, generally using transcriptions of audio-recorded sessions as data. This tracking process means reading between the lines of the patient's associations to discern those resisted aspects of the experience which the patient is simultaneously wanting to conceal and wanting to reveal. The heart of the coding scheme is this tracking process and the provision of certain guidelines for deciding what may or may not qualify as a disguised allusion to the transference. Incidentally, we are using the term "transference" loosely as interchangeable with the phrase "the patient's experience of the relationship," partly because we think we are dealing with transference when we are talking about the resisted aspects of the patient's experience, and partly merely for the sake of variety in communication. The term "transference" is a useful shorthand, although we recognize that it is laden with other connotations, including genetic implications, which the coding scheme does not deal with in any kind of direct way.

If he can reach some conclusion regarding what the patient is experiencing in the interaction and what he is resisting either becoming aware of or communicating or both, the judge is then also in a better position to evaluate the extent to which and how well the analyst picks up on these latent issues, interprets them, and encourages their further exploration.

3. Overview of the Variables

In a sense the system is rather simple, although perhaps it is deceptively simple. The judge codes the lines of a transcript of an audio-recorded session as he reads. The same system could be applied to sessions which the judge listens to, but we have generally used it with transcripts. As he reads, the judge identifies certain classes of communications and codes them as such, indicating the lines which are involved.[1]

Patient Variables

r, x, and xr: We code communications that are manifestly about the relationship with the therapist. These are signified by the lower case letter r. By implication, we take account of those associations that are manifestly about other experiences: about relationships with others or about thoughts and mental states that have no overt relationship to the analyst. By implication, we code these associations with the letter x. We say "by implication" because, in fact, we do not specifically code these associations. We assume that associations that are not coded are manifestly extra-transference associations. This is an important point of contrast between our system and the CCRT in which each "relationship episode" is coded separately and in detail (Luborsky 1977).

In addition to the r coding, there is a type of explicit reference to the relationship to which we give a special coding designated by xr. This coding refers to connections that the patient makes himself between extratransference and transference experiences.

Jxr and Jrr: At the heart of the system is the coding of disguised allusions by the patient to the relationship with the therapist. The allusions fall into one of two categories. The first are associations that are manifestly about extratransference issues (coded x implicitly) which the judge infers have latent meaning in the transference. This amounts to a sub-class of the larger class of x-associations. We indicate this kind of disguised allusion to the transference, as discerned by the judge, by the coding Jxr. In the case of Jxr, the judge has discerned a connection

---

[1] The coding form itself can be found in a previous publication (Gill and Hoffman, 1982b).

between something that is manifestly outside the transference and something in the relationship with the analyst. For example, the judge may infer that a motif which was introduced in an explicit way, that is, with an r association, has gone under the surface and has now been elaborated in a disguised way in associations that are manifestly not about the relationship. The latter associations continue to carry a theme which is of relevance to the interaction with the analyst and which was originally announced by the r. In other instances the extratransference associations may come first, and the judge codes them retrospectively as Jxr only after the issue surfaces explicitly. These two types of sequences will be discussed more fully in connection with the Specimen Hour.

The second type of disguised allusion to the relationship by the patient consists of associations that are *already* manifestly about the relationship which the judge infers have *other* latent, resisted meanings having to do with the interaction with the analyst. These associations are indicated by the letters Jrr. In this case, the judge is inferring that a communication which is about the relationship has other latent meanings which may be linked with a previous or, in some instances, a subsequent explicit communication about the relationship where the resisted issue is more apparent. Another way of speaking of this is to say that the two sets of communications about the relationship complement each other, with each illuminating that which is resisted in the other. Frequently, of course, one of the two sets has more of the resisted content than the other.

Bases for Coding Jxr and Jrr: Both kinds of inferences of disguised allusions to the relationship require justification on the part of a judge by reference to some relatively independent data. That is, as evidence that certain associations allude indirectly to the relationship with the therapist the judge must bring to bear some other data that are separate from the data that the judge is interpreting in this way. In accord with what we have said about the linking of x and r or r and r, these other data that have the status of evidence may take the form of a previous or subsequent explicit reference to the relationship by the patient. However, it may also take the form of some Significant Event (SE) in the interaction which the judge has observed but about which neither the patient nor the analyst have spoken. In the case of an r-basis, the judge argues, in effect, that it is reasonable to suggest that certain associations allude to the transference in a particular way on the grounds that the patient has explicitly said something else about the relationship which is consistent with this hypothesis. In the case of Significant Events in the interaction, the judge concludes that such an allusion is likely on the grounds that something else has occurred in the interaction which is closely related to the content of the associations coded Jxr or Jrr.

Sometimes the judge may notice an event or a quality in the interaction which he thinks may have impact upon the patient's experience before the occurrence can be demonstrated to have had such impact on the basis of subsequent data. In such instances, the judge codes his observation as a Potentially Significant Event or PSE. An example might be an announcement by the analyst that he is going on vacation or a particular kind of action by the analyst which the judge thinks might have an effect on the patient's experience subsequently, such as giving advice or speaking in terms which the patient might construe as critical or being silent for a long period of time. No meaning is actually attributed to these events unless or until the judge discerns an allusion to them in subsequent associations. If he never finds an allusion to them in subsequent associations, the Potentially Significant Events are nullified in the sense that they apparently have not impacted on the patient to the extent that the judge thought they might. The Potentially Significant Event simply gives the judge something to think about as a possible basis for understanding and coding subsequent associations. Conversely, when events in the interaction are not flagged in this way, they may still be utilized as bases for inferring disguised allusions to the transference. In such instances it is only when certain themes appear in the patient's associations that the judge's attention is drawn to previous events as probable sources of influence on the patient's experience. In such instances, the basis for the inference that certain associations allude to the relationship is called a Retrospectively Significant Event or RSE. Note that, formally speaking, RSE is the only SE basis of any consequence because every Potentially Significant Event or PSE is considered a likely significant influence only when the judge finds an allusion to it in subsequent associations. This point is of some importance in terms of theory of technique. It is in keeping with our view that events in the interaction do not carry "objective" meaning which will be common to all patients and that the "adaptive context" (Langs 1978) for the patient's associations can only be discovered retrospectively.

Strictly speaking, even an RSE only brings us to the point of a tenable hypothesis about the patient's experience of the relationship. In fact, validation of any proposed interpretation by the judge, whether Jxr or Jrr and whether with r basis or SE basis, depends to a large extent upon the patient's conscious responses to interpretations that the analyst actually offers. Such responses are exemplified by the "DSIR" and

"ENIR" codings discussed below in connection with the Specimen Hour.

The fact that the judge must provide evidence for his inference that associations carry latent transference meaning prevents a mechanical imposition of the principle of analysis of transference to the point that every association is construed as alluding to the relationship with the analyst. There can be many implicitly x-coded episodes in which the judge cannot discern any transference implications. The reasons that such implications may not be detectable are varied. It may be that the patient's resistance is such that the allusions to the transference are particularly obscure and the data become particularly opaque in this regard. Or it may be that the judge is simply blind to some possible allusion that is there and that another judge might pick up. Finally, it may be that the extratransference associations are not alluding to anything, in terms of their content, in the relationship with the analyst or at least that the strength of the patient's motivation to allude to such an aspect of his experience is weak. For example, the predominant feature of the patient's experience of the relationship with the analyst at a certain moment might be what Freud (1912b) referred to as the "unobjectionable" positive transference, so that the main thing to be said about what the patient is communicating is that he feels a sense of trust sufficient to convey some particular experience that he has had outside of the analysis with the hope that the analyst will be receptive, understanding, and so on. This aspect of the positive transference may well be something that need not be interpreted. It is important to note that even where the judge does discern a possible latent meaning about the relationship, coded Jxr or Jrr, there is no intended implication that the analyst should necessarily have interpreted that latent issue at that moment. The judge, in coding allusions to the transference, is not constrained by considerations of tact and timing. His sole job with regard to that particular task is to identify those communications in which it is plausible to hypothesize that there may be an allusion by the patient to some resisted aspect of his experience of the relationship with the analyst. Cumulatively, however, the judge may gradually develop the impression that certain important transference issues are being ignored or neglected or enacted in a transference-countertransference pattern of some kind without being interpreted. His judgment to that effect can be recorded on the global rating about which we will say more shortly.

Therapist Variables

The PERT scheme includes a set of codings for types of intervention by the analyst. These codings are designated with capital letters corresponding roughly in their meaning to the lower case letters that are used for coding the patient's associations.

The interventions which are about matters other than the relationship with the therapist are classified and coded with the letter X. Interpretations that are addressed to associations that are already manifestly about the relationship are also coded and are signified by the letter R. This coding also applies to interpretations of the patient's behavior in relation to the therapist, even if that behavior is not part of the actual content of the patient's associations. For example, if a patient has been late and the analyst offers an interpretation of that behavior the coding is R. We also have a coding for interpretations by the analyst of latent transference issues in associations that are not manifestly about the relationship with the analyst. We call these interpretations XR. In those instances when the interpretation seems to be designed primarily to shed light on experiences outside of the analytic situation on the basis of what has been explicated about the relationship with the therapist the coding is RX instead of XR. There is also a coding for interventions which are not in themselves interpretations but which encourage the exploration of some aspect of a patient's experience of the relationship. The analyst may simply invite the patient to speak further on a certain issue that he has referred to. For example, the therapist may simply ask "can you say more about that"? When that kind of invitation is extended with reference to issues in the relationship the intervention is noted and coded as an ER, referring to encouragement to the patient to elaborate further on some experience in his relationship with the analyst.

Although we have discussed Significant Events in connection with the patient variables Jxr and Jrr, they frequently do refer to various aspects of the therapist's behavior and in that sense could qualify as therapist variables. It is for this reason that Significant Events are represented in the coding scheme by the capital letters PSE and RSE.These variables represent the clearest direct reflection in the coding scheme of the notion that the therapist is continually contributing in important ways to the patient's experience and that these contributions must be taken into account whenever interpretations are formulated. Despite this special interest that we have in the influence of the therapist on the transference, Significant Events are broadly defined in the coding scheme and encompass unspoken aspects of the patient's behavior as well as unspoken aspects of the therapist's behavior. For example, a note at the beginning of a session to the effect that the patient is late might well be flagged by the judge as a Potentially Significant Event or PSE.

Global Rating

The PERT system includes a discursive clinical statement by the judge in which he outlines the principal transference issues that he has discerned in the hour and the extent to which they have been explored. He tries to assess the relative contributions of patient and therapist to that exploration and to point out those latent transference themes which may have been overlooked by both participants.

Following the clinical statement, the length of which may vary from about two-hundred-fifty to five hundred words, there is a quantitative rating of the degree to which the analyst addressed or encouraged exploration of the principal transference issues that the judge detected. The rating is from 1 to 5 with half points, so that it is, in effect, a nine point scale. The highest rating represents thorough or "extensive" exploration of transference issues.

When there are many Jxr or Jrr codings and few or no R, XR or ER codings, it is probable that the judge will be rating the therapist's contribution to the analysis of the transference low because the coding suggests that the analyst is missing opportunities for cogent interpretations. However, it is also possible that in some instances a therapist will have captured the heart of many of the latent transference meanings that the judge has considered with just one or two timely interpretations. In that case the rating of the analyst's work in the session would be high despite the fact that there may have been a good number of codings by the judge of disguised allusions to the relationship. In other words, there is no direct relationship between any of the codings at a microscopic level and the global rating. The judge is free to use his clinical judgment in a more intuitive way when rating the session in its entirety. In effect, it becomes an empirical question as to what the relationship is between the microscopic and macroscopic assessment of the hour.

Bear in mind that the judge should not penalize the therapist for not making transference interpretations when the judge himself finds that the patient's associations do not provide cogent evidence of allusions to the transference that may warrant interpretation. There may be sessions which are opaque enough so that the judge himself cannot discern what the latent transference issues may be if there are any. In such a case the judge may rate the therapist's performance high given the nature of the communications that he had to deal with. Even with these qualifications, however, there may be a bias built into the way the coding scheme was originally formulated (Gill and Hoffman 1982b) which favors a high frequency of interpretations. To offset this bias, we have considered the possibility of adding a rating of the extent to which transference issues have been explored "optimally" as distinct from "thoroughly" or "extensively." Such a scale would encourage the judge to take considerations of tact and timing into account in assessing the analyst's work. It would require that points be taken off when a relatively thorough exploration of transference has been accomplished at the expense of leaving the patient room to develop his own trains of thought. Such a scale would also be in keeping with a shift in emphasis in our thinking about analysis of transference that has occurred since the coding scheme was originally presented. Stated very briefly, this shift is one which makes the *way* the analyst conceptualizes and interprets the transference the central issue (see theoretical principle number 4 above) while stressing that from moment-to-moment a variety of considerations may override interpreting disguised allusions to the transference, calling instead for either no intervention or for another type of intervention (Gill 1984; Hoffman 1985, p. 165). However, the rating of the thoroughness with which the transference is explored still seems to us to be important and useful. In the first place, unlike rating how optimal the analyst's investigation of the transference has been, rating thoroughness is simpler and consensus should be relatively easy to achieve. Secondly, it is a meaningful variable that warrants empirical investigation in its own right.

The global rating leaves room for the judge to evaluate the quality of the interpretations that the analyst does make in addition to whether the analyst has taken advantage of or missed opportunities for interpretation. With some of our colleagues, efforts have been undertaken to develop scales for the rating of the quality of individual transference interpretations, taking into consideration "plausibility" and "timeliness" among other factors. Clearly, such scales would be an important addition to the PERT coding scheme.

4. Application of the PERT to the Specimen Hour

Introduction

We would like to illustrate the ways in which allusions to the transference are identified and coded according to our system by applying it to the Specimen Hour (this volume). We are selecting certain examples of the Jxr coding which struck us as particularly cogent, rather than every allusion to the transference that we thought we could discern.

We have selected a sequence of codings which includes two examples of "Retrospective Jxr" and one example of a "Straightforward Jxr." Following this particular sequence we will present one illustration of a Jxr coding for which a PSE (Potentially Significant Event) serves as the evidence or basis. We are not giving examples here of Jrr simply because there were none that we felt were particularly cogent in this hour. It may be helpful to the reader if we introduce the illustrations with a statement about the difference between Straightforward Jxr and Retrospective Jxr.[2] To describe the process from the judge's perspective, in a Straightforward Jxr, the judge comes across a reference to the relationship that is explicit at a certain point in the hour. He codes that reference as an r. Subsequently he finds some associations in which the theme that was referred to in the earlier statement, coded as r, seems to be elaborated in relation to some other context. On the basis of the preceding r, the judge now feels that he can infer that the extratransference associations carry latent transference meaning and he gives these x associations the Jxr coding. The sequence in the case of Retrospective Jxr is the reverse: the explicit reference to the relationship appears after the x associations to which the Jxr coding is given. At the point that the judge initially reads the x associations no Jxr coding is warranted since there is as yet no basis for it. Later on, however, when the patient refers explicitly to some aspect of his experience of the relationship, the judge recognizes, in retrospect, that a theme that appeared earlier in relation to others may well have carried latent meaning in relation to the analyst, and that latent meaning seems to be related in its content to the issue that has now surfaced more directly. The Retrospective Jxr coding is then given to the earlier lines that were implicitly coded x.

We have chosen in the examples that we are giving to state the possible latent meanings associated with the various Jxr's that we are proposing in the unspoken words of the patient, using the first person perspective. We are doing this, rather than putting the Jxr's in the form of possible interpretations that the analyst might offer to the patient, precisely because we want to emphasize the looseness of the connection between any particular Jxr coding and the possibility of an interpretation by the analyst at that moment. In other words, we are leaving open the question as to what the analyst should have said, how he should have said it, and when he should have spoken, although in our global assessment of the hour there will be some suggestions along these lines.

---

[2]The term "retrospective" is used in two contexts in the coding scheme. We speak of "Retrospectively Significants Events" (RSE) and of "Retrospective Jxr." These should not be confused.

Sequence of Jxr Codings with r-Basis

We are going to give several examples from this hour, each of which is related to the others in terms of the conflictual issues that seem to be involved. The examples we will give involve a sequence of communications which can be represented formally as (x_1), r_1, (x_2), r_2. We have x_1 and x_2 in parentheses to remind the reader that these communications are not formally coded as such. We will demonstrate how this sequence presented opportunities for what we felt were three compelling codings of Jxr. The first is a Retrospective Jxr. In this instance, r_1 serves as the basis for coding (x_1) retrospectively as Jxr. The second is a Straightforward Jxr in which r_1 serves as the basis for giving the Jxr coding to (x_2). The third is another Retrospective Jxr. Here, r_2 provides the basis for giving a retrospective coding of Jxr to (x_2). With the Jxr codings, the sequence becomes:

(x_1)
r_1
Retrospective Jxr coding for (x_1), with r_1 as basis
(x_2)
Straightforward Jxr coding for (x_2) with r_1 as basis
r_2
Retrospective Jxr coding for (x_2) with r_2 as basis

Two interesting overlapping patterns can be extracted from this sequence. In one, r_1 is pivotal in illuminating extratransference associations that precede and that follow it. We could represent this pattern as follows:

(x_1) <----- r_1 -----> (x_2)

In the second x_2 becomes the focus of illumination from both r_1 and r_2, and the pattern looks like this:

r_1 -----> (x_2) <----- r_2

The arrows that point to the left correspond with Retrospective Jxr codings.

These patterns are technically accurate in terms of the way the coding system works because the arrows point to the speech segments that are given the Jxr ratings; these are the associations that are interpreted in light of the explicit references to the relationship coded as r. However, the direction of illumination is never really one way from a clinical point of view. The communications always reflect on each other. The r is always interpreted in light of the x just as the x is interpreted in light of the r. What we find is an interweaving of meaning such that what was resisted in one context is expressed more openly in the other, and vice versa.

The following is the communication we are calling x_1:

x_1 (#16) In fact, unless it's business he's (father) still fairly strange on the phone. It's only occasionally, when there's been some real topic that he can talk about that's right there on his mind, that he isn't ill-at-ease on the phone. And usually if I get him when I'm calling he'll practically gasp, "Well, here's your mother,"or "I'll get your mother." And then, and then, once he's called her, if he's waiting for her to come, he'll talk to me, and then he can be fine. And, and (stomach rumble) it's just somehow he has to know that she's coming, so he's not stuck talking to me. (Sniff) But I also panic if I know sh-, when I call if suddenly I find out she's not there and I'm going to just have to talk to him. It seems a mutual kind of reaction at this point. (Sniff, pause, stomach rumble)

(#17) Because that sort of typifies our whole relationship. I think we're always (chuckle) panic stricken when we find we're going to be alone together with each other.

Sometime later the patient says the following regarding her experience of the relationship with the analyst. This is r_1:

r_1 (#53) I found it, I think I found it hard to come in here and lie down on the couch, with just you, being a man, in the room. But then that's, that could be any man, I suppose. (Pause)

(#54) I do suppose though, if, if uh, something occurred to me about you, even if it weren't a criticism, I don't know that I feel, I think I, I feel I can't talk about it, because it seems like kind of an intimate type of thing and, and I just am not, I don't know, I just never made personal remarks to anybody (chuckle) before I knew them for a long time.

What we are calling, for the purpose of illustration, r_1, would be broken down formally into two codings: one for the discomfort about lying down in a room alone with the analyst (#53), the other for the patient's inhibition about saying anything that seems personal to the analyst (#54). However, for our present purposes we will speak only of r_1 taken as a whole.

Thematically, it is not difficult to detect a connection between (x_1) and r_1. In both instances, the patient seems both anxious and inhibited regarding intimacy with a man. With the surfacing of the issue in r_1, the judge has reason to infer, retrospectively, that (x_1) which is about the father, has meaning that applies to the analyst. Hence, the coding of a Retrospective Jxr for (x_1). This is a good example of the way in which the two sets of communications, the one about the father and the one about the analyst, illuminate and enrich each other.

Although we have a special interest in resistance to awareness of transference, including escapes from the immediate interaction that take the form of displacements onto experiences with parents, we also recognize that the patient may resist becoming aware of aspects of his or her experiences with others (especially parents), and that some issues may surface more readily in relation to the analyst. Also we recognize that interpretations can sometimes legitimately move from the here-and-now to genetic prototypes, with the first shedding light on the second (RX). Thus, in this example, we could speculate that the possible sexual connotations in r_1, although probably resisted in themselves, may be more deeply resisted in (x_1) where the patient's relationship with the father is the subject.

Moving to our second example, the associations immediately following those of #54 are as follows:

> x_2 (#55) In fact, I was kind of horrified last night at myself. I had a course a_ after I left here and uhm, (sniff) it uhm, it's an art course for teachers (sniff) and we were working on rubbing things for texture. And at one point I noticed the professor's tie, which was a very nubby coarse woven one, and although it would have been too soft to rub, I just (chuckle) reached out and held it out and said, "Well, this has a wonderful texture," which it did. But I was horrified at myself, because I've just never done anything like that before. And then I was sure his reaction was horror too, that I had been so forward. I don't know what it was actually, but at the time I was sure it was just horror. (Pause)

These extratransference associations are what we are calling (x_2). Again, x as such is not formally coded in our coding form unless the judge feels that there is evidence of a possible allusion to the transference, in which case the coding is Jxr. In this instance the theme of (x_2) is about the very issue that was introduced in the previous reference to the analyst, that is, the issue of boldness with a man, and, perhaps, especially, sexual boldness. The judge concludes that a strong hypothesis would be that the impulse that is inhibited in relation to the analyst is revealed through a displacement onto the professor. Moreover, the reaction to the impulse in that interpersonal context, namely horror, also appears in a form that is proportional to the intensity of the wish. We have reason to speculate in light of (x_2) that not only would the patient be horrified, but that she also fears that the analyst would be horrified if she were more aggressive in the way that she approached him.

The latent meaning of #55 or (x_2) could be stated as follows:

> *Being here alone with you, a man, I feel the impulse to be forward with you, but I am horrified at that impulse and feel you too would be horrified if I pursued any kind of intimacy with you.*

Paragraphs 53 and 54, which we are calling r_1, would be cited as evidence to support this inference regarding the associations in #55 which we are calling x_2. And the coding of x_2 would be a Straightforward Jxr.

We have now completed the first sequence described earlier, (x_1)<--- r_1 --->(x_2), in which a pivotal explicit reference to the relationship serves as a basis for coding a previous and subsequent set of associations as Retrospective and Straightforward Jxr respectively. We now come to the last part of the overlapping sequence, r_1 --->(x_2)<--- r_2, in which two explicit references to the relationship both support related Jxr codings for (x_2). Because we have already dealt with the connection between r_1 and (x_2), (Straightforward Jxr), we have only the second part of the sequence to take up, the connection between (x_2) and r_2.

It is a little later in the session that the patient says the following, which is r_2:

> r_2(#61) Because that (chuckle) is, well even this I find hard to say, and it's, it's silly, but just in thinking about clothes and wearing what you want, uhm, just in, in noticing what you've worn since I've started coming and the, the variety and the freedom that you seem to have and, and I think I've been sort of envious of that. (Sniff) I feel very embarrassed (chuckle) saying that.

With the patient now expressing herself in a manner that she experiences as relatively bold in relation to the analyst and with her accompanying embarrassment, the judge has a basis to retrospectively interpret #55 as a paragraph in which this issue, which is muted in the transference, is elaborated vividly in a displaced form in relation to the professor. Now the latent meaning attributed to #55 might be:

> *I am anxious about an impulse I feel to be bold and seductive with you, even to touch you. Just commenting on your clothing feels a little like it felt when I reached out and grabbed the professor's tie. Also, I am concerned that you might be put off by my audacity.*

Again, it is important to recognize that though technically the Jxr coding is given to #55 while #61 is considered as the "basis," the two communications are illuminating of each other. In other words, it is not only that in light of what we find in #61 we can consider possible latent meanings of #55, but also that in light of what we find in #55 we discern what might be latent in #61.

The episode with the professor is a good illustration of the way in which a disguised allusion to the transference may be, simultaneously, a reporting of displacement in action outside the analytic situation. The interaction with the professor occurred after a session, a temporal juxtaposition which the patient's own report emphasizes ("after I left here"). So it seems tenable to suggest that when the patient grabbed the professor's tie, she was displacing onto him an impulse that she felt in relation to the analyst. In addition, however, the timing of the report of this event, just after the patient has spoken of her sense of inhibition with the analyst, suggests that at this moment in the session the experience with the professor comes to mind and is described as a displaced representation of an immediate conflict in her experience of her relationship with the analyst.

The two kinds of displacement, in action and in communication in the here-and-now, are not mutually exclusive, although the strength of the evidence for the hypothesis of acting out is not always as strong as it seems to be in this instance.

We should add that, theoretically and clinically, there is a more conservative hypothesis that often seems applicable. This more conservative possibility is that the patient is merely repeating patterns in various contexts inside and outside the analysis and that she quite naturally may speak of a series of instances of such a pattern in a particular session, including those which involve the analyst. In other words, according to this conservative hypothesis, there is no resisted, preconscious *intention to allude to the transference* through the report of experiences outside. Instead, there is a description of a series of experiences that happen to be comparable. When the analyst interprets something in the general form, "that sounds like something between us," he really leaves the question open as to whether there was such a communicative intention or not. Comparability alone is not strong evidence for the hypothesis that the patient is communicating something in a disguised form because of resistance. The latter hypothesis is based on more or less consistent *omissions* in what is said about the analyst regarding aspects of experience that are *included* in what is said about others. It is then that it becomes plausible to propose that not only are the issues comparable, but that what is resisted in one context is more openly expressed in another, and that the reporting of the outside events carries latent meaning that pertains to the experience inside the analytic situation.

Jxr coding with Significant Event as Basis

There is one final example of a Jxr coding in the Specimen Hour that we would like to present. Its importance lies in the fact that it makes use of a Significant Event in the interaction (PSE/RSE) as a basis for the Jxr inference and coding.

There is a sequence of associations occupying the first part of the hour, about one third to one half of the session, during which the analyst is silent. A series of "relationship episodes" is reported by the patient, including hostility and jealousy in relation to an aggressive, attention-getting rival teacher; an obsessional tendency in regard to making decisions, particularly in regard to potentially pleasurable experiences with her husband; inhibitions and anxiety in her relationship with her father; and feeling she was tactless and impulsive in stating the faults of one of her students to the child's mother. These episodes, occupying #'s 1 to 22 in the session, frequently include self-critical or self-interpretive commentary by the patient. For example #'s 5 to 7, 9 to 14, and 18 to 22 all end with self-critical and/or self-interpretive comments.

There follows the analyst's first intervention which is developed in the course of an exchange with the patient that includes some effort at clarification and some confrontation (#'s 23 to 45). The analyst points out that the patient looks to her husband for support, whereas she does not turn to him (that is, to the analyst) for the same, apparently because she expects none from him. The patient goes on to suggest that maybe she expects disapproval from the analyst (#'s 46 to 47). Then she associates to difficulties getting close to people and remarks that she needs to be critical of others before she can feel close to them. The analyst comments on the sequence of themes (#49) and then uses the opportunity to inquire as to whether the patient feels critical of him (#51). This intervention in our scheme would probably be coded ER rather than XR because it is offered in the spirit of a flyer rather than an interpretation that is grounded in some particular evidence. It is quite fruitful in that the patient now opens up and goes so far as to suggest that the analysis might be "a hoax" (#52). This brings us to #'s 53 to 55 which we have already discussed as r_2 and (x_2) in the earlier examples. The patient says that it is difficult to lie down with a man in the room (#53), and that she finds it difficult to talk about her reactions to the analyst because it seems too "intimate" (#54). Then there is the experience with the professor and his tie (#55). Finally, we come to #56 which reads as follows:

> (#56) Because several things have occurred to me while I've just been talking, shall I get off the other subject (chuckle)? (Sniff) I can't decide whether to – well, maybe I'll come back to it. Uhm, well, one thing is just a variation on my talking too much. When, at this same course last night, uhm – I'm, I'm usually very quiet when I'm, am new in a course and, and I don't like to say anything. But once I stop feeling that, once I've said something, whatever it is, then I just go the opposite way completely, and I get extremely aggressive. And at the time I don't realize I'm taking over, but then afterwards, if I think about it, I can see that I really did kind of take over or ins–, keep pushing myself into the conversation to the point where others might just say, oh well, I'm not going to bother trying to talk. And I do this, I've noticed, sometimes in conversations too, that I'll either try to anticipate what somebody's going to say and then continue on with what I'm thinking, or keep talking when I should stop because they're about to say something and then they won't, then they'll never say it. And that way I control the conversation. But the conversation might not get anywhere, or certainly nowhere near where it could have if I had stopped talking when it was time to. (Sniff)

The first few lines in this paragraph, in which the patient is hesitant about changing the subject, would be coded r in our scheme. The next associations are about the patient's tendency to swing from being extremely reticent, to taking over conversations to the point that she may actually block some kind of movement in the interaction. The explicit reference to her experience of the relationship at the beginning of #56 can serve as a basis for a Jxr coding for the ensuing extratransference associations. The latent meaning of the latter could be stated as follows:

> *Just now, when I changed the subject, I had the feeling that I was in danger of being overly aggressive and controlling as if to prevent you from saying something about what we were talking about before.*

Again, notice how the r is the justification in the coding scheme for coding the Jxr. At the same time the x is a vehicle for illuminating that which is left *unspoken* in the explicit reference to the relationship.

But all of this is by way of introducing the main point of this example which is to show how this last communication sheds light on the patient's experience of the relationship in the first part of the hour. Paragraphs 1 to 22 can be considered as a Significant Event in the process in which the patient speaks and the analyst is silent so that she, in effect, "controls" the conversation. Thus, in #56 we have an explication of what is enacted implicitly in #'s 1 to 22. In this light, a latent meaning of #56 could be stated as follows:

> *I have the tendency to do what I am describing with you. I think I did it when I came in today in the first half of the session. I felt I was taking over and controlling our interaction even to the point of beating you to the punch with interpretations of my own behavior.*

In the coding itself, the SE of #'s 1 to 22 (PSE if coded earlier and RSE if coded now) would be the basis for inferring that the extra-transference associations of #56 have latent meanings in the transference and warrant the Jxr coding.

It is noteworthy that this last example involves an issue that is also prominent in the other Jxr examples, namely, the conflict about aggressiveness with the analyst. The patient's way of being controlling may be both an expression of and a defense against certain "personal" feelings that she has about him. In being controlling she interferes with the chances that the conversation will "get anywhere" (#56). Perhaps, out of anxiety about the expression of her own aggressiveness and sexual inclinations toward the analyst, she ends up keeping her distance to an extent greater than what the analytic situation requires.

The analyst's interpretation of the patient's tendency to lean on her husband and to avoid allowing her needs to surface in the analysis is consistent with this view.

Although the patient's contribution to this pattern is quite strong, it is important to recognize that the analyst is participating in it as well. His silence is, in itself, an action which the patient can plausibly construe according to her own lights. For example, she may have imagined that for his part, the analyst might be saying to himself "Oh well, I'm not going to bother to talk" (#56). It is noteworthy that during the first 22 paragraphs there are several "pauses" (15-60 seconds) and, after #14, one "silence" (60 to 120 seconds), so that, in fact, the patient may be leaving room for the analyst to speak. Her subjective sense of the rhythm of her own speech and that of the analyst and her ideas about how he experiences her would be interesting to explore. Perhaps she feels that she has been controlling in the earlier sessions so that now the analyst has withdrawn and is sulking. But this is pure speculation.

5. An Example of a Possible Transference-Countertransference Enactment

As noted earlier, we have become increasingly interested during the past several years in the likelihood of enactment of transference-countertransference patterns in the analytic process and in the plausibility of the patient's conscious and unconscious ideas about the analyst's countertransference experience (Hoffman 1983), particularly what Racker (1968) refers to as "complementary counter-transference." In this session, the analyst's first intervention is a comment on the fact that the patient has turned to her husband with something that she has withheld in the analysis. The structure of the triangular situation that the analyst calls to the patient's attention is similar to the triangular situations that the patient described in the first part of the session in which she felt jealous of a rival teacher: "I become almost jealous of who she works with" (#2), and further, "I know that I want to have a response from the boys that, as long as I have it, then it's alright for her to have it too. But I, I know I respond very much to any time that she has a very warm response and, and I don't –" (#3).

What we are suggesting is that the analyst is in a position similar to what the patient described as her own as a teacher. Moreover, his confronting the patient on the fact that she omitted something the previous day that she hoped her husband would respond to with reassurance could readily be construed by the patient as evidence of the analyst's jealousy. In this context, the analyst is the one who is vulnerable and excluded. This kind of "projective identification" (Ogden 1982) may partially protect the patient from being the excluded, vulnerable party herself. We know, of course, that she is not entirely protected and that the other side of the coin is not far from the surface. She is extremely anxious about being "personal" with the analyst. In that sense, she may feel excluded from his personal life and is anxious about her impulse to somehow intrude herself into it. The point is that the theme of exclusion, jealousy, and conflict about trespassing repeats in various contexts with the patient sometimes in the role of the one who is the excluded party and sometimes the one who is excluding another. The analyst is inevitably drawn into this pattern, falling into positions complementary to those which are assumed by the patient.

The only coding in our scheme that may be warranted with respect to this pattern is the Potentially Significant Event or the Retrospectively Significant Event. The sequence in which the patient acts in such a way as to elicit an emotional response in the analyst could be coded as a Potentially Significant Event and ensuing associations could be examined to see whether they allude to this unspoken aspect of the interaction. At the point when the patient speaks of her jealous attitude towards the teacher, no Jxr coding can be given because there is no evidence at that point that such a pattern is also present in the analytic process itself. Whereas a subsequent explicit reference to the relationship could warrant a Retrospective Jxr, a PSE that occurs or crystallizes after the x material in question cannot justify such a coding. This is because Significant Events, as we have thought of them, *influence* the patient's *subsequent* experience and associations. They are not relevant to *prior* experience and associations in the same way. Perhaps a broader view of Significant Events is called for. In this broader view it would be possible to interpret that the patient may have sensed that she was in the midst of an unconscious attempt to enact a certain pattern and was alluding to it at a certain point, even though the pattern itself did not become apparent until later when the analyst himself took part in it.

We want to emphasize that we do not regard it as necessarily detrimental if the analyst inadvertently participates in a pattern which is actually a part of the transference itself. On the contrary, it may even turn out to be extremely useful in the long run, and may promote a depth of understanding that would not have been possible otherwise. What is important is that at some point the analyst and the patient be able to extricate themselves from such patterns of enactment and that the analyst be able to interpret what has gone on without denying his own contribution at the same time that he impresses upon the patient the extent to which he or she has had a significant role to play in shaping this aspect of the relationship (Bollas 1983; Ehrenberg 1982; Hoffman 1983; Levenson 1983; Racker 1968; Sandler 1976).

6. Disclosure of Suppressed Ideas about the Relationship (DSIR)

We have found that it is not uncommon, following a transference interpretation by the analyst or even a timely ER (that is an encouragement to the patient to elaborate on his or her experience of the relationship), for the patient to reveal some aspect of his experience of the relationship which had apparently been conscious but unspoken until that moment. The fact that the idea had been conscious is usually apparent from the manner in which the patient introduces the content of the idea itself. For example the patient may say "as a matter of fact, I was just thinking yesterday..." or "I was telling a friend of mine..." or "I did think to myself after I left last time..." or any number of other introductions which make it clear that the patient was aware at some point and had formulated in his own mind the very thought which he is about to verbalize to the analyst. We believe that this is an important phenomenon because it points to an aspect of resistance that is underestimated in our view in terms of its prevalence and its significance. What we have in mind is resistance to speaking of that which the patient is already conscious or at least of that which he has been conscious outside of the analytic situation.[3] What the analyst's intervention seems to do is free the patient to speak to him about an issue that the patient had been inhibited about speaking of before. We believe that frequently such disclosures are misidentified as evidence that, as a result of an interpretation, something that had been repressed has become conscious. In fact, what has happened is that the patient is now prepared to speak of something which he had been loathe to either formulate in his mind in the analyst's presence or to speak about openly. This shift occurs only after the analyst demonstrates that he is less defensive and less resistant himself than the patient may have imagined to hearing about the issue. One example of such a DSIR occurs in #52 of the Specimen Hour immediately after the therapist asks, in #51, whether the patient has had some criticisms of him. In #52, the patient says, tellingly perhaps, "I think if I had, I would have (chuckle) suppressed them too much to admit them." The patient may not be intending a precise use of the word "suppressed," but it does seem fitting because we are interested, in the case of DSIR, in suppressed as opposed to repressed thoughts. The patient goes on to say "I'm starting with one that's less (chuckle) personal, one that I'm sure *still is occurring to me* at times, although I don't think it functions as much in my thinking now as it might have – is uhm, sometimes wondering if all this really does get anywhere, and (sniff), you know, if it isn't some sort of a hoax." The italicized phrase makes it quite evident that the patient has had this thought before and is now free enough to "admit" it to the analyst.

---

[3]Freud (1905e, p. 17) classified resistance into three types: resistance to speaking of something conscious, resistance to becoming aware of something that is unconscious in the presence of the analyst, and resistance that is attributable to repression.

It is fortuitous, we think, that the first letters of the phrase "disclosure of suppressed ideas about the relationship" are almost the same as first letters of the word "desirable." We think that such a response to an intervention by the analyst is, indeed, desirable in that it brings to light something that the patient has been experiencing that has to do with the analyst and that the patient has been omitting from his or her associations because of some anxiety and the resistance that accompanies it. Something about the analyst's intervention in our view modifies the anxiety and the resistance so that these ideas can now be spoken about and explored. The phenomenon highlights the interactional dimension of resistance in that it is a change in the environment (that is, something in the analyst's behavior) that makes it possible, apparently, for the DSIR to occur. We think that the DSIR is a potentially useful variable to consider in psychoanalytic process research. We would expect to find a relationship between DSIR and preceding timely interventions by the analyst, either transference interpretations (XR and R) or simple expressions of encouragement to the patient to elaborate on some aspect of his or her experience of the relationship (ER).

7. Explication of New Ideas about the Relationship (ENIR)

We want to call the reader's attention to the fact that the paragraphs immediately following the DSIR of #52, namely, #53 and #54, constitute what we referred to in our earlier illustrations as r_1. Here the patient speaks of her discomfort lying down with a man in the room and of her difficulty being personal with him. The wording of the first idea "I found it hard to come in here and lie down on the couch, with just you, being a man, in the room" sounds like it might qualify as a DSIR because of the use of the past tense. However it is not as clear an example as the one in #52 where the statement is made explicitly that the idea had occurred to the patient before. In #54 the patient seems to be groping more for words to capture some aspect of her experience which she has not captured in words before. The indication that this is the case is in the words "I do suppose" and in the very halting manner in which the patient proceeds: "I do suppose though, if, if uh, something occurred to me about you, even if it weren't a criticism, I don't know that I feel, I think I, I feel I can't talk about it, because it seems like kind of an intimate type of thing and, and I just am not, I don't know, I just never made personal remarks to anybody (chuckle) before I knew them for a long time." We have labeled this kind of verbalization an "explication of a new idea about the relationship" or ENIR. This kind of verbalization also strikes us as extremely important clinically, and as a possible variable in psychoanalytic process research. The patient is actively trying to overcome resistance and give shape to an aspect of her experience of the relationship with the therapist in the here-and-now which is fraught with anxiety. The DSIR and ENIR variables were not included in our coding scheme as we presented it originally (Gill and Hoffman 1982b) and, in fact, we have not attempted any systematic studies either of interjudge agreement or of a hypothesis testing nature involving them. We do feel, however, that both DSIR and ENIR are fairly readily identifiable and that they can be useful both as intra-process dependent variables and as independent variables considered as components of the process that may contribute to a positive outcome.

8. Global Rating of the Specimen Hour

What follows is the consensus clinical statement by the authors about the Specimen Hour:[4]

> The session begins with a sequence of associations during which the analyst is silent. A series of "relationship episodes" is reported by the patient, including hostility and jealousy in relation to an aggressive rival teacher; obsessional tendencies when it comes to decisions, especially regard to potentially pleasurable experiences with her husband; inhibition and anxiety in her relationship with her father; and feeling she was tactless and impulsive in stating the faults of one of her students to the child's mother. The analyst, about a third to a half way through the session, offers two transference related interventions. In the first, he points out that the patient seeks reassurance from her husband but has omitted reporting certain experiences to the analyst as if she were avoiding leaning on him as she has claimed she intended to do. After some initial disclaimers, the patient acknowledges that she does want approval from the analyst and is afraid she will not get any. The second intervention is a suggestion that the patient may be inhibiting some critical thoughts about the analyst. These interventions are fruitful in that they open the door to the disclosure by the patient of several previously suppressed ideas about the relationship (DSIR's). One is that the had patient has had the thought that analysis might be a hoax. A second is that the patient feels uncomfortable about lying down alone with a man, the analyst, in the room. The patient also refers more generally to her

[4]This statement, having been prepared for publication, is longer and more elaborate than what the authors usually write-up in the course of routine codings of sessions.

avoidance of anything that seems too personal and, later, she expresses embarrassment in telling the analyst of her admiration and envy of his freedom in dress.

These explicit thoughts about the relationship are interwoven with several sequences of extratransference associations which seem to be alluding to resisted extensions of these issues in the transference. In particular, anxiety regarding the breakthrough of sexual and aggressive impulses is articulated vividly in relation to other people in a way which is readily interpretable as applying to the analyst as well. There is evidence that the very act of telling the analyst certain things, such as that she envies his style of dress, is experienced by the patient as a breakthrough of a forbidden impulse. Finally, some of the extratransference associations seem to allude to a pattern of interaction with the analyst, observable in the beginning of this session especially, in which the patient attempts to control the interaction by monopolizing the conversation. In this way the patient expresses her inclination to be aggressively dominant at the same time that she defends against her wishes for greater intimacy with the analyst. The analyst, himself, plays a role in this pattern in that he is silent for this part of the interview despite several pauses which may represent invitations to him to speak. It is possible that the patient experiences him as having withdrawn because of something about her own controlling behavior in this and/or previous sessions. These and other resisted and sometimes enacted aspects of the patient's experience of the relationship are not interpreted by the analyst. Hence, although he does make two significant and useful attempts to explore the patient's experience of the relationship, our rating of the analyst's contribution to the exploration of transference issues is only mediocre. In this instance the rating we gave was 3.0 on a scale of 1 to 5.

9. Comparison of the PERT with the CCRT and FRAMES

We would like to formulate what we see as the relationship between our coding scheme and Luborsky's (1977) Core Conflictual Relationship Theme and between the PERT and the method developed by Dahl and Teller (Dahl, this volume; Teller and Dahl 1981a, 1986) of analyzing a session in relation to what they call Frames.

The PERT and the CCRT

The PERT scheme provides primarily, a descriptive, qualitative account of the sequence of transference issues as they emerge in a session, both through direct and indirect communication. It also provides an assessment of the extent to which the therapist contributes to the explication of transference issues in the session, and there is a quantitative rating of the therapist's work. The fact that some of the variables that we code can yield numerical scores in the sense of the frequencies with which the codings appear is very much secondary. Also, it should be evident that the small x in our system is not comparable to a "relationship episode" with someone other than the analyst in the CCRT. This is not simply because the x coding is not actually made in our system but is implied, but, more importantly because the communications that come under the rubric of x are not differentiated according to theme or object as they are in the CCRT. We could have twenty consecutive pages of "x - material" in a transcript and clearly it would be misleading to say that this amounts to one "x-episode" that is comparable to one relationship episode in the CCRT. Nor is the x comparable in this regard to the r coding in our own system since each r does represent a specific communication by the patient on a specific relationship issue. If the theme changes during the course of communications that are explicitly about the relationship, a new, additional coding of r is warranted. That is not the case with the associations that are implicitly coded as x.

Also, we cannot emphasize enough the importance to us of making clear that communications implicitly regarded as x are *not necessarily* considered to be allusions to the transference. Actually, the main divisions within the patient's communications for us are not r and x, but rather, r and Jxr which is a subclass of x. That is, the main division is between explicit and implicit communications about the relationship, the implicit communications being inferred by the judge.

Another issue which we think is important is that the PERT, unlike the CCRT, is designed to search out not only the convergence of themes but the specific details of themes that are included in associations that are not about the relationship and that disappeared *as a function of resistance* in the associations that *are* about the relationship. In other words, we are interested in the detailed examination of points of convergence and divergence of themes depending upon whether the patient is speaking about the therapeutic situation or some outside situation. The PERT is much more molecular and detailed and more geared toward the tracking, not only of transference themes, but also of *resistance as it affects nuances of communication during the course of the session.* We think that if one focuses on the issue of resistance the difference between the CCRT and the PERT becomes clearer.

Another important difference between the systems is that the attempt by the PERT to capture at least some of the characteristics of transference-countertransference enactments that are observed by the judge but about which the patient does not speak explicitly has no counterpart in the CCRT. These are relationship episodes that are not in the manifest content of the patient's associations, but which the patient may allude to implicitly. We are particularly interested in the analyst's contributions to the transference through his own manner of relating. In the PERT these "contributions" would be coded as PSE or RSE and used as a basis for inferring disguised allusions by the patient to his experience of the relationship (Jxr and Jrr).

As we understand it, the CCRT was not originally designed as a way of getting at transference issues except in the sense that any theme and, certainly, any recurring theme can be hypothesized to have some bearing on the relationship with the analyst. But this is a very weak sense in which the CCRT is addressed to the transference. The search for recurring themes cannot be considered in itself the search for the transference themes.

From our point of view, the CCRT and the PERT complement each other in that the CCRT provides a systematic way of keeping track of and collating themes as they emerge in a session. Although it might be somewhat laborious, the systematic recording of "relationship episodes" should make possible a more reliable and comprehensive coding of disguised allusions to the transference, that is, of Jxr and Jrr. This would be a kind of systematizing of what the judge now does in the PERT when he "keeps in mind" various themes that have arisen in the hour and relates them to evidence in the form of r or SE in coding disguised allusions.

The PERT and Frames

Although we do not claim to have fully digested and understood the system developed by Dahl and Teller (Dahl, this volume; Teller and Dahl 1981a, 1986) for content analysis of psychoanalytic sessions, we would like to state what appear to be points of correspondence of the PERT and Frames. We believe that there are features of Frames that are very compatible with the PERT. In fact the PERT could be considered as a certain kind of application of Frames. We will not review the terms and the applications of the Dahl-Teller approach which is described elsewhere in this volume. Dahl (this volume) writes that "in cases where there is no evidence for a particular event in an instantiation, the value in the corresponding prototype event becomes the predicted value in the instantiation" (see page 56). What we are suggesting, given our particular clinical and research interest, is that the patterns of inclusion and omission of events associated with certain frames is often a function of resistance to awareness of transference and/or resistance to communication about the transference combined with the patient's inclination to overcome those resistances. We think that what we are looking for when we search out disguised allusions to the transference in the PERT amount to extratransference "prototype frames" that provide clues to the "defaults," due to resistance, in analyst related "instantiations." We think this describes precisely what we are doing when we code Jxr. In the case of Jrr, we look for prototype frames that are themselves about the transference which provide clues to defaults, due to resistance, in other associations that are also manifestly about the relationship with the analyst. The latter have the formal status, in the context of Dahl's system, of "instantiations."

It might help to clarify how these terms can be applied by looking again at one of the examples of a Jxr coding described earlier. The episode in which the patient grabs the professor's tie and then is horrified and is afraid that the professor is similarly horrified might be used as a prototype which has certain elements that are missing from, but can be read into, what the patient says about her experience of the relationship with the analyst. Without getting into it too formally, the episode includes an impulse to be forward and a reaction of anxiety. The impulse in this case is acted upon. In the relationship with the analyst the patient is much more inhibited. However, when she speaks to him about his manner of dress, she is taking a step which she experiences as rather personal and bold and she has a reaction of embarrassment which parallels the horror that she felt after she grabbed the professor's tie. So it is possible to read into the experience that is explicit in the relationship with the analyst the impulse to touch him, or more generally, to act impetuously in relation to him. We can also read into the patient's experience with the analyst an idea that he would be put off by this inclination to be forward with him; an inclination that the patient is usually inhibiting. What is missing from the experience with the analyst are the very ingredients that are elaborated upon in the experience with the professor, so that these experience with the professor give us the "default values" that can be applied to the experience with the analyst.

This is not to say that there may not be times when a frame will be more fully represented in associations that are manifestly about the interaction with the analyst in the here-and-now than it is represented in associations about another situation. In the first example of Retrospective Jxr that we have presented (see above p. 79), we commented that aspects of the patient's conflicts might find more overt expression in her relationship with the analyst than they would in her relationship with her father. It may be that as resistance to the awareness of transference is overcome there would be more instances in which the relationship between prototype and instantiation would be reversed. The prototypes for certain frames will be represented in interactions with the analyst and the instantiations in which certain events in the frame sequence are omitted will center on relationships with others, especially family members. Teller and Dahl (1986) write, "Ultimately, analysts would of course be interested in discovering childhood prototype frames that would provide clues to the origin of defaults in adult instantiations – the sources of both our adaptive and our neurotic expectations in life" (p. 796-797). What we are describing here is the opposite direction of discovery with here-and-now transference prototype frames providing clues to defaults in child-parent instantiations. This direction of discovery corresponds roughly, we think, with what Gill (1979, 1982) has defined elsewhere as the complement to resistance to awareness of transference, namely, resistance to the resolution of the transference. In the latter the patient is loathe to consider the possibility that his experience of the relationship with the analyst in the here-and-now, as it has been explicated, has significant origins in childhood experiences, including relationships with parents, siblings, etc.

Returning to our particular example, we can see that even in this one session there is more that surfaces to help us to see the factors contributing to the patient's conflicts in her relationship with the analyst than what comes to light directly with regard to the patient's experience of paralysis in her relationship with her father. We could hypothesize that the impulse to act impetuously, aggressively, and, perhaps, seductively that is suggested in the context of the patient's experience with the analyst might be a clue as to what is interfering and causing so much anxiety and awkwardness in the patient's relationship with her father.

Like the CCRT, Frames can be used in conjunction with the PERT scheme as a way of taking systematic account of all the data in a session for the purpose of tracking the patient's experience of the relationship with the analyst in the course of a session, part of a session, or a series of sessions.

In our view, one of the important omissions in Frames as described by Teller and Dahl is that it generally has been applied to the patient's associations without direct reference to the analyst's participation in the process. Although it seems to us that the method that Teller and Dahl have invented can be adapted to include the analyst, so far we see no evidence that there is any thought of doing so. In accord with the notion of an inevitable interplay of transference and countertransference, it would be useful to see prototype frames and instantiation of frames in which the analyst himself is directly involved, with some intervention or other behavior constituting evidence of one of the events in the sequence of events that make up a particular frame. An example from the Specimen Hour might be one based on the example of transference-countertransference enactment that we discussed earlier. The frame would have to do with a sequence involving jealousy and exclusion. The moment when the analyst "complains" about the patient's failure to turn to him for reassurance (whereas she had done so with her husband) would itself be evidence of an event in a sequence in which someone feels left out and hurt. The fact that in this particular context the analyst is cast in the role of vulnerable child, is consistent with the view that while certain patterns may be repeated over and over again, the patient may occupy a variety of different roles in those patterns, casting other persons, and the analyst in particular, into complementary positions. What we are saying here is in keeping with a comment by Teller and Dahl (1986) that "There are also variants in which another person, e.g. father or mother, replaces the patient as the subject of the action in a frame, as well as instances in which the objects of the action are variables, e.g. husband, parents or analyst ... Thus one can represent identifications in a formal way that until now has not been possible" (p. 795). We would add that the analyst may also be the subject of the action of a frame, and the patient the object.

Although, as we said earlier, the PERT can be considered as a particular type of Frame, there is a sense in which the patient's experience of the relationship with the therapist is supraordinate relative to all other contexts (or "categories") which generate and confirm the existence of Frames. This is simply because everything that is said in sessions is said to the therapist. We are not dealing with a literary text, but with a record of a particular interaction. Every word that is spoken is part of a particular event in the patient's life which is his experience of the analytic hour. Dahl and Teller do not seem to make anything of the difference between the analyst as the object and other objects that appear in the patient's associations. Such a distinction is warranted, not because of the special theoretical importance of the transference in psychoanalysis, but simply because of the fact that the reporting of experience in the session is always embedded in the experience of talking to the analyst. To put it in terms of "relationship episodes," all the episodes reported in the session are part of a supraordinate "relationship episode" which is constituted by the patient's experience of the session itself.

10. Conclusion

We have presented an overview of a method for coding the patient's experience of the relationship with the therapist (PERT) in psychoanalysis and psychoanalytic psychotherapy. We have illustrated the scheme by applying it to Specimen Hour. After illustrating the coding of a sequence of interrelated disguised allusions to the transference, we discussed the implications of the interplay of transference and countertransference for the PERT method. Also, two new process variables were introduced: disclosure of suppressed ideas about the relationship (DSIR) and explication of new ideas about the relationship (ENIR). We think these variables may be useful in the investigation of the immediate impact of transference interpretations as well as other aspects of process research.

Finally, we compared the PERT to Luborsky's (1977) Core Conflictual Relationship Theme (CCRT) and to Dahl's (this volume; Teller and Dahl 1981a, 1986) Frames. Among other differences, the PERT focuses upon the course of resistance as it affects communications about the immediate interaction in the hour, whereas the CCRT searches out thematic convergence. Also, the PERT includes assessment of the therapist's work in the session whereas the CCRT does not. The search for disguised allusions to the transference in the PERT can be viewed as a particular type of frame analysis in which aspects of what the patient reports about his experience of the relationship at any given moment are filled in by reference to other contexts where the full sequence of events associated with a particular frame are more fully represented. What is missing in terms of direct communication regarding the transference, that is the "defaults" in that communication, is ascribable to resistance. There is a sense in which the category of experience which comes under the rubric of "talking to the analyst" is supraordinate to all other categories in which other individuals are the objects of the patient's experience. This is simply because every utterance in the session is part of a supraordinate "relationship episode", which is the patient's experience of the session itself. Both the CCRT and Frames complement the PERT by providing a systematic way of mapping and keeping track of various themes in the course of an hour which have relevance to the coding of disguised allusions to the transference.

The Assessment of Transference by the CCRT Method

Lester Luborsky and Paul Crits-Christoph

1. Introduction

Ever since Freud introduced the concept of transference after the turn of the century (Freud 1912b), psychoanalytic clinicians have formulated it and reformulated it during the treatment of their patients. In their clinical writings they have attended to it even more than to the other two clinical factors that are considered curative, the therapeutic alliance and the internalization of the gains (Luborsky 1984). Despite its clinical centrality there has been no well researched operational measures of it on the basis of psychoanalytic sessions. It was only ten years ago that the advent of the CCRT measure (Luborsky 1977) began to fill that void. Now, in this volume are three of the most prominent current attempts to represent the transference: the CCRT, the PERT (Gill and Hoffman 1982b), and FRAME structures (Dahl, this volume; Teller and Dahl 1981a, 1986).

In this chapter we describe how the measure was discovered, how it works, an example from the Specimen Hour, its reliability and validity and future plans for it.

Fifteen years ago, in order to develop such a measure, Luborsky joined a group of clinical researchers who met once a week for several years – the Analytic Research Group of the Institute of the Pennsylvania Hospital. Although we made some progress and developed a measure of *amount* of transference (Luborsky et al. 1973), the group finally gave up the search and disbanded because their ultimate aim had been to discover a measure of the *content* of the transference, not just a measure of amount of transference.

Then several years ago Luborsky stumbled upon a content measure while occupied with what appeared to him to be another task. It happened in this way. After the helping alliance measure (Luborsky 1976) had been constructed he was exploring the question of how the helping alliance relationship measure might fit into a measure of the general relationship pattern. He looked into this question in much the way he had proceeded with the helping alliance measure. He read and reread psychotherapy sessions and then reviewed what he had been attending to in forming a concept of the general relationship pattern. First he saw he was giving special attention to the narratives of interactions between the patient and other people ("relationship episodes"), not only early episodes in relationship with the parents but current episodes in the relationship with the therapist. Relationship episodes are spontaneously told narratives found in almost all sessions. They are about other people, typically the father, mother, brother, sister, friends, bosses, and the therapist. He also noticed that his understanding of the relationship pattern within the narratives consisted of understanding these components: the patient's main wishes, needs or intentions toward the other person in the narrative, the responses of the other person, and the responses of the self. His inferences about the basic relationship pattern were primarily determined by the types of these components with the highest frequency across the relationship episodes. In fact, the combination of these highest frequency types of components constituted the main relationship pattern, the "Core Conflictual Relationship Theme" (CCRT). It was only later that experiences with the CCRT led him to realize that he had hit upon on an operational definition of the transference.

The method appears to have common elements with the TAT's scoring method and such appearances are not entirely deceiving. Some of the categories of the two are similar; for example, the wishes are similar and the expected responses from others is similar; it is called "Press" in the TAT. But there are major differences. In the CCRT, (1) the narratives are presented by the patient or subject as real narratives not fantasies, and (2) the principal inferences are about the few most recurrent organizing themes or mental schemas, not as in the TAT about a large array of all kinds of themes. In fact, the CCRT may belong to a family of conceptualizations of relationship patterns which includes Tomkin's (1979) concept of a nuclear script, Meichenbaum and Gilmore's (1984) concept of core organizing principle and similar concepts reviewed by Singer (1984). Despite the similarities in terms of concepts, the CCRT method is the most advanced in terms of representing a guided clinical judgment system for evaluating the transference concept, with some evidence for reliability and validity as described below (Luborsky et al. 1985 and Luborsky et al. 1986).

2. The CCRT Procedures

The CCRT measure is described in detail in a guide to the method (unpublished but available upon request, Luborsky 1986)[1]. The first step in the method is to identify the relationship episodes in the session. This is typically done by independent judges before the transcripts are given to the CCRT judges. A minimum of eight relationship episodes are usually used as a basis for scoring the CCRT.

The CCRT judge reads the relationship episodes in the transcript and identifies the types of each of the three components in each episode:

a) the patient's main wishes, needs, or intentions toward the other person,
b) the expected or actual responses of the other person; and
c) the responses of the self.

The CCRT represents the types of components with the highest frequency across the sample of relationship episodes.

The judge first identifies the wishes, responses from others and from the self in each of the RE's and from these makes a preliminary CCRT formulation (steps 1 and 2) and then the same judge re-identifies and re-formulates (steps 1' and 2'):

Step 1: Identify the types of wishes (W), responses from others (RO), and response from self (RS) in each relationship episode (RE).

Step 2: Formulate a preliminary CCRT based on the highest frequencies of each of the types of each component.

Step 1': Re-identify, where needed, the types of W, RO, and RS based on the step 2.

Step 2': Re-formulate, where needed, based on the recount of all W, RO, RS in step 1'.

---

[1]In the meantime a German version has been published by Luborsky (in Luborsky and Kächele 1988)

The CCRT judges work independently of each other. Judges are trained by first reading the CCRT guide and trying several practice cases, receiving feedback from the research team about their performance after each one. Although we have preferred to use experienced clinicians as judges, some graduate students have also performed well as judges because the task does not require that the judge be committed to a particular school of therapy and clinical understanding is more crucial than clinical experience.

3. Examples from the Specimen Hour

Two experienced independent CCRT judges evaluated the CCRT for the Specimen Hour. Before they applied their CCRT scoring 11 relationship episodes had been independently identified in this session. For purposes of simplifying this presentation the 11 relationship episodes were abbreviated so that they could all be shown in Figure 1. The two CCRT judges showed good agreement with each other on their CCRT formulations. Their combined formulation is briefly summarized at the center of the outer ring of 11 episodes. The wish that appears most frequently in these episodes is the wish to be assertive in the sense of wanting to exert control, to be dominant and to be better than the other person. The next most frequent wish is the wish for reassurance. The wish for reassurance is typically associated with the episodically uncontrolled expression of her most frequent wish for control or dominance of others. The other person is expected to or actually responds negatively – the other person dominates, controls, disapproves and does not reassure. The negative responses from the self include: feeling an absence of control over herself, self blame, annoyance, anger, upsetness – with the last three of these being the most frequent.

The CCRT approach can be applied by trained CCRT judges as it was in the example just given, or it can be applied more informally by the therapist during the course of the session. The therapist must decide when the CCRT components are close to being experienced and when it is desirable technically to interpret them.

4. Reliability of the CCRT (Agreement among Judges)

Even in the first trials of the CCRT method (Luborsky 1977) considerable agreement among judges was found. In Levine and Luborsky (1981) 16 graduate psychology students judges individually scored the

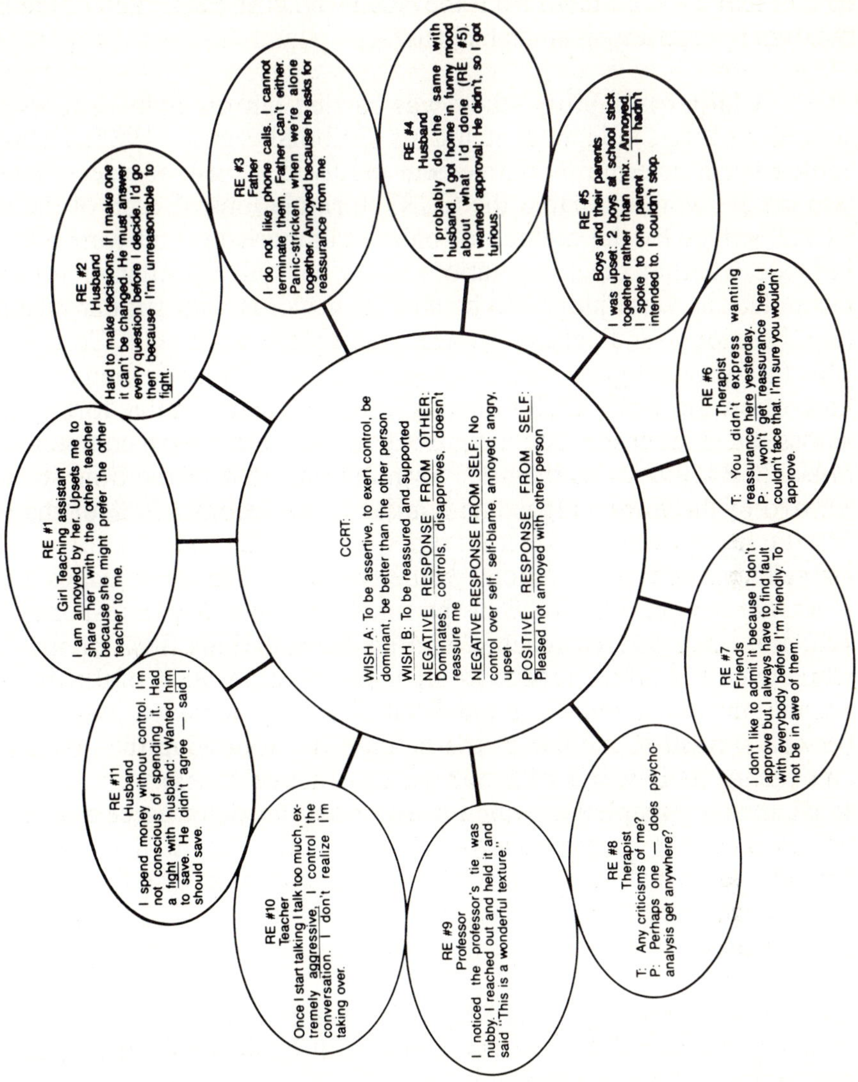

Figure 1 RE's and CCRT for Specimen Hour

CCRT for one patient (Mr. B.N.). When the scoring of each of these judges was compared with composite scoring of research judges (who also individually scored the CCRT) good agreement was found (average correlation of .88). Furthermore, agreement was shown by the method of "mismatched cases" – agreement was greater when the components to be compared were drawn from the Mr. B. N. case itself rather than from two other purposely mismatched cases.

A larger reliability study was carried out on eight patients each scored by three independent judges (Luborsky et al. 1985; Luborsky et al. 1986). Determining agreement involved the use of a second set of two judges who compared the CCRT formulations of each of the three CCRT judges by the method of paired comparisons and were asked to indicate whether the formulations were basically similar or different. Formulations were judged to be similar if words with similar meanings (e.g. "anxious" and "afraid") were used by the different CCRT judges. This task showed good interjudge agreement (96%). We then calculated how often the three CCRT judges came up with similar formulations across the eight cases. The data revealed that on the wish component the three CCRT judges had similar formulations 75% of the time (6 out of 8); two of the three judges had similar formulations 100% of the time. For the negative response from other, 63% of the time the three judges arrived at similar formulations, while two out of the three judges arrived at similar formulations 88% of the time. For the negative response from self, the three judges reached similar formulations 38% of the time, while two of the three reached similar formulations 88% of the time. We should emphasize that for good reliability to be achieved judges should be well-trained in the use of the method (by following the manual and comparing their work with our set of practice cases). A much larger study is near completion which shows good levels of agreement (Crits-Christoph et al., in preparation)

5. Validity

Two kinds of validity were tried. An example of the most usual type, which is the correlation of the measure at hand with a more standard measure, will be presented first.

Validity (1): CCRT "improvement" versus standard improvement measures.

To assess the validity of the CCRT we related it to other measures. Using data from the study of eight patients (Luborsky et al. 1986), we hypothesized that change in the CCRT from early to late in treatment should be related to independent measures of the outcome of treatment. The measure of change in CCRT was the difference score between the early-in-treatment pervasiveness of each CCRT component (i.e., the percentages of relationship episodes that contained each main wish, negative response from self, negative response from other, positive response from self, and positive response from other) and the late-in-treatment pervasiveness of the same CCRT components. Two independent outcome measures were selected as criteria, one from the perspective of the patient, the Hopkins Symptom Checklist total score, and one from the perspective of an external clinical judge, the Health-Sickness Rating Scale (Luborsky 1975). Both measures were obtained at the beginning of treatment and at termination. Change in the pervasiveness of the main negative R was significantly correlated with change in Health-Sickness Rating Scale, $r = -.81$, $p < .05$, as was change on the main wish, $r = -.73$, $p < .05$. Change in the main positive RO was significantly correlated with change on the Symptom Checklist, $r = -.79$, $p < .05$. The direction of all of these correlations was as expected: increase in the frequency of positive components or decrease in negative components of the CCRT was associated with more favorable outcomes. A study by Baguet, Gerin, Sali and Marie-Cardine (1984) has also shown a relationship between change on the CCRT and change on the Health-Sickness Rating Scale.

Another kind of validity also has been explored. It is validity defined as meaningful relationships of the CCRT to other phenomena:

Validity (2): Correspondence of the CCRT with Freud's Observations of Transference:

A more indirect way of examining the validity of the CCRT is to compare its results with nine observations Freud (1912b) made about transference. This comparison is based on a study of eight patients' psychotherapy sessions (Luborsky et al. 1985; Luborsky et al. 1986). Each patient's CCRT was scored by three independent judges on a minimum of ten RE's drawn from two sessions early in treatment and by three different independent judges on ten RE's from two sessions late in treatment (about one year later). Each of Freud's nine observations were translated into operational definitions and these were examined for the degree to which they applied to the CCRT results. At this point Freud's observations will only be briefly listed; details can be found in Luborsky et al. (1985, 1986): (1) each patient has one transference pattern; (2) each patient has a special form of transference pattern; (3) the pattern applies to "the conduct of his erotic life;" (4) the transference pattern is composed of a portion that is kept out of awareness and a portion that is in awareness; (5) the pattern "is constantly repeated – constantly reprinted afresh – in the course of the person's life;" (6) the pattern "is certainly not entirely insusceptible to change;" (7) the relationship with the therapist in the course of treatment becomes like the general transference pattern; (8) the transference pattern derives from the "combined operation of his innate disposition with the influences brought to bear on him during his early years;" (9) the transference is evident both inside and outside of the treatment. We were able to make an operational definition for most of these and found that for them the CCRT findings and the operational definition of Freud's observation appear to be consistent.

6. Plans

A high priority for further development of the CCRT is more studies of reliability, validity, and comparisons with other measures. Much of this will be accomplished through analysis of a sample of 43 patients from the Penn Psychotherapy Study. Within the next three years we hope to publish a definitive guide to the method and to the research using the method. These are the specifically planned studies to be carried out during this period:

1. Further Reliability Studies: These studies will be based on the 43 cases each evaluated by three judges. We have found that the paired comparison method is a way to deal with providing a quantified estimate of the similarity of the scoring of the judges with each other. Since the categories used for each patient are tailor-made descriptions to fit each patient, a paired comparison system of judgment of these descriptions by independent judges judging degrees of similarity is a first approximate solution to the need to provide a quantified reliability estimate.

2. More Simplified and Reliable CCRT-Scoring Methods: Since the usual CCRT scoring is by tailor-made categories for each patient and such categories not only are time consuming to score but they engender problems in reliability, we have been refining a set of uniform pre-set categories. We intend to compare the usual CCRT tailor-made scoring with a combination scoring in which the judge first does the usual CCRT scoring and then consults the pre-set category list and translates each of the CCRT categories into the best-fitting pre-set category. The combination system seems to us to be a prudent one to achieve the scoring of the pre-set categories. In the next stage of this research we will venture to try an unassisted system. CCRT judges will select the most applicable categories from the pre-set category list without having first done their own tailor-made categories. We do not expect the results of the direct-use-of-pre-set-categories to be as reliable as the results of the combination system, but we will see.

For the pre-set category list (Edition #1) we used a normative sample of 16 cases: 8 from the Penn Psychotherapy project and 8 from other research centers. The set of categories in the Edition #1 is built on an empirical basis, i.e., it is an assemblage of the categories that best describe the core theme components in the RE's of our sample of 16 patients. Edition #2 to be developed in the same way in the next two years will be on a normative sample of 60 cases.

The principles for selecting the categories and organizing them are as follows: (1) the categories chosen are those that most frequently appear in the 16 cases in the normative set. (2) The categories are the ones that are most readily discriminable from each other, that is, they are fairly clearly non-overlapping. (3) The adjectives used within each category are fairly synonymous. (4) The words selected for the categories in each of the three types of component lists are the same wherever possible e.g. wish: "not be dominated;" response from other: "dominates;" response from self: "feels dominated."

Our plan is to have two independent judges apply Edition #1 to the set of 43 cases drawn from the Penn Psychotherapy project. We will then evaluate the agreement in the ways described above.

Based on the application of the combination system in three cases we have some impressions of the findings: (1) The translation of the tailor-made categories into the pre-set categories could usually be readily done. (2) The tailor-made categories tend to capture more completely the special flavor of the category as it applies to the particular patient. (3) The pre-set category system is convenient and relatively rapid to use as compared with the tailor-made system and is an obvious asset for simplifying the job of assessing interjudge agreement.

3. Further Validity Studies: Our plan is to apply both kinds of validity studies in the enlarged sample (N = 43) to permit (1) the comparison of change in the CCRT vs change in the health-sickness rating scale (as described earlier) and (2) the comparison of Freud's observations and about transference with the CCRT findings.

4. Further Comparison of the CCRT Measure with Other Measures: The measure that potentially has most in common with the CCRT is the Patient's Experience of the Relationship with the Therapist method (PERT) (Gill and Hoffman 1982b; Hoffman and Gill, this volume). This guided clinical judgment method uses transcripts of psychotherapy sessions and offers guidelines for the frequency of communications regarding the patient's manifest experience of the relationship with the therapist as well as presumed implicit references to the experience. It has two main divisions: (1) experiences of the relationship that are manifestly about the relationship with the therapist and (2) experiences of the relationship that are not manifestly about the relationship with the therapist and have no specific designation. A comparison of the two methods is underway in which the PERT method and the CCRT method are being applied to the same sessions.

5. Further Simplified Assessment Methods: A questionnaire method for establishing general relationship patterns has been developed by Horowitz et al. (1983) which should be compared with the CCRT. It includes interpersonal behaviors mentioned as problems in psychiatric interviews; it is an "inventory of interpersonal problems" (IIP). The questionnaire has good internal consistency and test-retest reliability. We will evaluate 20 patients by both the IIP and the CCRT. We do not expect the IIP to tap into the transference pattern as clearly as the CCRT but the proposed study offers chance to see the strengths and liabilities of the two methods.

A Comparison of Three Transference Related Measures Applied to the Specimen Hour

Lester Luborsky

1. Introduction

My aim is to compare and contrast the three transference related systems most represented in this volume: CCRT, PERT and Frames. My discussion will be mainly devoted to examining the Specimen Hour from the three systems' vantage points and then drawing conclusions about their inter-comparisons. Moreover, I have discovered that even for those of us who are most intimately acquainted with each of the measures, discerning the commonalities across them is a strenuous exercise. The energy that needs to go into this is a function of the effort that must be made to overcome the potential near-sightedness of partisanship for a particular measure. It also is an effort to fulfill the difficult-to-meet requirement that the systems be applied to the same material in order to be able to see their differences and commonalities.

Therefore, for doing this task it is helpful to review Figure 1 (see page 103) with the 11 relationship episodes (RE) for the Specimen Hour. The CCRT research has demonstrated that clinical judges who follow our guided clinical judgment system can reliably agree about the CCRT within these relationship episodes (Crits-Christoph et al., in preparation). I have depicted this CCRT as a central template in the center of a core circle. The type of wish that appears most frequently is, to be assertive, in the sense of wanting to exert control, to be dominant and to be better than the other person. The next most frequent wish is the wish for reassurance. Typically the wish for reassurance is associated with the episodically uncontrolled expression of her most frequent wish for control or dominance of others. The expected or actual negative responses from the other person are that the other person dominates, controls, disapproves and does not reassure. The negative responses from the self include feeling an absence of control over herself, self-blame, annoyed, angry, upset; the most frequent of these is annoyed, angry, and upset. After the therapist identifies the CCRT, since it is a potentially transference-related theme, the therapist then must decide when and which of these theme components needs to be interpreted.

The PERT system applied to Hour 5 would identify a JXr i.e., a judged experience of the relationship with the therapist, probably in the third, fourth or fifth RE. Even though in the PERT system there is no systematic delineation of REs, as there is in the CCRT system, many of the PERT scores happen anyway to occur in relation to REs, as can easily be seen in the review of Gill and Hoffman (1982b) in Luborsky et al. (1986). The PERT system might suggest the same response as the therapist gave in RE 6.

Some evidence is now available indicating that the PERT system and the CCRT system similarly identify the basic relationship pattern that underlies transference. Luborsky and Crits-Christoph (this volume) report results of paired comparisons showing that the two method's summary description of the transference are more similar for matched pairs than for "mismatched" pairs (even though the PERT system had provided relatively little information in their descriptions about the transference related material).

An examination of Hour 5 in terms of the FRAME system suggests that many of the Frames are event sequences that are part of the relationship episodes. For example, Frame B (see page 54 f.) labeled SUPPORT, especially describes RE #4 in relation to the husband. The sequence there is very much like the sequence that is described in similar terms in the CCRT. In the CCRT one wish is for reassurance; in the Frame it is "wants support." The Frame terms and the CCRT terms are also similar and the response from self in the CCRT and in the Frame terms – "expresses hostility" – are identical. A more complete and systematic comparison needs to be done and there is ample data from Hour 5 to do this.

2. Stability of the Measures Over Time

Each transference related measure, the CCRT, PERT and Frames, tracks aspects of a relationship pattern that has considerable stability over time. In fact for the CCRT we have some data that demonstrates the stability of the main conflictual relationship pattern and by implication, of the transference pattern (Luborsky et al. 1986). I will illustrate this with a sample from the Specimen Hour compared with a much later sample taken from session 1028. In the later session the relationship episodes are recognizably similar to the ones in Hour 5. The main changes in the later session are more comfort and ease in recognition by the patient (and therapist) of the main theme and more positive responses from others and to self. In the later session, for example, there is a relationship episode about the husband. It refers directly to similar material in Hour 5. In this later session, however, while the RE again reflects the wish to dominate, control and express anger to the husband and the expected response from him of anger but then a new response from self is also evident of feeling loving, of recognizing that the sequence of other feelings is familiar and surmountable.

Another relationship episode in the later session reflects what appears to be at first a new theme. It is an old wish to be pregnant by the father and now by the therapist. One consequence of the involvement in the wish is feeling disappointed in the response from the husband because he has a lesser position in comparison with father and therapist. Further examination of the RE suggests that the narrative is a further specification of a wish that was recognized consistently in earlier sessions, to assert her need to get a response from a man. Earlier it appeared to be mainly to get a reassuring response, later it is to get a loving, sexual response and also get pregnant by and have a child by father and analyst. The response from self to the wish is a positive one. It reflects familiarity with the theme, acceptance of it and the capacity therefore to mend the relationship with the husband by recognizing the wish toward father and analyst as an unreasonable restriction on her loving response to the husband.

What these brief examples reflect is that the therapist's and patient's continual re-examination of the transference pattern in each session does not result only in stereotypically re-recognizing the original relationship pattern. It also sets the stage for an expansion in the connotations and connections through working through. The mental set of the therapist is not just satisfaction with re-recognition of a recurrent formulation, but it is attunement to the current information and then understanding anew specific form of the relationship pattern and transference in each session (as pointed out by Marshall Edelson, personal communication, 1984).

3. The Interrelationship of the Transference Pattern and Symptoms

Each of the transference measures has something to contribute to the understanding of the appearance of symptoms. As an example the CCRT is especially able to provide this understanding in the Specimen Hour.

In that session the collision of the opposed wishes may give an impetus to the appearance of the symptoms. The opposed wishes are (1) the wish to dominate, demand and exert control in order to get a positive response from the other, versus (2) the wish to get reassurance and help. In addition, each of these wishes strongly collides with the expected response from the other person, who is expected to reject the wishes. For this patient the opposition of these wishes is the framework in which one of the main symptoms, the sexual inhibition, can be better understood.

These transference pattern methods are only one source of information about the symptom. Certain recurrent behaviors in the session whose context can be examined may also bc informativc. These behaviors probably occur at moments of special tension. The two recurrent behaviors that are very frequent for this patient are stomach noise and chuckles. An inspectional analysis was carried out (obviously it will require independent judgment as well) of the context in which these two behaviors occur. The design was set up in the way that symptom-context studies are typically set up (Luborsky 1970), i.e., each time the behavior appears an examination was made of the 100 words the patients speaks just before it and just after it. I found that for the stomach noises the context particularly includes expressions of assertiveness and anger and signs of upsetness about these. For example, at the end of paragraph 18 of the transcript, "I got furious at him" is temporally associated with an outbreak of this symptom.

The other recurrent behavior, the chuckles, tends to occur around somewhat similar contents but these are responded to in a different way. The contents are (a) pleasure at being able to challenge the therapist (e.g. by insightful statements of her own), (b) embarrassment at challenging the therapist, (c) insightful statements that she provides about herself but with pride and embarrassment at the pride – these are combinations of (a) and (b) e.g. in paragraph 11, "Sometimes my advice is pretty good" and this statement is followed by embarrassment.

The context for both of these behaviors, the stomach noise and the chuckles, despite their differences tends to focus on the central conflict of asserting the wish to dominate, control, challenge yet still be able to get a positive response from the other person.

4. Conclusions about Commonalities and Differences

A partisan for any one of the three systems could say "my system is better than the other system." That conclusion is true in part and not true in part. The summary in Table 1 makes clear in what ways these systems have been developed and in what ways they have not yet.

Table 1 Comparison of Assessment Development of Three Transference Related Measures: CCRT, PERT and Frames

	Transference Potential		Transference Activation		Adequacy of Utilization by T.	
	Clinical	Guided	Clinical	Guided	Clinical	Guided
CCRT	X	X+	X	–	X	Xa
PERT	X	–	X	X	X	–
FRAME	X	X	X	X	X	–

Clinical = unguided clinical judgment
Guided = guided clinical judgment
X+ = guided clinical judgment plus evidence for reliability and validity
Xa = guided system for evaluating the adequacy
Transference Potential = A relationship pattern that is likely to be experienced in the relationship with the therapist
Transference Activation = Patient's experiences in the relationship with the therapist
Adequacy of Utilization = Can the measure be used to evaluate the adequacy of T's intervention?

The operative word is "yet" – in time each of them can develop the currently undeveloped aspect. Each of the three systems is compared in the table in terms of the nature of the assessment of (a) the transference pattern, (b) the transference *experience* within that pattern, and (c) the adequacy of the therapist's therapeutic interventions based on the evidence from the transference experience.

In the table we see within each of the three systems a clinical analysis is attempted for (a), (b) or (c). Then, in addition, some of the methods, for example the CCRT, provide a guided clinical judgment system that permits the collection of objective evidence on reliability and validity. For the PERT system, the relationship pattern is analyzed by clinical judgment only and no guided clinical system has yet provided evidence on reliability and validity; for the transference experience a guided system is available but nothing yet by way of evidence of its validity and only one small sample showing reliability for the total number of PERT scores in a session. (Agreement on the locations of each PERT has not been reported.) The Frame system is also still in an early stage of development, in terms of objective guidance systems. However, each of these systems embodies some reasonable approximation between the concept of transference and their particular measure of it. But there might be some differences of opinion about how closely they approximate the concept. Apropos of that, I was amused by an experience I once had. I heard two men telling riddles to each other. One riddle seemed very appropriate to our difficulty of matching the transference concept with each operational measure of it. The first man, Sam, said: I have a riddle for you. What is it that is green, hangs on a wall and whistles? The second man, Joe, sitting next to him, thought a while and said: I don't know, what? Sam: A herring. Joe: A herring isn't green. Sam: So you paint it green. Joe: But it doesn't hang on a wall. Sam: So you hang it on the wall. Joe: But it doesn't whistle. Sam: So who cares if it whistles.

5. Summary of the Commonalities and Differences

1. All three measures were fashioned to serve as clinical judgment methods for evaluating relationship patterns and transference experiences within these patterns. The construction of these measures is part of a recent world-wide interest in the development of measures of relationship schemas (Luborsky et al. 1986).

2. Beyond being clinical measures, they are "guided" clinical measures. The word guided in this instance means guided by a system that potentially can be reliably applied. According to Holt (1978), guided clinical systems tend to provide more effective measures with greater predictive potential than unguided clinical systems.

3. All three measures tend to attend to relationship episodes. The CCRT does this more explicitly and uniformly than the others.

4. Only the CCRT has much evidence for both reliability and validity of assessing the transference potential.

5. Some degree of integration of all three of these systems may be advantageous for each of them. A start on this direct was made by the combination of CCRT and PERT (Luborsky 1984, Appendix 4).

Application of the CCRT: A Measure of Adequacy of Therapist's Interpretation and a Measure of Patient's Self-Understanding

Paul Crits-Christoph and Lester Luborsky

1. Introduction

One of the central concepts in the theory of the curative action of psychoanalytic psychotherapy is the power of transference interpretations for augmentating self-understanding (Luborsky 1984). Despite the importance of transference interpretation and patient self-understanding to theory, there have been few attempts to empirically investigate these aspects of psychoanalytic psychotherapy. It is the purpose of this chapter to present two psychotherapy process rating scales: (a) adequacy of therapist's response to transference, and (b) patient's self-understanding. We will first review relevant research and then describe the beginnings of our new quantitative approaches based upon the Core Conflictual Relationship Theme Method (Luborsky 1977).

Before proceeding with the description of our psychotherapy process measures, it is important to define some of our main concepts. Transference is a term used in a variety of ways by clinicians. Often, transference is defined as the patient's distorted attitudes and feelings specifically toward the therapist. This pattern is seen as originating from early conflictual relationship with significant parental figures. We use the term transference in a broader sense to refer to the maladaptive relationship patterns that are evident in relationships outside of the therapeutic situation as well as with the therapist. Freud (1912b) seemed to have this latter definition in mind when he stated, "It is not a fact that transference emerges with greater intensity and lack of restraint during psychoanalysis than outside it." (p. 101)

We should also say a few words about our use of the concept of self-understanding. The term "insight" is a more commonly used one, but our preference is for self-understanding because it is a broader term. An important distinction can also be made between self-understanding as knowledge about one's self versus "emotional insight." Assessment of self-understanding as knowledge about one's self runs the risk of tapping into patients' over intellectualized self views rather than "real" understanding. The term "emotional insight," however, is often used to describe the process of being in touch with and experiencing one's emotions (Hohage and Kübler, this volume), rather than the acquisition of understanding about specific content that was previously outside of awareness. Our interest is primarily in the latter phenomena.

2. Research on Therapist's Response to Transference

A variety of studies have attempted to measure the amount of emphasis on transference interpretation during psychotherapy sessions. Usually these measures consist of ratings or content coding systems scored by clinical judges. Those studies are reviewed below.

One of the many variables judged by the paired comparisons method in The Menninger Foundation Psychotherapy Project (Kernberg et al. 1972) was "Focus on Transference." Judges used process notes and other test and interview data collected at termination to evaluate this dimension. Results indicated that for high skill therapists treating patients with low initial ego strength, high focus on transference was associated with better global improvement at follow-up.

Malan (1976b) used therapists' process notes to document an association between the frequency of transference interpretations and treatment outcome. These findings were extended by Marziali (1984), who examined the frequency of transference interpretations using audio recordings of sessions. The frequency of interpretations with therapist-parent links and therapist-parent-other links correlated significantly with several psychodynamic outcome scales.

The earliest precise analysis of the immediate effects of transference interpretations within psychodynamic psychotherapy sessions was by Garduk and Haggard (1972). Using a sample of four cases, they compared the immediate effects during the 5 minutes after transference interpretations versus after noninterpretations. Interpretations were shown to elicit more defensive associations, more transference-related material, more understanding, and more affect than were noninterpretations.

Luborsky et al. (1979) examined the immediate preconditions and consequences of 16 transference interpretations for each of three patients in psychoanalysis. There was a clear parallel between the positivity of the immediate response to interpretation and the outcome of the three treatments.

Similarly, Silberschatz (1984) examined the immediate impact of transference interpretations in three cases. The accuracy of transference interpretations were rated by using the Plan Diagnosis Method (Rosenberg et al. 1986) to independently describe patients' psychodynamic themes. For each patient, Silberschatz found high correlations between the accuracy of interpretations and scores on the Experiencing Scale (Klein et al. 1970) which was applied to the segment of patient speech following interpretations.

Despite the promising findings reported in these studies, many questions remain. No attention has been paid to the development of a psychometrically sound scale of the accuracy or adequacy of interpretation. Aside from the Silberschatz (1984) report which was based on only three cases, no study has employed an independent measure of the content of the transference on which clinical ratings could be based. Judges were allowed to define the transference as they saw fit. In contrast, the measure we have begun to develop is a guided clinical rating. The judge assesses the extent to which the therapist accurately addresses transference as defined by an independent criterion: The Core Conflictual Relationship Theme (CCRT) (see the chapter by Luborsky and Crits-Christoph for a full description of this method). Guided clinical ratings have frequently been found to have better predictive validity than unguided ratings (Holt 1978). It is this use of a guided clinical rating that we feel represents an important methodological advance.

3. Development of a Measure of Adequacy of Therapist's Response to the Transference (ATRT)

Our measure of adequacy of therapist's response to the transference is a set of guided clinical ratings. The rater uses the CCRT formulation for the particular session as a guide in judging the adequacy of the therapist's interpretations.

The validity of these ratings, of course, depends upon the extent to which the CCRT method is a measure of transference. Recent results (Luborsky et al. 1985; Luborsky et al. 1986) have supported this proposition. In fact, the CCRT method has produced data which is consistent with nine of Freud's observations about transference (Luborsky and Crits-Christoph , this volume).

The rating scale of adequacy of the therapist's response consists of three items that correspond to the three main components of the CCRT method. After reading a given session and becoming familiar with the independently derived CCRT formulation for that session, the judge then rates the accuracy of the therapist's responses to (1) the main wish component of the CCRT, (2) the main response from other component, and (3) the main response from self component.

4. Reliability

The accuracy of therapist's response scale has been applied thus far to a pilot sample of 12 sessions drawn from the treatments of patients in psychoanalysis and psychoanalytically oriented psychotherapy.

The per judge reliabilities for the ratings of therapist response to (1) the main wish, (2) main response from other, and (3) main response from self were: .66, .60, and .81, respectively. For the pooled judges ratings, the coefficients were .79, .75, and .90, respectively. For the sum of the three items, the per judge agreement was .72, and the pooled judge reliability, .84. Finally, the internal consistency reliability (combining judges scores for each item) was .92.

These data suggest that judges can agree reasonably well as to when the therapist's interpretations are accurate, i.e., match the content of the independently derived CCRT. In addition, the high internal consistency figure indicates that when therapists are accurate on one component of the CCRT, they tend to also be accurate with the other components. This may reflect differences in general skillfulness of therapists, or, alternatively, accuracy may vary from session to session, independently of therapist's skill.

5. Problems and Questions for Future Research

We are currently in the process of utilizing our ATRT scale of accuracy of interpretations to predict the treatment outcomes of 43 patients in psychoanalytic psychotherapy. Our experiences so far with the scale have raised a number of practical and theoretical concerns. First, we have recognized that although CCRT formulations usually are expressed in terms of the highest frequency of each of three components, lesser frequency themes may still be important for the therapist to address. We have, therefore, expanded our rating scales to include assessment of the accuracy of the therapist's response to lesser frequency themes as well.

A second issue involves the nature of the sample to which these ratings can be applied. In order to successfully predict the outcomes of psychotherapy, the sample used must contain an adequate range of therapist's general level of accuracy of interpretation. Fortunately, our sample of 43 patients drawn from the Penn Psychotherapy Project (Luborsky et al. 1980) appears to contain a sufficient range of skillfulness among the therapists. Similarly, the choice of which sessions in the treatments are sampled is important. Sessions chosen must be representative of how each therapist worked with each patient and should contain a certain minimum number of interventions by the therapist on which ratings can be based. This latter point raises the question of the appropriateness of ratings of this type for research on psychoanalysis per se, as opposed to psychodynamic psychotherapy. The relative fewer therapist responses present in a classical psychoanalytic treatment may make it more difficult to judge the therapist's general level of accuracy. On the other hand, our experience with the application of the rating scale to the 12 pilot sessions, half of which were sessions of psychoanalysis, indicated that judges can make reliable inferences as to a therapist's accuracy of responding, even when the number of therapist interventions is low.

An additional potential problem that may arise particularly in applying the scale to psychoanalysis concerns the level of inference about a patient's relationship pattern that is made by the CCRT judges versus the therapist. The CCRT judges rely only upon patient material present in the few sessions which they score. Therapists, however, can make inferences at deeper levels because they are familiar with the subtleties of patients' themes from material in previous sessions. Ultimately, these questions relate to the validity of the rating scale, and remain to be answered by the results of our studies in progress.

6. Research on Self-Understanding

Most research on self-understanding and insight has been in the context of determining its predictive power for the outcome of psychotherapy. Specifically, such studies are aimed at determining whether patients who come to treatment with high levels of self-understanding or patients who develop self-understanding in the course of treatment have better outcomes. In a review of studies of factors influencing the outcomes of psychotherapy (Luborsky et al. 1971), five of such studies were found for non-hospitalized non-psychotic patients.

The earliest study was by Raskin (1949). Patient statements were rated for insight and understanding. Change in insight was found to be highly correlated with outcome for a sample of 10 patients. In another study, Rosenbaum et al. (1956), found that pre-treatment level of insight as judged by the therapist was not related to outcome. In a brief abstract Zolik and Hollon (1960) report that insight significantly predicted outcome of treatment. More recently, Morgan et al. (1982), measured insight with a 10-item rating scale applied by clinical judges to two sessions from early in treatment and two sessions from late in treatment for 20 patients. Level of insight correlated moderately but non-significantly with outcome. Finally, O'Malley et al. (1983), had judges rate "self-examination and exploration of feeling" from early psychotherapy sessions. Significant prediction of a therapist outcome measure was obtained, but no significant findings were present for patient or clinical observer measures.

In addition to the above rating methods, a "self-observation" content analysis scale has been described by Cartwright (1966). The scale has two parts, one for therapist's statements and the other for patient's responses. The therapist's statements are classified into one of the eight categories according to their relation to the patient's job of observing himself. These range from "non-observation statements" to "interpretations." The patient's six categories of responses were: (1) non-self, (2) focusing, (3) self as object, (4) self as presently experienced and not fixed, with appropriate affect, (5) observing an immediate experience, (6) integration of self-observation. These scoring categories were applied to four cases; for each case the sessions selected were all of the first interview, every fifth interview thereafter, plus the last interview. The four patients were two female patients in treatment with two male therapists, one a psychoanalyst and the other a client-centered therapist, and two male patients in treatment with two male therapists, likewise, one an analyst and the other client-centered. The data indicated that although each therapist of the matched patients behaved quite differently, patients responded quite similarly in terms of the six self-observation categories. It was found that matched patients can reach high levels of self-observation response to either analytic or client-centered techniques (although client-centered theory did not specifically deal with self-observation as a variable necessary to the change process). It appears from these four cases, therefore, that the level of self-observation reached by the patient depends more on what he brings to treatment than on specific techniques followed by the therapist – this, of course, is restricted to the comparison of client-centered and analytic treatments, both of which have in common a high level of therapist's clarification responses.

Although some positive findings are evident in the above studies, the results have been inconsistent. Several investigators employed single item ratings of insight and often no reliability data was presented. One of the studies, O'Malley et al. (1983), used a measure of the extent to which the patient was attempting to self-explore rather than a measure of the amount of acquisition of self-understanding per se. Only two of the five predictive studies actually consisted of psychodynamic psychotherapy. The main point, however, is that all of these existing measures of self-understanding are unguided clinical ratings. As with the measure of accuracy of therapists' response, the measure that we have recently begun to develop is a guided clinical rating based upon the Core Conflictual Relationship Theme.

7. Development of a New Measure of Self-Understanding: Self-Understanding of CCRT

The 13 items for the Self-Understanding Scale were derived from the guidelines provided in Luborsky's (1984) manual for Supportive-Expressive Psychotherapy. The items (each rated on a five point scale from no understanding to very much) tap the patient's self-awareness of different facets of the core theme (wish, response from self, response from others), awareness of the CCRT in the patient's relationship with the therapist, with others outside of treatment, and in past relationships, the extent to which the patient understands the relationship of the CCRT to his or her main symptom, and a few other areas.

Two judges applied this scale to the pilot sample of transcripts of 12 whole sessions mentioned previously. The judges were instructed to read the transcript of each session, then read the independently derived CCRT evaluation for that patient in that particular session, then re-read the transcript with the CCRT in mind, and, finally, rate the 13 self-understanding items.

In order to examine whether the same amount of information about self-understanding could be derived from ratings of brief segments – thereby significantly reducing the research time involved – we had two other judges rate the items on 250 word segments, one drawn from each of the 12 sessions. We also wondered whether focusing on a smaller amount of clinical material might increase the reliability of the scale. These segments were selected from the part of the session immediately after and including the therapist's main interpretive statement for that session (2 independent judges had 92% agreement in selecting the main interpretation of each session). We reasoned that the material following the therapist's main interpretation might include the best clues as to the patient's level of self-awareness of the core theme.

Material from the Specimen Hour 5 can be used to illustrate more concretely the nature of the Self-Understanding Rating Scale. The session was first scored by the Core Conflictual Relationship Theme Method. Results indicated that a wish for reassurance, direction, and approval was present, although this wish was not the most dominant one. At one point in the session, the patient says, "I do seek reassurance whenever I talk, even here." Judges would use this statement to rate this session as high (e.g. 5 on the 1 to 5 rating scale) on self-understanding of this wish, and also high on self-understanding of the theme in relation to the therapist.

8. Reliability

Table 1 presents the reliability data for the obtained ratings on the 12 sessions. As can be seen, adequate interjudge and internal consistency reliabilities were obtained for the ratings of whole sessions. The pooled judge reliabilities indicate that 2 judges are a sufficient number, with their combined ratings to be used for the subsequent research applications of the scale. The level of internal consistency reliability and examination of the item-total correlations indicated that all 13 items were adding to the measurement of the overall dimension.

The reliabilities of the ratings of brief segments are slightly lower, but still adequate. The correlation between the ratings from sessions and those from brief segments, however, is only modest (r = .44). Without knowing which set of ratings has greater validity it is difficult to make a choice as to the better methodology (segments versus sessions). Our bias at this point is to stay with the whole sessions approach until we have some indication that we can get by with smaller units (both types of ratings can in fact be obtained).

Table 1 Reliability of Self-Understanding Scale

Whole Sessions			
	Interjudge		Internal Consistency
	Per Judge	Pooled (2 judges)	
	.66	.80	.97
Brief Segments			
	Interjudge		Internal Consistency
	Per Judge	Pooled (2 judges)	
	.61	.76	.88
Correlation of Sessions Ratings with Segments Ratings: r = .44			

9. Problems and Questions for Future Research

Despite achieving adequate levels of reliability with our new scale, several questions remain concerning the application of the measure. The three main problems are: (1) what constitutes good evidence for the existence of a certain degree of self-understanding? (2) how often should we measure self-understanding over the course of treatment? and (3) what form of outcome criteria should be used in assessing the predictive utility of the measure?

(1) What constitutes good evidence for the existence of a certain degree of self-understanding?

It is not clear from our method what type of patient statements are used by the judges to signify the presence of a certain level of self-understanding. To what extent do judges rely on explicit statements versus a more inferential judgment as to what a patient is or is not aware of at a given time? Knowledge of these "indicators" of self-understanding would be important in developing a manual for the use of the scale by others. Towards this end, we have begun to have our judges write down the evidence they use to make their clinical ratings. Once we compile a list of the types of evidence used by raters, we can conceivably construct a more objective "counting signs" method of scoring self-understanding, rather than having to rely on ratings. In our past research on the helping alliance (Morgan et al. 1982; Luborsky et al. 1983), we followed this approach of beginning with a rating method and subsequently developing a "counting signs" method.

(2) How often should we measure change in self-understanding over the course of treatment?

Clinical theory holds that understanding increases as treatment unfolds. For research purposes, this implies that it is necessary to assess self-understanding at multiple points during treatment rather than in one simple measurement. Figure 1 illustrates this point vividly.We applied our scale to three sessions each of two patients in psychoanalysis (Ms. A. and Mr. D.). Early in treatment (about session 15) both patients had about equal levels of self-understanding of their CCRT's. Later in treatment, however, one case (Mr. D.) had a substantial gain in self-understanding while the other did not (Ms. A.).

Incidentally, the analyst for the Mr. D. case rated the treatment as moderately successful, but the Ms. A. case had been rated by her analyst as only very slightly successful. Whether discrimination of successful versus unsuccessful cases can be achieved in a larger sample with our measure of self-understanding remains to be seen.

The question of which sessions to select for assessment of self-understanding is clearly important. In short-term dynamic therapy, gains in self-understanding might be evident in the first few sessions. In the analytic cases shown here, little progress had ben made by session 15. Ideally, we would have a baseline level of self-understanding of core themes that is determined before treatment starts. We could then measure change in self-understanding to any point in the treatment process. Measuring pre-treatment level, however, means building into our research design a preliminary interview or test that would yield such information.

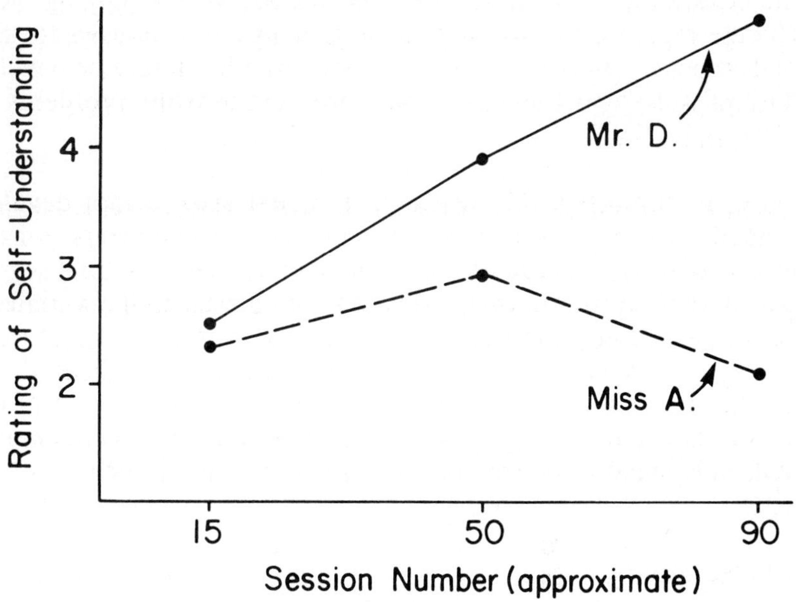

Figure 1 Change in Self-Understanding Over Time in Two Patients in Psychoanalysis

A final related question here is whether self-understanding increases in gradual increments or whether there are "key" events in treatment (Rice and Greenberg 1984) where there are large advances in self-understanding. If there is a consistent, gradual change, the selection of which specific sessions to rate is not crucial. On the other hand, if episodic change is the rule, many sessions might first have to be screened to identify where key events are occurring.

(3) What form of outcome criteria should be used in assessing the predictive utility of the measure?

Theoretically, gains in self-understanding of core conflicts should be associated with general symptom reduction. It is more likely, however, that a greater association would exist with improvement on the specific relationship conflict than on a global outcome scale. The question, then, is what would be the measure of change in specific relationship problems? It is tempting to use the CCRT method itself as this measure of change in specific relationship conflicts. The possibility of contamination between the predictor (self-understanding of CCRT) and the criterion (change in CCRT) would exist here. Applying the CCRT change measure to different sessions than the ones used for the self-understanding measure is one solution. Another might be developing a patient self-report measure of core relationship problems (Crits-Christoph 1986).

In summary, this research is a first step toward developing a guided measure of self-understanding. The scale appears to have adequate reliability and can be applied to whole sessions or brief segments of psychotherapy transcripts. Questions remain as to the validity of the scale, particularly in terms of its relationship to outcome of treatment. The few cases that we have to date, however, seem to indicate that we are on the right path in this regard. If successful, this program of research will begin to fill the gap between the widespread clinical emphasis on self-understanding and the paucity of research in this area.

10. Summary

Two new measures derived from the CCRT are described here: (1) A measure of the adequacy of the therapist responses to transference, and (2) a measure of the patient's self-understanding. These methods were tested on a pilot sample of transcripts of sessions and found to have adequate reliability and promising indications of usefulness in an area that has had great need for such measures. These measures will help to test the theory of the curative action of psychoanalytic psychotherapy, which holds that transference interpretations have a special power for augmenting self-understanding.

Testing Hypotheses of Psychotherapeutic Change Processes*

George Silberschatz, John T. Curtis, Polly B. Fretter, and Thomas J. Kelly

1. Introduction

How the therapist influences the process and outcome of psychotherapy is a widely debated topic in the psychotherapy research literature. Despite a large body of research (see Parloff, Waskow, and Wolfe 1978; Schaffer 1982 for reviews) surprisingly little progress has been made in understanding how the therapist contributes to the success or failure of psychotherapy. In this paper we will present the argument that the lack of progress is due to (1) inadequate conceptualization of how therapist interventions affect particular patients, and (2) imprecise, overly global methods of evaluating therapist behaviors. In particular, the relevance or suitability of the therapist's behavior to the particular problems and needs of a given patient has not been adequately assessed.

We will briefly review some of the literature on how the therapist influences psychotherapy and discuss some of the methodological problems in these studies. We will then describe a new conceptual approach developed by Weiss (1986), for understanding how therapist behaviors affect patients and show how this approach leads to more precise methods of assessing the therapist's contribution to psychotherapy. Research studies of psychoanalysis and of brief dynamic psychotherapy using this approach will be presented and a procedure for testing alternative psychoanalytic hypotheses about how the therapist's behavior affects the patient's progress will be described.

*Preparation of this chapter was supported by a grant from the National Institute of Mental Health (MH35230) and by the Research Support Program of Mount Zion Medical Center.

2. Background

Most theories of psychotherapy assume that the therapist plays a significant role in the change process and that specific therapist behaviors and techniques constitute effective ingredients of the treatment. Psychoanalytic theories place a strong emphasis on the therapist's facilitating patient insight through interpretation: "Insight through interpretation is the supreme agent in the hierarchy of therapeutic principles characteristic of analysis" (Bibring 1954, p. 747). The interpretation of transference is thought to be a particularly potent intervention by many psychoanalytic writers (e.g. Gill 1982; Greenson 1967; Loewald 1960, 1971; Macalpine 1950; Malan 1963, 1976a, 1976b; Stone 1967). Nonetheless, empirical evidence for the efficacy of specific therapist techniques (including interpretation) is lacking or inconsistent (Clairborn 1982; Gomes-Schwartz 1978; Luborsky et al. 1980; Parloff et al. 1978). For example, Garduk and Haggard (1972) showed that in psychoanalytic therapy interpretations increase patient productivity more than non-interpretations. However, in another study (Sloane, Staples, Cristol, Yorkston, and Whipple 1975), the opposite was found to be true: patients who received more interpretations showed *less* improvement at outcome than did patients who received fewer interpretations.

The failure to demonstrate the differential effectiveness of one therapy technique over another has led some investigators to focus on so-called "non-specific factors" that are thought to operate in all helping relationships (e.g. Frank 1982; Strupp 1978b). These non-specific variables include therapist behaviors that facilitate an accepting, therapeutic atmosphere (e.g. therapist warmth, friendliness, empathy, encouragement). While early studies of these variables seemed promising (Rogers 1957; Truax 1963; Truax and Mitchell 1971), more recent studies have failed to demonstrate a consistent relationship between these non-specific factors and treatment outcome (e.g. Gomes-Schwartz 1978; Luborsky et al. 1980; Mitchell, Bozarth, and Krauft 1977; Orlinsky and Howard 1978; Parloff et al. 1978).

Some reviewers have suggested that the difficulty measuring the therapist's influence is due to the inadequate methodology employed in most studies of the psychotherapeutic process (Elliott 1983, 1984; Fiske 1977; Gottman and Markman 1978; Greenberg 1986; Parloff et al. 1978; Schaffer 1982). According to these reviewers, most psychotherapy research is based on the erroneous assumption that there is little variability between or within patients, therapists, and treatments. Kiesler

(1966) referred to this assumption as the homogeneity myth and showed how this false assumption has weakened most studies of psychotherapy (see also Gottman and Markman 1978). Just as patients and therapists differ substantially, so too does the meaning of various process events. A prevailing assumption in much of the previous literature is that:

> . . . given client or therapist behavior is either 'good' or 'bad' without regard to the context in which it appears. This fits poorly with the observation of experienced therapists that a given kind of therapist response or client performance seems to be crucial at one point and irrelevant or even detrimental at another. (Rice and Greenberg 1984, p. 10).

A strategy which avoids the uniformity assumption involves identifying clinically significant critical incidents or key events within therapy sessions. This method, initially applied to psychotherapy research by Luborsky (1967, 1970; Luborsky and Auerbach 1969; Luborsky, Singer, Hartke, Crits-Christoph, and Cohen 1984) in his "symptom-context" studies, has been successfully applied in a number of psychotherapy process studies (e.g. Elliott 1983, 1984; Fretter 1984; Gassner, Sampson, Weiss, and Brumer 1982; Greenberg 1982, 1986; Horowitz, Sampson, Siegelman, Wolfson, and Weiss 1975; Mahrer 1985; Rice and Greenberg 1984; Silberschatz 1978, 1986; Silberschatz, Fretter, and Curtis 1986a). With this type of approach – recently designated the "events paradigm" in process research (Stiles, Shapiro, and Elliott 1986) – the investigator identifies significant episodes within the therapy session (e.g. the patient's describing a particular problem or conflict) and evaluates the extent to which the therapist's intervention facilitates problem resolution. The events model of research is:

> . . . geared to the goal of understanding. Rather than assuming a given kind of process to have equal significance at any point in therapy, this new approach relies on the segmentation of therapy into different episodes or events in order to understand process in the context of these clinically meaningful units. This approach of breaking therapy down into classes of recurring events prevents one from being swamped by the data through a selective focus on those episodes in the therapeutic interaction that hold promise of illuminating the change process. (Rice and Greenberg 1984, p. 11)

The events approach asks, "Which specific therapist interventions, introduced in which momentary therapeutic contexts, will lead to which immediate and subsequent impacts (outcomes) for the client?" (Stiles et al. 1986, p. 174).

The focus on key change episodes in therapy is a clear advance over previous homogenized approaches to psychotherapy research. However, the events approach does not address another methodological problem evident in most studies of how therapist's behaviors influence psychotherapy – namely, the quality or suitability of the therapist's behavior. The events paradigm may lead an investigator to focus on critical incidents in therapy – for instance, significant transference re-enactments – but it does not provide a framework for determining whether the therapist's interventions in response to these key episodes are well suited to the patient's particular needs. For instance, if a patient fails to respond to a therapist's interpretation it could be because interpretation as a technique is ineffective or because the particular interpretation (or line of interpretation) is not pertinent to that patient. Thus, what is needed is a procedure for evaluating the "goodness-of-fit" between the therapist's behavior and the patient's particular problems and treatment goals.

3. A Framework for Determining the Suitability of Therapist Behaviors

How does one develop a measure of suitability? Some investigators have proposed that variables such as therapist "skillfulness" (Schaffer 1982) or "generic helpfulness" (Elliott 1984) can be rated using broadly defined, "generic" rating scales. However, such a broad approach does not recognize that interventions that are helpful to one patient may not be helpful to another. The helpfulness of an intervention can not be meaningfully determined without first knowing the specific needs of a particular patient. Thus, assessing the quality or suitability of therapist behaviors requires:

(1) identifying what the patient's problem(s), need(s), and therapy goal(s) are; and

(2) determining whether any given intervention appropriately addresses the patient's problem(s) or facilitates the attainment of the goal(s).

The concept of suitability used by the Mount Zion Psychotherapy Research Group (Weiss, Sampson, and the Mount Zion Psychotherapy Research Group, 1986; see also, Curtis and Silberschatz 1986; Silberschatz and Curtis 1986; Silberschatz et al. 1986b) is based on a theory developed by Weiss (1986). Weiss has proposed that psychopathology stems from unconscious pathogenic ideas or false beliefs that are typically based on traumatic childhood experience. According to Weiss, patients enter psychotherapy with an unconscious plan for solving problems and disconfirming pathogenic beliefs. The patient's plan may be thought of as an unconscious strategy for disconfirming certain pathogenic beliefs by developing greater understanding of them in the therapy and by testing them in the relationship with the therapist.

In testing a pathogenic belief, the patient carries out a trial action which is intended to provide information about the belief. For example, a patient whose parents were bothered by his autonomous strivings might develop the belief that his autonomy is harmful or upsetting to others and thus might stifle certain desires and needs. This patient might test the belief that his autonomous behaviors are harmful by behaving independently in the therapy (e.g. by coming up with his own insights, being late to sessions, ignoring the therapist's comments) to see if the therapist can comfortably tolerate these behaviors. If the therapist does not become defensive or act critically toward the patient, he passes the test; that is, the therapist's behavior disconfirms the patient's false idea that his autonomy would hurt the therapist. On the other hand, the therapist might fail the test by acting in a way that the patient would experience as being hurt by or critical of his independence. Such a response would tend to confirm the patient's pathological expectation that it is dangerous to act autonomously and to disagree. This example of testing illustrates one prominent way in which patients may work to disconfirm pathogenic beliefs. Tests may vary according to their relevance to central pathogenic beliefs; *key tests* are those tests that are most critical to the patient because they are central to the pathogenic beliefs which the patient is working to disconfirm (Silberschatz and Curtis 1986).

According to Weiss's theory, the therapist's attitudes, overall style of response, and particular interventions can help the patient relinquish pathogenic beliefs. Therapeutic styles or interventions that are consistent with the patient's unconscious plan are considered to be "plan compatible," while interventions that are counter to the patient's plan are "plan incompatible." A therapist can help a patient disconfirm a pathogenic belief by passing the patient's test or by intervening in a plan-compatible fashion; therapeutic progress tends to follow such plan-compatible interventions. Interventions which are incompatible with the patient's plan or fail a patient's test tend to be followed by therapeutic retreat. Studies by the Mount Zion Psychotherapy Research Group have shown that patients' plans can be reliably inferred (Bush and Gassner 1986; Caston 1986; Curtis, Silberschatz, Sampson, Weiss, and Rosenberg, 1988; Rosenberg, Silberschatz, Curtis, Sampson, and Weiss 1986), and that formulations of patients' plans can be used to assess the suitability of therapist behaviors (Fretter 1984; Silberschatz 1986; Silberschatz et al. 1986a).

The work of the Mount Zion Psychotherapy Research Group (Weiss and Sampson 1986) thus provides a framework for assessing how the therapist's behavior influences the patient's therapeutic progress. It suggests two different types of significant events in therapy – patient initiated events (key tests) and therapist initiated episodes (interpretations) – when therapist interventions are likely to be instrumental in effecting change. Weiss's theory provides a conceptual framework for assessing the goodness-of-fit between therapist behaviors (passing/failing tests, plan-compatible/plan-incompatible interventions) and the patient's particular problems and goals. We will now report several studies that illustrate how these concepts have been applied to studies of psychoanalysis and brief dynamic psychotherapy.

4. An Empirical Study of Significant Events in Psychoanalysis

The Patient's Tests of the Analyst

As noted, Weiss (1986) has identified the testing of the therapist by the patient as one type of critical incident or significant event in psychoanalytic therapy. The therapist's response to the patient's tests is thought to play a decisive role in the process and outcome of therapy: if the therapist's response to the patient's test is perceived by the patient as disconfirming a pathogenic belief (passing the test), the patient will feel relieved, reassured, and is likely to feel less anxious and more productive in the therapy. If the therapist's response confirms the pathogenic beliefs (fails the tests), the patient is likely to feel distressed and may show signs of therapeutic retreat.

A study (Silberschatz 1978, 1986) designed to test this hypothesis was carried out on the verbatim transcripts of the first 100 hours of a tape-recorded psychoanalysis. The patient, Mrs. C, a 28-year-old professional woman with an obsessive-compulsive personality structure, sought treatment because of her inability to enjoy sexual relations with her husband. The analysis, carried out by an experienced (Freudian) psychoanalyst, was completed long before this study was planned. The method for the study involved three steps: (1) identification of the patient's key tests (significant events); (2) ratings of the degree to which the analyst's response to these tests would be perceived by the patient as disconfirming the belief which the patient was testing (passing/failing the test); and (3) assessment of the patient's behavior and affects immediately before and after the test in order to determine whether the patient changed in the predicted direction.

The first step entailed selecting a pool of all possible tests. Nine judges read verbatim transcripts of the first 100 hours of Mrs. C's psychoanalysis and selected all instances in which the patient attempted to elicit a response from the therapist. It was assumed that many tests would have this form and that such instructions would help judges select a large pool of potentially relevant test episodes. In all, 87 such instances were identified. Typescripts of the patient's attempts to elicit a response as well as the therapist's interventions (which included silences) were then prepared. Three psychoanalytically trained judges (who were familiar with the concept of testing) read a formulation of Mrs. C's plan (which had been reliably developed as part of a separate study; see Caston 1986) and identified which of the pool of incidents represented the patient's key tests of the analyst. A sample of 46 episodes was selected by all three judges as instances of key tests.

The second step used four experienced psychoanalysts who were familiar with the clinical application of the testing concept. These judges read the plan formulation and then independently rated (on a 7-point scale) the extent to which the analyst had passed or failed each key test.

The immediate effects on the patient of the therapist's passing or failing a test were assessed using several patient measures: ratings of the patient's level of experiencing (i.e., degree of involvement and productivity; see Klein, Mathieu, Gendlin, and Kiesler 1970), boldness, relaxation, and an affect classification system which measured the patient's level of fear, anxiety, love, and satisfaction (Dahl 1978, 1979b; Dahl and Stengel 1978). A segment of speech preceding the test sequence (pre-segment) and a segment of speech following the test sequence (post-segment) were rated on each of the measures by different groups of judges. The segments (approximately six minutes of patient speech) were presented in random order without any context and with the judges unaware whether the segment was a "pre-test" segment or a "post-test" segment. Reliabilities for all of the above ratings were adequate, ranging from .65 to .94.

Correlations between the ratings of the therapist's intervention (the degree to which he passed or failed a key test) and changes (residualized gain scores – Cohen and Cohen 1975) in each of the patient measures indicated that the patient became significantly more involved, more productive, and more relaxed when the therapist passed a key test (Table 1). These results support the hypothesis that the patient was reassured by the therapist's passing tests and that the patient's satisfaction was demonstrated by her becoming less anxious, more involved, and more productive in the analytic work.

Table 1 Correlation between the Degree to which the Analyst Passed the Patient's Tests and Changes in the Patient Measures for the Key Tests

Measure [a]	r
Experiencing	.33*
Boldness	.32*
Relaxation	.35*
Love	.37*
Fear	-.34*
Satisfaction	.15*
Anxiety	-.29*

[a] $N = 46$.

* $p < .05$, two-tailed test

(Data for this table are taken from Silberschatz, G. et al. (1986b). Testing pathogenic beliefs. In J. Weiss, H. Sampson, and the Mount Zion Psychotherapy Research Group, *The Psychoanalytic Process: Theory, Clinical Observation, and Empirical Research.* Guilford: New York.)

The results of this study on patient tests also have implications for identifying key events. Correlations between therapist behaviors and the patient's immediate responses were not significant for the larger sample of 87 instances (i.e., those episodes broadly defined as the patient's attempts to elicit a response). However, correlations were significant for the subsample of episodes which were *directly pertinent* to the patient's plan – i.e., the sample of 46 *key* tests. This pattern of findings suggests that significant events in psychotherapy must be identified in a case-specific fashion and cannot be adequately identified using broad criteria (e.g. patient demands). A clinical formulation of the patient's particular problems, needs, and treatment goals is needed to identify events that are most significant for a given patient.

5. An Empirical Study of Alternative Hypotheses of the Psychoanalytic Process

Selection of key events in psychotherapy sessions is inevitably based on theories of psychotherapeutic change. Just as the practicing clinician bases his interventions on a conceptual framework, psychotherapy researchers have argued that empirical studies of psychotherapy must be guided by theory (e.g. Bergin and Lambert 1978; Gendlin 1986; Strupp 1986; Yeaton and Sechrest 1981). In a review paper on dimensions of successful treatments, Yeaton and Sechrest (1981) pointed to the importance of powerful theories in practice and in research studies: "What we need is good theory, in the sense of an understanding of the mechanisms relating the causes and the problems as well as the presumed manner by which the treatment alleviates the problem" (p. 157). A well articulated theory both delineates significant events and specifies the kinds of therapist interventions during those key events that are likely to be helpful. This degree of specificity is necessary to test a theory.

Within psychoanalysis, Weiss (1986) has identified two distinct models that meet the above criteria for testability. Because the two models differ in their predictions about how a patient responds in a particular situation, it is possible to test empirically which theory better fits observation. We will briefly describe an empirical study which tested these competing hypotheses in a psychoanalytic case (Silberschatz 1978; Silberschatz, Sampson, and Weiss 1986b).

The study focused on an event frequently observed in psychoanalytic treatment: the patient's transference demands – those instances in which the patient, either overtly or covertly, makes a demand on the analyst to respond to him in some particular way. The patient may, for example, demand affection, special attention, advice, criticism, punishment, rejection, or humiliation. A central aspect of the psychoanalytic theory of therapy is that the analyst should maintain an analytic or neutral stance and should not accede to the patient's demands. There are, however, two fundamentally different theories regarding the nature of the patient's transference demands. These theories contain different explanations for the therapeutic value of the analyst's not acceding to the patient's demand and make different (opposite) predictions about how the patient is likely to behave if the analyst does or does not accede to the demands.

The first explanation is based on what Weiss (1986) has termed an Automatic Functioning (AF) model. According to this model, the patient makes a transference demand in order to gratify an unconscious wish. When the analyst does not accede to the patient's demand, the patient's unconscious wish (transference longing) is frustrated. As a result, the wish is intensified and is pushed into consciousness. The other explanation is referred to by Weiss (1986) as a Higher Mental Functioning (HMF) model. According to this model, when a patient makes a demand of the analyst he does so primarily to test a pathogenic belief. For example, the patient may demand advice from the therapist to test the distressing pathogenic belief that the therapist, like a parent in childhood, wishes to run his life. If the therapist does not accede to this demand, the patient will feel reassured, more relaxed, and more productive in the therapy.

Both the AF and HMF models agree that the analyst should maintain a neutral stance in response to the patient's demands. However, they differ sharply in explaining how the analyst's neutrality is helpful to the patient. In fact, these two models make opposite predictions about the patient's affective response. According to the AF model, a patient would be likely to feel unhappy, distressed, upset (frustrated) by the analyst's neutrality. This hypothesis was explicitly stated as one of the formal predictions made in the Menninger Foundation Psychotherapy Research Project:

> . . . patients whose neurotic needs are not gratified within the transference respond to this frustration with regressive and/or resistive reactions, and/or painful affects . . . (Sargent, Horowitz, Wallerstein, and Appelbaum 1968, p. 85)

By contrast the HMF model predicts that the patient is generally reassured by the analyst's not acceding to the demand (because doing so disconfirms a pathogenic belief), and that the patient's satisfaction is often demonstrated by his becoming more relaxed and productive in the session.

Because the two models differ in their predictions about the patient's response to the analyst's neutral stance, it was possible to test empirically which model better fits observation. Is the patient frustrated and distressed as the AF model predicts, or is the patient generally satisfied and relaxed as the HMF model predicts?

In order to compare the AF and HMF hypotheses, it was necessary to identify instances of the patient making transference demands which fit the criteria of *both* models – that is, instances which psychoanalysts who utilize AF concepts would identify as the patient seeking to gratify a key unconscious wish, and which psychoanalysts applying HMF concepts would identify as the patient posing a key test of the analyst. The analyst's responses to the patient's transference demands were rated by AF psychoanalyst judges for the degree to which they were neutral, in the sense of frustrating the patient's wish, and by HMF psychoanalyst judges for the degree to which they "passed or failed" the patient's tests. A passed test is one in which the analyst's response is likely to disconfirm the pathogenic belief which the patient is testing; a failed test is one in which the analyst's response is likely to confirm the pathogenic belief. Finally, the patient's behavior immediately before and after each response was compared (using several patient measures) in order to test the predictions of each model.

The verbatim transcripts of the first 100 hours of a tape-recorded psychoanalysis were the primary data for this study (the same data utilized in the testing study described above). Nine clinical raters read through these transcripts and identified all instances of the patient's transference demands. Eighty-seven transference demands were identified (these included attempts by the patient to elicit approval, affection, guidance, punishment, etc.). Typescripts of each of the segments were prepared; they included the patient's transference demand (or control segment) and the analyst's response (which in some instances was silence).

Five psychoanalyst judges accustomed to applying the AF model in their clinical work and four judges accustomed to applying the HMF model independently rated the analyst's interventions. The AF judges rated each analyst's intervention (on a 7-point scale) for its degree of neutrality from the AF perspective – that is, the degree to which the analyst frustrated the patient's wish. Similarly, the HMF judges rated the extent to which the analyst passed or failed the patient's test. Interrater reliabilities were satisfactory for both ratings.

The next step in this study entailed identifying those transference demands which were pertinent to *both* the AF and HMF models. Three AF judges identified those instances in which the patient was attempting to gratify a key unconscious wish, and three HMF judges identified all instances of key tests. Each judge made his selection on the basis of a case formulation written from his perspective (i.e., AF or HMF). A total of 34 transference demands were identified by both groups of judges as significant events or key transference episodes to which their theories applied. Data analyses were based only on the 34 overlapping instances that were identified as both key wishes and key tests.

To test the predictions of the AF and HMF models, the patient's behavior before and after each of the 34 key incidents was rated on several process scales. Segments of patient speech (averaging about six minutes in length) immediately before (pre-segment) and immediately after (post-segment) the transference demand were rated independently by different teams of judges on the Experiencing Scale, the Boldness Scale (the patient's capacity to boldly confront new material), the Relaxation Scale (a measure of associative freedom and relaxation), and an affect classification system (Dahl 1978, 1979b; Dahl and Stengel 1978) which measured the patient's level of fear, anxiety, love, and satisfaction. All of these ratings were made with satisfactory levels of interjudge reliability.

The results of this study are summarized in Table 2. Predictions derived from the HMF model were supported while predictions of the AF model were not. All seven correlations in Table 2 are in the direction predicted by the HMF model and are opposite to the direction predicted by the AF model. Four of the seven correlations are statistically significant. These findings indicate that when the analyst did not accede to the patient's key transference demands the patient did not feel frustrated or upset; rather, the patient became more relaxed and spontaneous, more bold in tackling issues, and more positive in her attitude toward others. These results support the view that when the patient expressed a transference demand, she was testing a pathogenic belief. By not acceding to these demands, the analyst's behavior provided reassurance against the danger associated with the patient's pathogenic belief.

6. Studies of Brief Psychodynamic Psychotherapy

In both of the studies described above, the significant events studied were patient initiated episodes (the patient's transference demands or key

Table 2 Correlation between Ratings of the Therapist's Behavior and Changes in the Patient Measures for Segments Identified as both Key Frustrations

Measure [a]	r	Predicted by AF	Predicted by HMF
Experiencing	+.23	-	+
Boldness	+.41*	-	+
Relaxation	+.35*	-	+
Love	+.36*	-	+
Satisfaction	+.15	-	+
Fear	-.31	+	-
Anxiety	-.34*	+	-

Note.

AF = Automatic Functioning Paradigm.

HMF = Higher Mental Functioning Paradigm.

+ or – = sign of the correlation predicted by the theory.

[a] N = 34.

* $p < .05$, two-tailed test

(Data for this table are taken from Silberschatz, G.et al. (1986b). Testing pathogenic beliefs vs. seeking transference gratifications. In J. Weiss, H. Sampson, and the Mount Zion Psychotherapy Research Group, *The Psychoanalytic Process: Theory, Clinical Observation, and Empirical Research.* Guilford: New York.)

tests). A recent study carried out by Fretter (1984; Silberschatz et al. 1986a) focused on therapist initiated events – namely, therapist interpretations. The study was designed to show that suitability of interpretations would be a better predictor of immediate (in-session) patient progress than type of interventions. The suitability of the therapist's intervention was defined as the compatibility of the intervention with the patient's plan – plan compatibility. The type or category of intervention studied was the transference interpretation.

The verbatim transcripts of the brief (16 weekly sessions) psychodynamically-oriented psychotherapies of three cases were the primary data for this study. The research design involved 6 steps:

(1) locating all therapist interpretations;
(2) identifying all transference and non-transference interpretations;
(3) rating the plan compatibility of interpretations;
(4) measuring the patient's behavior (in-session productivity) immediately before and after interpretations;
(5) assessing changes in patient behavior (from pre- to post-interpretation); and
(6) comparing the extent to which the category of the interpretation (transference vs. non-transference) and the plan compatibility of the interpretation predicted these change scores.

The data were analyzed separately for each case in a repeated single-case design.

Malan's intervention typology (Malan 1963, 1976b; Marziali 1984; Marziali and Sullivan 1980) was used to categorize all therapist interpretations as either transference or non-transference interpretations. To assess the plan compatibility of the interpretation, previously developed plan formulations of each case were employed (Curtis et al., in press; Rosenberg et al. 1986). A group of clinical judges (experienced psychologists and psychiatrists who were familiar with the plan concept) read the plan formulation and then rated each interpretation for the degree to which it was compatible with the patient's plan (Plan Compatibility of Intervention Scale – PCIS). Excellent inter-judge reliabilities were obtained.

Immediate patient progress was evaluated by applying the Experiencing Scale (Klein et al. 1970) to pre- and post-interpretation segments of patient speech. Six judges independently rated segments of patient speech that immediately preceded (pre-segment) and immediately followed (post-segment) each selected interpretation. These segments – approximately 3 to 5 minutes of patient speech – were isolated from the transcripts and presented to the judges in random order. Rater bias was controlled by keeping judges blind to the status of the segment (pre- or post-segment) and to therapy outcome.

The results of this study showed that transference interpretations did not further patient progress more than non-transference interpretations. That is, none of the patients showed significantly greater levels of experiencing following transference interpretations than following non-transference interpretations. By contrast, Plan Compatibility scores were significantly correlated with the EXP (residualized gain) scores for each case. Interpretations judged to be plan-compatible tended to be followed by an increase in the patient's level of experiencing, whereas interpretations judged to be incompatible with the patient's plan tended to be followed by a decrease in the patient's level of experiencing.

These results are consistent with the findings obtained in studies of psychoanalysis. These findings, together with results obtained in the patient testing studies described above, suggest that simple assessment of events in psychotherapy – be they patient initiated or therapist initiated – is unlikely to yield consistent results unless the meaning of such events for a particular patient is taken into account. For instance, a patient who grew up with an overly involved and intrusive parent could be hindered by frequent transference interpretations if they were experienced by the patient as intrusive and thus closely parallel to the way in which the patient had been traumatized as a child. For this kind of patient, a heavy focus on transference would clearly be unsuitable and could possibly be detrimental. A case-specific method for assessing the suitability of the therapist's behavior is needed to assess the effectiveness of any particular interpretation.

7. Methodological and Theoretical Implications

The studies reported here – as well as others carried out by the Mount Zion Psychotherapy Research Group (see Weiss and Sampson 1986) – support the value and feasibility of studying significant events in psychotherapy and of testing theories about the meaning of these events. The identification of significant events provides a useful strategy for studying psychotherapy and has the potential to bridge the wide gap between the practice of psychotherapy and research on psychotherapy (Stiles et al. 1986). However, the results described above suggest that key events need to be identified in a case-specific fashion so that the meaning of the event can be assessed. Strupp (1986) noted that analyses of psychotherapy process must be "relatively specific for the individual patient-therapist dyad" (p. 126). He concluded that for psychotherapy research to advance, research methods must be geared to the specific dynamics of particular patient-therapist interactions. Although others in the field have drawn similar conclusions, empirical studies using such case-specific methods are extremely rare. The studies reported here illustrate how such methods can be applied to study psychoanalysis and brief psychotherapies.

The studies summarized in this paper illustrate the importance of testing theories of psychotherapeutic change. As noted, most theories of psychotherapy are too abstractly stated and hence can not be easily tested. The theory proposed by Weiss (1986) stipulates how the patient's problem develop (pathogenic beliefs based on childhood trauma), how the patient works in therapy to master problems (efforts to disconfirm pathogenic beliefs), and how the therapist helps or hinders the patient's therapeutic progress (passing or failing tests and plan compatibility of interventions). The theory is based on what Weiss has termed the Higher Mental Functioning Paradigm and is consistent with recent developments in cognitive psychology and cognitive science (e.g. Abelson 1981; Gardner 1985; Mandler 1984; Neisser 1976; Schank and Abelson 1977; Simon and Newell 1970). The studies described here and elsewhere (Weiss and Sampson 1986) provide empirical support for the theory and show how the predictions based on this theory can be tested against other theories.

The accuracy and usefulness of a theory may be argued from many different vantage points. Freud noted that:

> As a rule, however, theoretical controversy is unfruitful. No sooner has one begun to depart from the material upon which one ought to be relying, than one runs the risk of becoming intoxicated with one's own assertions and, in the end, of representing opinions which any observation would have contradicted. For this reason it seems to me to be *incomparably more useful to combat dissentient interpretations by testing them upon particular cases or problems.* (Freud 1918b, p. 48; emphasis added)

Despite Freud's recognition of the importance of systematically studying case material, it is only recently that psychoanalysis has begun to go beyond the informal case study method. As Wallerstein and Sampson (1971) noted, it has generally been quite difficult for psychoanalysis to combine rigorous scientific methods with the complexity of its explanatory concepts, perhaps because objective research tends to sacrifice clinical relevance for rigor. This paper illustrates that controlled research methods can be added to the more traditional methods of clinical observation without sacrificing clinical relevance.

Developing an Instrument for Characterizing Psychotherapy Techniques in Studies of the Psychotherapy of Borderline Patients*

Harold W. Koenigsberg, Otto F. Kernberg, Lawrence Rockland, Ann Appelbaum, Arthur Carr, and Paulina Kernberg

1. Introduction

A recent methodological advance in psychotherapy research has been the introduction of manuals to operationally define the treatment under study. Such manuals describe the prototypic form of the treatment, but can not insure that treatment actually delivered corresponds to this ideal form. Even with clearly defined treatments, deviations from the described treatment are apt to occur for several reasons. Passage of time after the initial training period may allow a drift in technique – a problem that becomes even more serious in studies of long term psychotherapy. In addition, as Mintz, Luborsky and Auerbach (1971) have shown, the actual employment of therapeutic techniques is determined by patient as well as therapist factors. Thus, a treatment defined in the abstract may take a substantially different form in the actual patient encounter. While this may be clinically advantageous in some situations or harmful in others, it complicates efforts to study a defined therapeutic approach.

An instrument to measure the therapeutic techniques actually employed is necessary to insure that the treatment under study is actually the treatment specified. In addition to its usefulness for monitoring the application of the intended techniques, an instrument for measuring techniques would also provide useful empirical data about the relative timing and mixture of techniques in actual treatment situations. In this chapter we will describe the development of such an instrument, the

*An earlier version of this manuscript was presented at the annual meeting of Society for Psychotherapy Research, Lake Louis, Canada, June 1984 and appeared in the *Journal of Nervous and Mental Diseases*. The authors thank Allison Orr-Andrawes, M.D., Charles Gardner, M.D., John Urbach, M.D., Gretchen Haas, Ph.D., John Clarkin, Ph. D., Frank Yeomans, M.D., and Andrew Lotterman, M.D. for their contributions to this work. Howard Hunt, Ph.D. provided valuable statistical consultation.

Therapist Verbal Intervention Inventory (TVII), for use in a study of the psychodynamic treatment of patients with Borderline Personality Disorder (BPD), report on its reliability, and present preliminary data on its ability to distinguish "supportive" and "expressive" psychotherapy.

Several instruments for measuring technique have been described in the psychotherapy research literature. Some are tailored to specific forms of treatment, particular patient populations, or problem areas. Strupp (1957) has described a multidimensional system for analyzing psychotherapeutic techniques. Interventions are classified along five dimensions: (1) Type of Therapeutic Activity, (2) Depth-directedness, (3) Dynamic Focus, (4) Initiative, and (5) Warmth-Coldness. Included within the first dimension are seven categories of technique: Exploratory Operations, Clarification, Interpretive Operations, Structuring, Direct Guidance, Minimal Activities, and a miscellaneous category. Strupp and colleagues (1966) introduced a number of therapist variables into a therapy rating instrument developed by Bellak and Smith (1956). Among the therapist variables are five specific technique measures: frequency of interventions, frequency of interpretations, depth of interpretation, initiative, and support. The choice of these particular variables was "intuitively derived" (p. 369). Harway et al. (1955) developed a seven point scale to measure depth of interpretations. The measurement of five specific confrontative interventions is described by Mitchell and Berenson (1970). Rounsaville, Chevron and Weissman (1984) developed scales to measure the extent to which a particular form of psychotherapy, Interpersonal Therapy (IPT), was employed in the treatment of depressed patients. Hoyt and co-workers (1981) designed a Therapist Action Scale (TAS) which measures twenty-five operationally defined therapist actions employed in the brief psychotherapy of patients with stress response syndromes.

While many of these instruments tap sets of essential psychotherapeutic techniques, some achieve poor interrater reliabilities and others are tailored to specific therapy models. In developing a scale for our study of dynamic psychotherapy of BPD patients, it was necessary to address a number of design issues.

2. General Considerations

Selection of the specific techniques to be included in the instrument should be governed by research objectives. Early technique scales selected techniques rather arbitrarily on the basis of the intuitive judgment of the investigators. Since a limited number of techniques may be included in any instrument, decisions must be made about which to include and which to exclude. Interventions considered essential in one model of therapy, however, may be seen merely as adventitious remarks from the the perspective of a different model. While an atheoretical approach to data collection might appear desirable, any systematic selection of categories for observation implies an underlying theoretical framework. The choice of techniques must take into account the treatment model under study and the theoretical framework underlying that treatment. All techniques necessary to define the particular therapeutic approach must be included. Since treatments may also be described in terms of interventions that are disallowed, the monitoring instrument must be designed to identify instances of such techniques as well.

A second issue in the development of a technique instrument is the choice of the conceptual level at which the interventions will be described. Two factors must be balanced – the need for a reliable rating system vs. the need for clinically meaningful constructs. Description in terms of operationally defined concrete therapist behaviors should enhance interrater reliabilities, but if carried too far, runs the risk of divorcing observation from clinical concepts.

An approach must be selected for quantification. Several strategies are available; techniques may be rated as simply present or absent, instances of use may be counted, or the use of an intervention may be measured in terms of its clinical valence within context of the session. Harway et al. (1955) have shown, for example, that "depth of interpretation" is rated differently if judged on the basis of individual therapist remarks summed over an entire session than if assessed by an overall rating the same interview. A session may be powerfully influenced by a succinct phrase uttered once.

An additional consideration is the size of the session segment to which the instrument will be applied. Short sampling units may have the advantage of increasing interrater reliabilities and of enhancing the resolving power of the instrument for identifying fine structure within the treatment. The use of sampling units that are too small, however, may break interventions into clinically meaningless fragments. Strupp and co-workers (1966) attributed the low reliabilities that they obtained with their scale to the use of too large a time unit for sampling, a full session. In a comparison of 4 minute segments and entire sessions, Mintz and Luborsky (1971) have shown, on the other hand, that reliable ratings of certain variables, e.g. "optimal empathic relationship," could not be made on the basis of short segments.

3. Desired Features for the Therapist Verbal Intervention Inventory (TVII)

For the purposes of our study of the dynamic psychotherapy of patients with Borderline Personality Disorder, we require an instrument that addresses the full range of interventions used by psychodynamically oriented therapists in treating patients with severe character pathology. While various approaches have been proposed for the treatment of borderline patients (Kernberg 1975, 1982; Masterson 1976; Zetzel 1971) most draw from a set of basic exploratory and supportive interventions. A useful summary of these interventions has been formulated by Rosen (1974). Kernberg (1984) has proposed that purely expressive, purely supportive, or mixed supportive-expressive approaches may have differential effects. To permit testing of this hypothesis, we have attempted to develop an instrument that distinguishes these approaches.

The TVII has been designed to identify the techniques characteristic of these forms of psychotherapy. In doing so, it includes the techniques which characterize psychoanalytically-oriented psychotherapy in general. The instrument thus should have applicability for studying dynamic psychotherapy as it is used with many types of patients.

The existing instruments, described above, have been developed for use with healthier patients than those to be treated in our study. Our instrument differs in the inclusion of a number of interventions that may be called upon in work with patients of lower ego strength. Thus, limit setting, direct correction of distorted perceptions of the therapist, intervention in the patient's life situation, enlisting the aid of others, and deviating from a neutral therapeutic stance were all included in our instrument.

In addressing the question of the conceptual level at which the techniques are described, we sought to balance a need for reliability with a need for categories that relate to the clinical literature. Experimental studies of psychotherapy can be valuable in providing empirical grounding for abstract theory. To achieve this, the experimental categories should be designed as bridges between raw experiential data and accepted clinical constructs. For this reason, we have chosen to define our categories at a level of abstraction somewhat above that of operationally defined therapist behaviors. This choice was made in the belief that raters with some clinical sophistication could reliably rate interventions at an intermediate level of inference. The reliability studies described in this article afforded an opportunity to test this assumption.

Since the impact of a particular technique within a session depends not only upon the number of times the technique is invoked, but also upon phrasing, timing, overall context and other factors, we have chosen to rely upon the raters' clinical judgment of the "relative emphasis" placed upon a particular technique within the sampling unit. The extent to which each technique is utilized is quantified on a scale from 0 (absent) to 5 (maximally present). Drawing from the experience of Strupp et al. (1966) and Mintz and Luborsky (1971), we have chosen 15 minute segments as sampling units. We have restricted the instrument to verbal interventions. We seek to measure interventions as they are invoked by the therapist, independent of their effect upon the patient; thus the TVII instructions specify that the techniques are to be rated without regard to the patient responses. Since an individual statement by the therapist may serve several functions at once, TVII raters are permitted to score a given intervention in more than one category.

4. Development of the Instrument

Items for inclusion in the TVII were derived from review of related instruments (Harway et al. 1955; Hoyt et al. 1981; McNair and Lorr 1964; Mitchell and Berenson 1970; Rounsaville et al. 1984; Strupp 1957; Strupp et al. 1966), a survey of interventions described in the psychodynamic literature (Rosen 1974), and the clinical experience of the authors. An initial version of the scale was designed and distributed to eleven clinicians experienced in dynamic psychotherapy. This group included two clinical psychologists and nine psychiatrists with a range of 5 to 28 years of post-training clinical experience; six group members were psychoanalysts. The group applied the instrument to videotaped psychotherapy sessions. They viewed treatment sessions of four BPD patients conducted by three therapists. Group discussions of these sessions led to refinement of the instrument. Items relating to reiteration of the basic treatment contract and to arranging the practical details of treatment were added. In addition the rating instructions were clarified.

The authors developed a manual for the instrument, which provided definitions of the items and illustrative clinical examples.

5. Assessment of the TVII in Expressive Therapy

The individual items of the instrument were assessed for interrater reliability and agreement. In addition, a study was carried out to determine whether the instrument could be taught to an independent group of raters who had not participated in its development. This work is reported in detail elsewhere (Koenigsberg et al. 1985) and will be briefly summarized here.

Study 1: Interrater Reliabilities – Experienced Clinicians

Eight members of the research team, who had participated in the design of the instrument, applied the TVII to videotaped segments of psychotherapy sessions. These raters were experienced clinicians (6 psychiatrists and 2 clinical psychologists with from 5 to 28 years of postgraduate clinical experience). A total of 11 segments were rated. The segments were 15 minute portions of 45 minute interviews, drawn from the recorded treatments of two patients by one of the authors (O.F.K.). Both patients carried diagnoses of personality disorders. Each treatment was characterized by the treating therapist as an "expressive psychotherapy" in which relatively few supportive techniques were employed.

For each intervention, the frequency of its use throughout the 11 segments was determined by averaging, over the raters, the proportion of segments in which the rater scored it as present. The frequencies of occurrence for the 35 TVII items are displayed in Table I. The distribution of frequencies indicates that 16 techniques were used less than 20 percent of the time, while the remaining techniques were rather evenly distributed in frequency of use from 30 percent to 100 percent. The 16 infrequently used techniques group into two classes. Ten are supportive techniques: advice, sympathy, encouragement, cognitive support of defenses, emotional support of defenses, correcting transference distortion, deviating from neutrality, limit setting, intervening directly in the patient's life, and enlisting the assistance of others in intervening. Four are techniques that would be expected more often in expressive (insight) psychotherapy: clarification, confrontation, interpretation of childhood events, and genetic reconstruction (linking past, present and transference).

Table 1 Interrater Reliabilities and Agreements for TVII Items in Two Studies

TVII ITEM			Research Group Freq	Research Group Finn's[a] r	Independent Raters Freq	Independent Raters Finn's[b] r	Independent Raters T[c]
1a.	Provides factual information	- concerning external reality	39%	.76	36%	.90	.68
1b.		- concerning practical arrangements of treatment	13%	.99*	21%	.96*	.68
1c.		- concerning general psychological processes	30%	.81	11%	.93*	.84
2.	Gives advice		16%	.85	0%	--	--
3a.	Seeks clarification	- of the transference	74%	.58	64%	.80	.68
3b.		- of external reality	41%	.72	93%	.80	.53
3c.		- of the patient's childhood	7%	.95	0%	--	--
3d.		- of the present defenses	53%	.58	32%	.87	.68
3e.		- of the patient's internal reality	74%	.71	71%	.64	NS
4.	Offers sympathy		7%	.97	4%	.99*	1.00
5.	Offers encouragement		9%	.89	4%	.99*	1.00
6a.	Confronts	- in the transference	94%	.71	68%	.87	.68
6b.		- in the external reality	49%	.44	46%	.64	.37
6c.		- in the patient's childhood	6%	.98	0%	--	--
6d.		- in the present defenses	85%	.55	29%	.81	.53
6e.		- in the patient's internal reality	84%	.48	39%	.42	.53
7.	Supports defense cognitively		2%	.98	14%	.95*	1.00
8.	Supports defense emotionally		3%	.99*	0%	--	--
9a.	Interprets	- in the "here-and-now" of the transference	82%	.57	32%	.83	.68
9b.		- in the external reality	34%	.56	25%	.73	.68

Table 1 (Continued)

	Research Group		Independent Raters		
	Freq	Finn's[a] r	Freq	Finn's[b] r	T[c]
9c. - in the patient's childhood	8%	.93	0%	--	--
9d. - in the patient's defenses	71%	.56	39%	.65	.37
9e. - in the patient's internal reality	63%	.69	11%	.85	.84
9f. - in linking the observations of a), b), c), d), and/or e) with assumed unconscious past (genetic reconstruction)	15%	.83	0%	--	--
10. Stresses reality to reduce transference distortion	56%	.71	25%	.93*	.84*
11. Reduces transference distortion by deflection onto extra-transferential objects	5%	.95	0%	--	--
12. Deviates from technical neutrality	6%	.84	0%	--	--
13. Intervenes to reinstate technical neutrality	0%	--	0%	--	--
14. Sets limits within the hours	9%	.83	0%	--	--
15. Directly intervenes in patient's life	6%	.80	0%	--	--
16. Intervenes in patient's life by enlisting the aid of others	0%	--	0%	--	--
17. Reinforcement of treatment contract	64%	.73	21%	.96*	1.00*
18. Focus on external reality	47%	.75	100%	.88	.84*
19. Focus on transference	97%	.74	75%	.82	.53*
20. Therapist's relative verbal activity	100%	.82	100%	.78	.53*

[a] All Research Group Finn's r values are significant at $p < .01$, df=77, except those marked *.

[b] All Independent Raters Finn's r values are significant at $p < .01$, df=21, except those marked *.

[c] All T values are significant at $p < .05$ except those marked *

This distribution of techniques is consistent with the therapist's report that he was conducting an expressive treatment and with the fact that exploration of childhood antecedents and genetic reconstruction customarily occur in the later phase of such treatments (Kernberg 1975). Since the raters were not blind to the therapist's intended technique in this study, the agreement between the TVII ratings and the therapist's stated technique may be artifactual and should not be taken as evidence of validity. This issue is reexamined in the second study, reported below, where the raters were blind to the therapist's intention.

For each variable, Finn's r gives the agreement among the raters across the 11 segments on the presence or absence of that variable (Finn 1970). It takes account of the possibility of chance agreement. The Finn's r values are presented in Table 1.

Study 2: Interrater Reliabilities – Independent Raters

A second study was undertaken to determine if an independent group of clinicians with less extensive clinical experience could be trained to use the TVII reliability.

Three raters who had not participated in the development of the TVII were trained by one of the authors (H.W.K.) in use of the instrument. Two raters were in their first year post psychiatry residency and one was a third year psychiatric resident. Training consisted of an initial review of the TVII and its manual, followed by practice rating of videotaped segments. The raters were encouraged to make notes of the specific interventions that formed the basis of their ratings. These interventions were reviewed and the scoring discussed. The raters received about five hours of training, before the reliability testing began.

Scoring was based on seven 15-minute psychotherapy segments. The patient was a woman with a character disorder and the treatment was characterized as a brief expressive psychotherapy by the treating therapist (O.F.K.). The raters were blind to the therapist's description of his technique. Segments were drawn at random from the first eight sessions.

Occurrence frequencies for each of the 35 techniques were calculated as above and are reported in Table 1. Seventeen techniques had a frequency of occurrence of less than 20 percent. These items were identical to the low frequency items in Study 1, with two exceptions: providing factual information about general psychological processes replaced factual information about treatment, and interpretation addressing the patient's internal reality was added. The low frequency of these items, with the exception of the last, is consistent with the early phase of an expressive psychotherapy. The TVII, then, correctly characterized the treatment, a finding supportive of the validity of the instrument. The low occurrence rating for the last item may be explained by the fact that the raters consistently reported difficulty in identifying interventions that addressed "internal reality."

Interrater reliabilities were calculated using Finn's r.[1] The results are displayed in Table 1. All but one of the values ranged from .64 to .99; the single low reliability of .42 was associated with the item "confrontation in internal reality." Since a spuriously high interrater agreement is possible for techniques rarely used, the high r value for this technique should be viewed with caution.

We have also examined the interrater agreement achieved with the TVII, using the approach of Lawlis and Lu (1972) and the value, T, defined by Tinsley and Weiss (1975). For our six point rating scale, we consider raters to agree if they come within one scale point of each other for a given rating. In calculating the extent of agreement, the probability for chance agreement has been conservatively estimated, using the values provided by Lawlis and Lu (1972) for a 5-point scale. Where chi-square indicates that the agreement is significantly different from chance, we have calculated the T values. These are displayed in Table 1.

6. The TVII Applied to Supportive Therapy

With the achievement of acceptable interrater reliabilities in our pilot studies with expressive psychotherapy sessions, we applied the instrument to a broader range of treatments conducted by a number of different therapists. The therapies examined were characterized as "supportive" or "mixed supportive-expressive" by the treating therapists. These treatments were conducted by psychoanalysts with experience and special interest in supportive psychotherapy.

On the basis of early experience applying the TVII to these treatments, we empirically identified a number of additional supportive interventions that had not been included in the original TVII. These included techniques in which the therapist explicitly offers himself as a

---

[1]Finns' r (Finn 1970) is an estimate of the reliability of judges assigning items to a set of categories.

model, directly fulfills the patient's stated or inferred wishes, seeks help or advice from the patient, discloses information about himself, and actively discourages certain behaviors, attitudes, or feeling states. These techniques were defined operationally and incorporated into version 2 of the TVII.

Study 3: Reliability of Version 2 of the TVII

We examined the reliability of the expanded version of the TVII by obtaining ratings of 16 segments of "supportive" and "mixed supportive-expressive" sessions conducted by three different therapists and involving five different patients. Three experienced members of the research group rated the sessions. Interrater reliabilities were calculated using Finn's r. These values are displayed in Table 2, along with the frequencies of use of each intervention. Finn's r values for techniques endorsed as present in fewer than 20 percent of the segments are enclosed in parentheses since low frequency interventions may have spuriously high interrater reliabilities. Excluding the infrequent interventions, reliabilities range from .97 to .64.

Study 4: A Comparison of "Expressive" and "Supportive" Sessions

In order to determine whether psychotherapy sessions identified as "expressive" and "supportive" by the therapists could be distinguished in terms of the interventions identified by the TVII, we compared the frequency of use of 27 specific techniques in the two types of treatment. We report here on some preliminary findings from a comparison of eight segments taken from "supportive" psychotherapy sessions with eleven segments from "expressive" psychotherapy sessions. The "supportive" segments were drawn from three psychotherapies conducted by two different therapists (A.A. and P.K.). The "expressive" segments were drawn from psychotherapy sessions of two patients conducted by the same therapist (O.F.K.). All therapists were psychoanalysts with over ten years of experience.

Table 2 Interrater Reliabilities for TVII - Version 2

TVII ITEM		Research Group	
		Frequency (%)	Finn's r^d
1.	Informs, instructs, educates:		
	a) External Reality	25	.94
	b) Psychological Processes	21	.90
2.	Informs, instructs re treatment:		
	a) General conditions	23	.95
	b) Arrangements	33	.97
	c) Behavior between sessions	6	(.97)*
	d) Behavior within sessions	10	(.96)
3.	Seeks clarification:		
	a) Transference	35	.86
	b) External reality	98	.72
	c) Childhood	13	(.91)
	d) Defenses	48	.63
	e) Internal reality (affects, fantasies)	77	.71
4.	Reinforces treatment contract	2	(.99)*
5.	Accepts, confirms, suggests, praises:		
	a) Defenses	33	.77
	b) Superego	13	(.97)*
	c) Therapeutic alliance	4	(.96)
	d) Positive transference	4	(.99)*
	e) Negative transference	4	(.96)
	f) Feelings states	73	.70
	e) Actions	42	.72
6.	Dissuades, criticizes, rejects, prohibits:		
	a) Defenses	10	(.91)
	b) Superego	4	(.99)*
	c) Positive transference	4	(.96)
	d) Negative transference	6	(.97)*
	e) Destructive attitudes behavior	8	(.92)
	f) Feeling states	4	(.96)
	g) Actions	13	(.89)
7.	Sets limits:		
	a) Within session	0	0
	b) Outside session	0	0

Table 2 (Continued)

		Research Group	
		Frequency (%)	Finn's r^d
8.	Offers sympathy	6	(.98)*
9.	Expresses hopefulness	10	(.96)*
10.	Confronts:		
	a) Transference	29	.94
	b) External reality	19	(.93)
	c) Childhood	4	(.99)*
	d) Defenses	27	.86
	e) Internal reality	35	.80
11.	Intervenes in patient's life:		
	a) Collaterals	0	--
	b) Medication	0	--
	c) Direct help	0	--
12.	Explains deviation from technical neutrality	0	--
13.	Stresses reality of relationship:		
	a) Response to negative feelings	8	(.93)
	b) Response to positive feelings	0	--
14.	Interprets:		
	a) Transference	21	.91
	b) External reality	17	(.87)
	c) Childhood	15	(.96)
	d) Defenses	33	.74
	e) Internal reality	33	.67
	f) Linking above with past	13	(.94)
15.	Directs focus away from therapist	6	(.94)
16.	Reveals information about self:		
	a) Factual data	17	(.94)
	b) Feeling states	15	(.98)*
	c) Confirms patient's perceptions	8	(.98)*
17.	Accepts help from patient	2	(.99)*
	GLOBAL ASSESSMENTS:		
18.	Focus on external reality	98	.76

Table 2 (Continued)

		Research Group Frequency (%)	Finn's r[d]
19.	Focus on transference	42	.85
20.	Therapist verbal activity	100	.88
21.	Deviation from technical neutrality	27	.81
22.	Restore technical neutrality	0	--
23.	Fulfills patient's wishes:		
	a) Stated	15	(.94)
	b) Inferred	29	.81
24.	Offers self as model	15	(.94)
25.	Supports defenses	31	.76

[d] All Finns's r values significant at p <.05 except those marked *.
( ) = Item endorsed <20% of the time.

The frequency of use of each intervention in each treatment was defined as the ratio of the number of segments of that treatment in which a rater scored the technique as present divided by the total number of segments of that treatment and averaged over all raters' assessments. The frequency of use of each of the 27 techniques examined is plotted for each type of therapy in Figure 1. This provides a graphic TVII profile of each form of treatment. The chi-square statistic was used to identify significant differences in the frequencies of use of each technique between the two types of treatment. Significant differences ($p < .05$) were identified for thirteen of the interventions.

The "supportive therapy" used significantly more support of defenses (technique 6), clarification in the external reality (technique 11), and overall focus on the external reality (technique 26). "Expressive therapy" used more clarification of the transference (technique 10), confrontation of the transference (technique 15), confrontation in the external reality (technique 16), confrontation of defenses (technique 18), confrontation in the internal reality (technique 19), interpretation of the transference (technique 20), interpretation in the external reality (technique 21), interpretation of the defenses (technique 23), interpretation of internal reality (technique 24), and overall focus on the transference (technique 27).

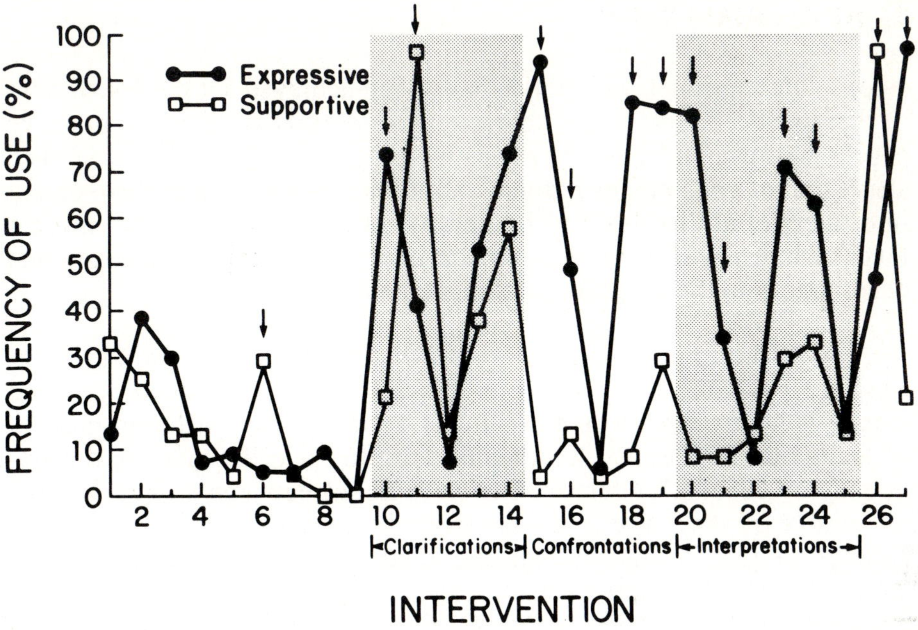

Arrows indicate significant differences ($p < .05$).

Key to Type of Intervention:

1. Provides Information about Treatment Arrangements, 2. Provides Information about other Reality Issues, 3. Provides Information about Psychological Processes, 4. Offers Sympathy, 5. Encourages/Hopefulness Expressed, 6. Supports Defenses, 7.Deflects Focus Away from Therapist, 8. Sets Limits in Sessions, 9. Intervenes in Patient's Life, 10. Clarifies Transference, 11. Clarifies External Reality, 12. Clarifies Childhood Experiences, 13. Clarifies Defenses, 14. Clarifies Internal Reality, 15. Confronts Transference, 16. Confronts External Reality, 17. Confronts Childhood Memories, 18. Confronts Defenses 19. Confronts Internal Reality, 20. Interprets Transference, 21. Interprets External Reality, 22. Interprets Childhood Experiences, 23. Interprets Defenses, 24. Interprets Internal Reality, 25. Interpretation linking any of items 20 - 24 above, 26. Overall Focus on External Reality, 27. Overall Focus on Transference

Figure 1 TVII Profiles of Supportive and Expressive Psychotherapy Sessions.

7. Discussion

Acceptable interrater reliabilities have been achieved for the assessment of therapeutic interventions characteristic of expressive and supportive psychotherapy. These interventions were defined at a level of inference above that of concrete operational definition. Thus it is possible to obtain interrater reliability for psychotherapy variables defined at a middle level of inference. Such an approach is of use in linking experimental observations to the language of clinical theory.

Our preliminary work suggests that the TVII-version 2 can distinguish psychotherapy sessions characterized as "supportive" and "expressive" by the treating therapists by identifying different profiles of technique for the two treatments. Significant differences in the frequency of 13 of 27 interventions were noted between supportive and expressive therapy. The findings reported here are preliminary; they are subject to the limitation that the instrument has been applied to expressive psychotherapy sessions conducted by one therapist and supportive treatments carried out by two therapists. We can not separate the generic technique from therapists' individual styles with this small sample of psychotherapists. Nevertheless, the differences identified – more focus upon the transference and use of confrontation and interpretation in the expressive treatment and more focus upon external reality and support of defenses in the supportive treatment – are consistent with the treating therapists' own conceptualizations of their treatments.

The TVII appears to be a potentially useful tool for monitoring pychotherapeutic techniques in ongoing studies of the treatment of patients with severe personality disorders. We have been able to train therapists at the advanced resident or immediate post-resident level to use the TVII to rate videotaped sessions reliably. Further work with a variety of treatment approaches applied by a range of therapists is necessary to confirm its construct validity.

Artificial Intelligence as a Basic Science for Psychoanalytic Research*

Virginia Teller

> The empirical field of psychoanalysis as a science is defined by its objects of study. These objects of study are symbolic forms and symbolic processes: the works of man and their modes of construction. Such forms and processes are unique, species-specific, quintessentially human (Edelson 1977).

Can the field of Artificial Intelligence provide the foundations for a basic science of psychoanalysis? My answer to this question is a resounding 'yes'. Developments in Artificial Intelligence and the related field of Cognitive Science in recent years have direct bearing on a number of problems being studied by psychoanalytic researchers. The discussion that follows, which is aimed at providing a basis for these claims, focuses on four aspects of the issue. Section 1 defines the goals of the fields of Artificial Intelligence and Cognitive Science; Section 2 describes some potential contributions that these fields can make to psychoanalytic research; and Section 3 presents a case study of the usefulness of this approach drawn from my own research. Section 4 and 5 bring the computer into play first with the introduction of a pattern-directed inference system and then with a survey of computational models of the psychotherapy process.

1. The Goals of Artificial Intelligence and Cognitive Science

An interesting perspective on the goals of artificial intelligence (AI) can be obtained by examining definitions of the field given in introductory

*I wish to thank Hartvig Dahl, Merton Gill, Michael Hölzer, and Horst Kächele for valuable comments on earlier versions of this paper, the preparation of which was supported in part by PSC-CUNY Research Award 665235.

textbooks. Winston (1984) describes AI as "the study of ideas that enable computers to be intelligent." In his view the central goals of the field are (1) to make computers more useful and (2) to understand the principles that make intelligence possible. According to Rich (1983) AI is the study of how to make computers do things that, at present, people are better at. And my personal favorite (source unknown) defines AI as an attempt to get computers to exhibit behavior that would be considered intelligent if a human behaved the same way. What these definitions of AI share is, first, a commitment to the goal of making computers smarter and easier to use and, second, the belief that the way to accomplish this is to build computer systems that exhibit aspects of human intelligence.

The class of problems that AI tackles requires *symbolic* rather than *numeric* computation. Numeric problems are typically difficult for humans to solve but relatively easy for computers. Examples are counting and sorting tasks, statistics, and a variety of "number crunching" computations performed routinely in the sciences and engineering. Many kinds of symbolic computation, however, are performed with relative ease or even automatically by humans, but have proved extremely difficult for computers. Sensory perception (e.g. vision), understanding and producing natural language, expert reasoning, commonsense judgment, theorem proving, games, learning, and clinical intuition – all of these are tasks in which symbols rather than numbers are manipulated.

Unlike numeric processing, which is primarily quantitative, symbolic processing requires qualitative, logical, and inferential reasoning. Traditionally, of course, symbolic problem solving was thought to be a uniquely human ability. Since AI aims at constructing computers that can solve symbolic problems, one product of AI research will be symbolic processing machines that work with ideas and knowledge in ways that are analogous to the ways humans reason with the ideas and knowledge they possess.

Over the years the levels of success achieved by AI workers in their efforts to build computer systems capable of equaling human performance in the area of symbolic computation have gradually improved from severely limited to quite remarkable. One of the hurdles that has had to be surmounted is the fact that, owing to their complexity, reasoning in these domains almost always proceeds under conditions of uncertainty and incomplete knowledge. It is often unfeasible, if not impossible, to seek an optimal solution to a particular problem such as the next move to make in a chess game, the understanding of an English sentence, or the diagnosis of a patient seeking medical treatment. As a result researchers in this field are forced to content themselves with less than perfect answers in many cases. Simon (1981) coined the term "satisficing" – a blend of "satisfactory" and "sufficient" (sufficing) – to describe this situation.

Even with this limitation, impressive results in AI have frequently been attained at the expense of generality. A program that performs nearly flawlessly within a particular, narrowly circumscribed domain will flounder outside of its area of expertise. A chess program knows nothing about how to play checkers or backgammon; a system that understands English does not know a word of Spanish; a program knowledgeable in eye disease lacks rudimentary knowledge of psychiatric evaluation.

Whereas Artificial Intelligence has existed for about thirty years, the newer field of Cognitive Science has emerged only in the last ten. In the United States formal recognition came first in 1977 when the journal of that name appeared and was further solidified in 1979 with the establishment of the Cognitive Science Society. Cognitive Science is an aggregation of scientists studying various aspects of the human mind. The collection of researchers who consider themselves cognitive scientists are drawn primarily from the fields of cognitive psychology, linguistics, artificial intelligence, philosophy, mathematics, and neuroscience. The area of greatest interest for psychoanalytic researchers lies at the intersection of these two fields, AI and Cognitive Science.

2. What AI and Cognitive Science have to Offer Psychoanalytic Researchers

Lacking a basic science of its own throughout the nearly one hundred years of its existence, psychoanalysis has repeatedly sought in the natural, physical and social sciences formalisms that might allow the principles, tenets and beliefs of the field to be structured into a coherent scientific theory. In the course of these endeavors, psychoanalysts have borrowed concepts, models, even whole theories, from such disciplines as psychology, linguistics, philosophy of science and physics.

Edelson (1977) warned of the dangers of delving too lightly into a foreign discipline, whether a near neighbor of one's own or a distant cousin, and advised the researcher of the commitment necessary both to achieve mastery of a new field and to keep up with subsequent developments. The consequences of failing either to attain an adequate grasp initially or to keep up with changes include the risk that the researcher, influenced by outdated doctrines, may apply misguided ideas to his work.

With these caveats in mind, I shall propose in this section a conservative rather than a wholesale borrowing from the fields in question and trace in the next section exactly how and where these ideas might profitably be applied in psychoanalytic research. The major contribution that AI and Cognitive Science can make to psychoanalytic research as I see it can be stated succinctly:

> These two disciplines offer tools for representing (literally: *re-presenting*) the data of psychoanalysis in ways that shed light both on the process of therapy itself and on the cognitive structures and processes that underlie the ability of the patient and the analyst to engage in this special form of discourse.

I take "the data of psychoanalysis" to mean verbatim transcripts of recorded psychoanalytic sessions. These contain, on the part of the patient, free association discourse and, on the part of the analyst, interventions based on his or her current understanding of the patient's discourse. By "tools" I mean ideas, notions, concepts, models, and theories, some embodied in computer programs, concerning human cognitive capacities in general and, more specifically, the structure of discourse and the intentions (i.e., wishes and beliefs) that lie behind utterances.

Perhaps this abstract pronouncement will become more concrete if I illustrate with an example from the research that I have been engaged in with Hartvig Dahl for six of the ten years we have worked together. If asked how the AI/Cognitive Science paradigm has informed our work I would pinpoint two principle sources of enlightenment. The first of these is the development in Cognitive Science of a new view of concepts that is best known as "prototype theory", the leading advocate of which is Eleanor Rosch (e.g. Rosch 1978; see Smith 1985). The heart of the theory states that:

(1) A concept is mentally represented in part by a prototype, i.e., by properties that are true of some concept instances but not all, and

(2) An object will be categorized as an instance of a concept to the extent it is similar to the concept's prototype. Since instances can be expected to vary in their similarity to the prototype, some instances will be more prototypical (or simply more 'typical') members of a concept than others.

Our second source of inspiration came from AI work in knowledge representation, which deals with the problem of how to structure information in computer programs so that an intelligent system can draw inferences from it. For many years formalisms based on first order predicate logic held sway but gradually more elaborate schemata such as semantic nets, scripts, and frames have become popular. In particular, Marvin Minsky's "frame theory", which proposes frames as a fundamental means of knowledge representation in computer programs (Minsky 1975), has much in common with Rosch's prototype theory.

According to Minsky, a frame is a data structure for representing a stereotyped situation, like a child's birthday party. There are stereotyped expectations called "defaults" associated with such parties, and these are specified in the frame. For a birthday party these might include *Sunday best* as the dress for a little girl and *ice cream and cake* as food. When a description of a specific birthday party fails to mention food or dress, the default expectations from the frame, which may be thought of as a prototype, can be assumed.

3. Prototypes and Frames

What is the precise nature of psychoanalytic clinical inference? What competence underlies a psychoanalyst's ability to construct an interpretation? In our efforts to address such questions we embarked upon an intensive study of #18, 19 and 20 of the Specimen Hour as a way of discovering exactly what this patient was telling her analyst. As we unraveled this segment of discourse, we were lead, in part by the notions of categories, prototypes and frames, to postulate first *category maps* and then *event sequence frames* as forms of re-presentation (Teller and Dahl 1981a, 1984, 1986).

The method we have developed involves constructing prototype frames and searching transcripts for repetitions of the prototypes. The process begins when we can identify in the transcript a report by the patient of an event in her life that appears to be a characteristic behavior pattern. These usually take the form of brief narrative episodes where the patient relates in reasonable detail a particular incident with a particular person, e.g. "I had a fight with my husband last night. It all started when ..." We also require some indication that the episode is self-typical and not just an isolated occurrence. The prototype frame describes the sequence of events in the episode as a series of predicates, each of which summarizes manifest statements made by the patient. The patient's statements, in effect, constitute the justification for the prototype frame. The prototype gives an abstract, structural description of a self-typical behavior pattern and specifies the order of events that must occur each time the pattern is repeated. When repetitions are discovered, evidence, again in the form of manifest patient statements, must be obtained for each event in the frame. If evidence is lacking for an event, the predicate from the prototype can be assumed by default.

Most of the prototype frames we have constructed are inductive generalizations from particular incidents. However the prototype developed in the illustration below is derived from a generalization that the patient herself makes about her own behavior.

The passage from which the CRITICAL-FRIENDLY prototype is constructed occurs in #48 of the Specimen Hour, which is the fifth hour of the psychoanalysis of a young married woman:

> And this makes me think of uhm, (stomach rumble) friendships I've had with other people and, something that I don't like to admit, because I don't approve of it (chuckle), so I can't imagine anybody else would, but I seem to have to find fault with just about everybody that I'm friendly with to some degree whether it's just a small degree or a larger degree. And, even though in a way I might feel inferior to them, and I imagine I feel inferior to a lot of people, I still have to find fault with them and maybe criticize them to David (husband), I don't know. I always have to openly criticize them, but in any case I have to kind've done that and then I can go on to a re–, a, some kind of friendly relationship with them. And until I've done that I can't really accept them as somebody that I want to be at all close to in any way at all. And, and if I can't, if I find I can't be critical of them in some aspect, then I just can't seem to be around them at all. I, I, I don't know, it's more than sort of being, well, it's not being in awe of them. It's just feeling very uncomfortable, I guess, with them.

The prototype CRITICAL-FRIENDLY frame with the three-event sequence shown in Figure 1 is accompanied by manifest patient statements that justify each event. In this prototype the patient states explicitly not only that when she thinks of friendships she *has to be critical* (C) before she *can be friendly* (F), i.e., 'If C then F', but also 'If not C then not F'. The prototype representation restricts the class of predicates that can match the prototype events, states the sequence in which these events must occur (though not the order they are reported in the discourse), and illustrates the contingent nature of the behaviors, namely that *if* the patient wishes to be friendly, *then* she must be critical and *only then* can she be friendly. Most importantly the prototype serves as a hypothesis about the patient and constitutes a prediction that the same

FRAME (Summary Predicates)

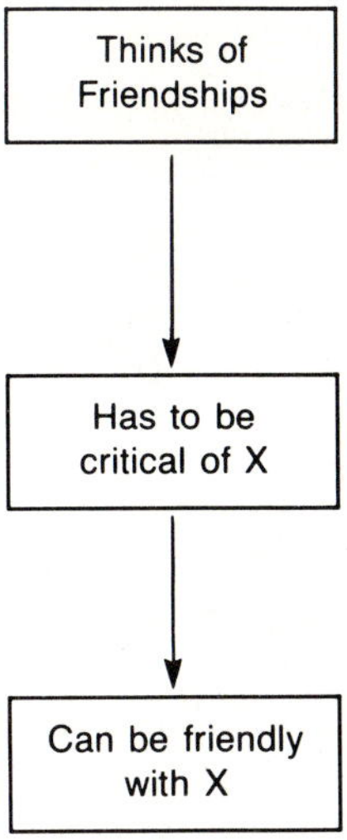

SUMMARY OF JUSTIFICATION (Primary Predicates)

Thinks of Friendships:

1. P has friends. [*And this makes me think of friendships I've had with other people. . .*]
2. People in general want to have friends [group-typical behavior.]

Has to be critical of X:

1. *I seem to have to find fault with just about everybody that I'm friendly with to some degree. . .*
2. *I still have to find fault with them and maybe criticize them to David.*
3. *I always have to openly criticize them.*
4. *If I. . .can't be critical. . .then I just can't. . .be around them. . .*

Can be friendly with X:

1. *. . .I have to kind've done that and then I can go on to a, re-, a, some kind of friendly relationship with them.*

WARRANTS FOR GENERALIZATION
(Additional reasons for taking the deduction from P's own generalization seriously):

1. Present tense verbs: *makes, think, seem, have, criticize, can, can't.*
2. Plural nouns: *friendships, people, them, everybody.*
3. Self-typical behavior: *always.*

Figure 1 Prototype of the CRITICAL-FRIENDLY Frame

pattern will occur again. The warrant for making this generalization is also implicitly supported by the set of linguistic properties shown in Figure 1.

Data supporting the prediction of the prototype occurs in the form of reports of partial or complete instantiations of the frame elsewhere in this or other sessions. In fact there are four repetitions of the CRITICAL-FRIENDLY frame in the Hour 5. Although the detailed evidence for each instantiation cannot be given here, Table 1 summarizes

Table 1 Instantiations of the CRITICAL-FRIENDLY Frame

EVIDENCE FOR:	[1] ASSISTANT	[2] TWO BOYS IN SCHOOL	[3] STUDENT REPORTS	[4] ANALYST
Thinks of Friendships	YES	NONE	NONE	Requires an Inference
Criticizes X (To Y:)	YES Analyst	YES Analyst	YES Parents	YES Analyst
Can be Friendly	YES	NONE	NONE	YES

the status of the evidence for the events in the repetitions. The reader is invited to examine the relevant portions of the Specimen Hour to verify this summary. When there is no evidence for or against the occurrence of a particular event, the predicate from the prototype can be assumed.

The first three instantiations are described below:

(1) #4 to #10: P criticizes her assistant for being loud, noisy, boisterous, insensitive and unfeeling, then wonders what the function of friendly advice is, if you're a good friend of somebody.

(2) #19: P complains about two boys in school who are disruptive and together too much.

(3) #22: In her student reports, P put all her energies into pointing out the negative things.

The prototype occurs in #48, and immediately afterward the analyst remarks:

> / So your thoughts turned from thinking about whether I would approve or disapprove of things you say to what you've just been talking about. There any connection? Does it follow perhaps that uh *you have some criticisms of me* that have occurred to you? / (emphasis added)

The fourth instantiation arises when the patient replies with a criticism:

> (Pause) I think if I had, I would have (chuckle) suppressed them too much to admit them. (Clears throat, sniff, pause) Uh, perhaps one – *I'm starting with one* that's less (chuckle) personal, one that I'm sure still is occurring to me at times, although I don't think it functions as much in my thinking now as it might have – is uhm, sometimes *wondering if all this* really does get anywhere, and, you know, if it *isn't some sort of a hoax.* But that's partly because I was brought up to think of it as being something that really *didn't do any good* for anybody and *just costs a lot of money.* I don't think that occurs to me as much now. (emphasis added)

A few minutes later (#61) the patient says a friendly thing:

> Because that (chuckle) is, well even this I find hard to say, and it's, it's silly, but just in thinking about clothes and wearing what you want, uhm, just in, in *noticing what you've worn* since I've started coming and the, *the variety and the freedom that you seem to have* and, and I think *I've been sort of envious* of that. (Sniff) I feel very embarrassed (chuckle) saying that. (emphasis added)

Then talking about colleagues at work (#62), she continues:

> ... *it's really sort of a gesture of friendship,* I guess, to anybody, that *if you like something somebody has on, acknowledging it.* (emphasis added)

The analyst's transference intervention asserts that what the patient says is true of her relationships with other people will apply to him as well. A leap of inference is scarcely required to arrive at this conclusion. It follows directly from the structure of the preceding discourse, which contains not only a clear prototype, but also three partial instantiations. And the transference prediction is confirmed as the patient proceeds to reenact the CRITICAL-FRIENDLY frame first by claiming that psychoanalysis is a hoax and then by paying the analyst a compliment as a "gesture of friendship." Dahl (this volume) reports how the hypothesis and prediction embodied in the CRITICAL-FRIENDLY frame were corroborated in an independent study he discovered only recently, although it was carried out several years before we began this line of research.

Our meticulous examination of a single psychoanalytic session has enabled us to take a significant step toward demystifying the psychoanalytic process. The main results can be summarized as follows:

(1) Objective patterns and structures are present in the discourse of a patient in psychoanalysis. These can be discovered (e.g. by a careful listener) and are not merely constructed according to the disposition of the analyst. Techniques for finding such structures in verbatim transcripts are described in Teller and Dahl (1986).

(2) Repetition is the key to understanding free association discourse. It is the phenomenon that makes psychoanalysis a possible rather than an impossible profession. A patient repeats herself "in other words," reporting over and over the adaptive as well as the maladaptive behavior patterns. As we have claimed elsewhere, the cast may change, the situations vary, but the plots endure with structural tenacity.

(3) To a large extent, the reasoning process involved in making inferences from free association discourse appears to be informed, astute common sense. The ability to detect repetition, for example, derives from one's capacity to judge similarity, extrapolate missing information, etc. Common sense, of course, is not the sole factor accounting for psychoanalytic clinical inference. Other factors must be added to this capacity, for example, specific knowledge about psychoanalytic theory and treatment.

4. Pattern-directed Inference

Pattern-directed inference systems are computer programs that look for interesting or important situations that occur as patterns in input or memory data and use these patterns to guide overall activity by selecting and triggering appropriate responses. Although their internal structures vary widely, all include as basic components (a) a source of input, (b) a knowledge base, and (c) an inferencing mechanism to direct the reasoning process. PDIS's have been implemented for a variety of applications, including speech understanding, expert systems for medical diagnosis, and the investigation of cognitive processes such as concept formation, problem solving, and inferential reasoning (cf. Waterman and Hayes-Roth 1978).

If one imagines carrying out extensive, practical studies along the lines suggested in the preceding section, one is likely to be daunted by the arduous nature of the task. The problem cries out for a technology that would automate the process of scanning the patient's discourse for instantiations of prototype frames. These frame structures have several properties that make them excellent candidates for pattern-directed inference:

(1) Frames are orderly, contingent event sequences
(2) that are invariant across objects (people) and situations (behavior settings),
(3) whose prototype predicates can be used to fill in missing information in partial instantiations, and
(4) that, in principle, can be detected by an analyst listening to a patient or even by a computer programmed to search for repetitions in free association discourse.

To date, however, pattern-directed inference systems have been characterized by two limitations: first, when natural language input is used, a PDIS generally accepts only well-formed, grammatical English utterances, and second, a given PDIS typically operates only within a well-defined and circumscribed subject domain. A challenging goal would be the development of a PDIS that would overcome these limitations. Two basic questions are: Can a computer program operate intelligently on extended, spontaneous English discourse? And can such a system, in addition, perform across the broad range of subject domains found in speech "from the couch"?

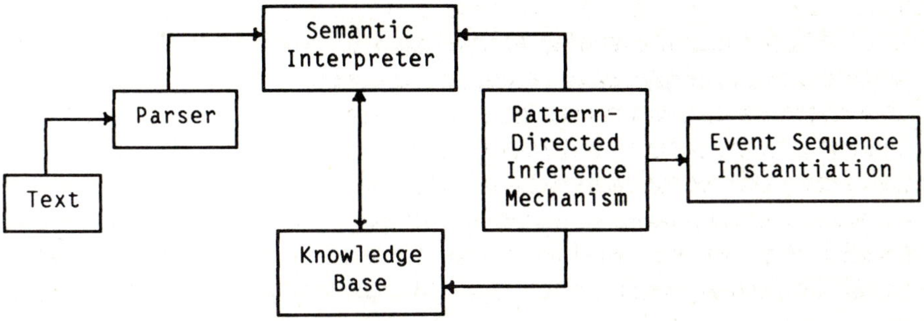

Figure 2 General Organization of a Pattern-Directed Inference System for the Detection of Repetitive Event Sequences in Psychoanalytic Discourse

The task of the PDIS would be to take free association discourse as input and identify instantiations of prototype frames. The general organization of this system is shown in Figure 2. The parser and the semantic interpreter, interacting with the knowledge base, successively derive the syntactic structure and semantic representation of the input discourse. The pattern-directed inference mechanism then compares semantic representations with patterns stored in the knowledge base and judges which, if any, of the input utterances qualify as instantiations of prototype frames. A successful PDIS would ultimately:

1. Accept as input the transcribed discourse of a psychoanalytic patient.
2. Operate with a knowledge base containing at least two different kinds of information: (a) a set of prototype event sequence frames known to be characteristic of the patient, and (b) a set of situation frames similar to Schank and Abelson's (1977) scripts representing typical behavior settings in the patient's life, e.g. kitchen or bedroom at home, classroom at school, analyst's waiting room, etc.
3. Search the input discourse and recognize repetitions of any of the prototype patterns that appear in different settings and are described in different words.
4. Justify each instantiation by citing evidence from the text to support the existence of the events in a sequence.
5. Produce results that are comparable to human judgments of the same material.

Constructing a system that successfully performs these tasks will require extending the state of the art in artificial intelligence. Nonetheless there is reason to be optimistic about the chances of making headway. One reason, pointed out by Hayes-Roth et al. (1978, p. 597), is that "the PDIS formalism derives much power from its factorization of complex problems into manageable, largely independent subprograms." Modularity is one of the most important features of a PDIS. Consequently work can proceed on several fronts at once, and progress in one area need not hinge on progress elsewhere. Moreover in the case of the data structures we have described it is advisable to start modestly and work incrementally, initially using only two or three frames and limiting the knowledge base to the situation frames necessary for the three paragraphs already exhaustively analyzed. The knowledge base can be expanded gradually to accommodate the entire session and eventually other sessions as well. At the current, early stage of this project, portions of the PDIS have been borrowed from existing natural language systems and are being adapted for our purposes.

The program of research suggested here tackles fundamental, unresolved problems in both artificial intelligence and psychoanalytic research. In psychoanalysis the hermeneuts are pitted against the would be scientists. There is no question that a working PDIS would be a boon to those trying to reclaim the field for science. It would be a tool for empirical investigations and provide a means of testing the claim that patterns like those I have described are discovered rather than constructed. Moreover its very existence would constitute a form of evidence in favor of the existence of patterns to be discovered and thus would lend support to the possibility that analysts can indeed find them.

In AI one particularly thorny problem, sometimes referred to as the frame selection problem, arises during natural language processing when the correct context for an utterance must be inferred from ambiguous discourse, i.e., the correct behavior setting for a narrative must be selected when the knowledge base contains several such domains. It is one thing to make correct inferences in a restricted domain consisting of only one or two settings, but the multiple behavior settings implicated in even a modest amount of patient discourse pose serious difficulties. Even a partial solution would be a significant breakthrough.

5. Computational Models of the Psychotherapy Process

A pattern-directed inference system that could find instantiations in text of the frame structures described above would follow in the tradition of computer programs that simulate some aspect of the behavior of patients or therapists. Undoubtedly the best known of these – and probably one of the most famous programs of all time – is Weizenbaum's (1966) ELIZA. When running in DOCTOR mode, ELIZA assumes the role of a nondirective Rogerian therapist, responding to input from a person at a terminal in a noncommittal manner, often simply by reformulating the input statement as a question. Intended as an illustration of how gullibly humans interact with computers, ELIZA has no knowledge of natural language and relies on keyword lookup and simple pattern matching techniques to produce replies.

Efforts to create more realistic patient verbal behavior have been the focus of Colby's work, most notably in his PARRY programs, which simulate the conversation of a paranoid male in a psychiatric interview (Colby 1981; Teller and Dahl 1981b). In terms of the mechanisms used to understand the interviewer's queries, PARRY differs little from ELIZA. Literal pattern matching gives a rough idea of the input, and an appropriate response is composed from a repertoire of over 1,800 canned utterances. Nonetheless, PARRY embodies sets of beliefs about the real world and goals to be realized. Perhaps its most interesting feature is a simple method of scaling a small set of emotions (the level of anger, for example, may range from 0 to 10) so that the intensity reflects the state of its interactions with the interviewer and influences the course of the interview. Moreover, within the limited context in which the program operates, PARRY has succeeded in convincing many psychiatrists that they were interviewing a human psychiatric patient.

Less attention as been given to ERMA, the product of Clippinger's (1977) ambition to model the discourse of a female patient in psychoanalysis. The one halting paragraph that ERMA produces includes the false starts, hesitations and disfluencies that are characteristic of actual transcripts of psychoanalytic discourse. Underlying ERMA's ability to "speak" like a human patient is a multiple agency cognitive model. Control in the system resides in the interaction of five separate modules, each designed to perform particular high level functions: LEIBNITZ (knowledge base), CALVIN (superego), FREUD (introspection), MACHIAVELLI (means-ends analysis) and CICERO (discourse). These modules interact by interrupting each other to get an idea, reflect on it, censor it, plan its expression and oversee its realization as the utterance of a patient in conflict trying to put off telling the analyst a taboo idea. Leuzinger (1984) used Clippinger's model as the framework for studying cognitive processes involved in treatment recommendations and for studying the changes of dream-handling in five patients over the course of their analyses (see Leuzinger-Bohleber and Kächele, this volume).

The contribution of the PDIS outlined above to this area of research would be unique. This can be seen if we compare this hypothetical PDIS with the projects just mentioned on three attributes: the presence of intelligent mechanisms (e.g. for understanding natural language); the role or point of view assumed by the program; and the type of output produced. The results are shown in Table 2.

The PDIS can be thought of as simulating the behavior of a psychoanalyst listening to and drawing inferences from the discourse of a psychoanalytic patient. Does this make the PDIS a computational model of a psychoanalyst? This is a thorny question that cannot be answered briefly. The proposed PDIS embodies several principles of cognitive processing deemed to be crucial to the psychoanalytic enterprise but completely lacks other types of knowledge that may be equally important, for example, knowledge that can be gained only through

Table 2 Comparison of Computational Models of the Psychotherapy Process

	Intelligence	Role	Output
ELIZA	no	therapist	generate reply
PARRY	some	patient	generate reply
ERMA	yes	patient	generate discourse
PDIS	yes	therapist	analyze discourse

psychoanalytic training or years of experience in treating patients. In addition, the design of the system leaves it to humans to find the prototype frames and only calls for the computer to identify repetitions. This is in fact a necessary limitation, since the process of detecting prototypes in transcripts is, at this point, scarcely understood at all. No computer can be programmed to perform a task for which there exists no principled description. Suffice it to say that, despite the usefulness of the computational approach in my research, there is absolutely no prospect that such a system could ever replicate the expertise of a human analyst.

Whether or not the PDIS is regarded as a computational model, this attempt to recast notions about psychoanalytic clinical inference into the terms of another discipline follows in the spirit of Freud's own work, most notably in the Seventh Chapter of *The Interpretation of Dreams*, where the model described in neurological terms in the Project is restated in psychological terms. If Cognitive Science were available then, Freud might well have created an AI model instead. My point here is not to indulge in idle speculation but rather to emphasize that with the conceptual and computational tools available today, we as researchers have an opportunity to achieve for psychoanalysis what Freud himself could not. This opportunity should be seized and exploited to its utmost.

Part II.

The Evolution of Single Case Study Methods

Audio-Recordings of the Psychoanalytic Dialogue: Scientific, Clinical and Ethical Problems

Horst Kächele, Helmut Thomä, Wolfgang Ruberg, and Hans-Joachim Grünzig

1. Introduction

The tape-recording of psychoanalytic sessions should by now be standard procedure for those who are prepared to undertake serious empirical research on the psychoanalytic process. However, the number of those who expose themselves to this procedure is still small, nearly as small as the number of those willing to engage in the careful scrutinizing of what they do when practicing psychoanalysis. Glover's 1936 (1955) questionnaire investigation into the prevailing techniques among British psychoanalysts has to be looked upon more as an opinion poll than as actual empirical research.

There are many reasons why analysts are so reluctant to use tape-recording in their practice. First of all, since Freud's (1916/17) warnings against the presence of a third person are often extended to the presence of a recorder or of microphones in the consulting room, it is instructive to look at Freud's exact wording. He stated that the patient "would become silent as soon as he observed a single witness to whom he felt indifferent" (p. 18). It is clear that this statement cannot be used as an argument against the tape-recording of sessions.

Freud could not have known in 1916 that human inventiveness would one day produce a very unobtrusive instrument – the tape recorder. As we know, it gives an unmistakably correct account of the verbal exchange that is superior to any recollection by the analyst, including detailed notes written after the session or – as Freud preferred – late in the evening. Since Freud was trained to follow the rules of the natural sciences, we assume that he would have welcomed new ways to assure accurate observation and data collection in the psychoanalytic situation. When he pleaded for training analyses it was in part meant to reduce analysts' distortions in their understanding of their patients' free associations. Although this was not only an utopian but a misleading ideal for psychoanalysis we believe that it was offered in the same spirit in which we suggest that tape-recording and transcribing the dialogue offers a powerful tool for investigating the exchange between patient and analyst – to the extent that this is expressed in their language. Although much more does indeed happen on an unconscious and emotional level, it is the final aim of the psychoanalytic process to translate or to interpret, that is, to put into words the patient's unconscious wishes and defenses. And these words are the starting point for further investigations.

It is our experience that after a certain time the treating analyst gets accustomed to the tape-recording. And his evenly hovering attention is no longer distracted by his inadvertent attempts to select certain passages for later note taking, to say nothing of the shorthand and seemingly accurate notes that some analysts, e.g. Wurmser (personal communication) have taken. As the first analysts to start, in 1968, tape-recording psychoanalytic sessions in Germany we were very interested in systematically collecting and examining our own clinical experiences with recording. We therefore planned a formal investigation on which we shall report after we first consider certain related problems.

We begin with Freud's warnings against the presence of a third person in the consulting room. Indeed, a great many "third persons" become potential intruders if the dialogue between analyst and patient is recorded and transcribed. The analyst protects the patient in this situation in two main ways: first, by obtaining informed consent, and second, by protecting the patient's anonymity. By now it is a well established fact that only very few patients refuse tape-recording if everything is properly explained. The patient is told that, if he agrees: (1) the sessions will be tape-recorded and made accessible to the patient himself, the treating analyst and the scientific community, (2) it is up to the patient to decide whenever he wants the recording machine turned off and/or if he wishes to stop the recording altogether, and (3) the analyst assumes an active responsibility for protecting the patient's anonymity.

Protecting the patient's identity and his secret, is readily accomplished by such devices as using codes in the transcripts, by systematically limiting access to such transcripts to bona fide clinicians and researchers who themselves assume the treating analyst's responsibility to maintain confidentiality, and by carefully disguising publicly presented and published patient material. Because it is each analyst's individual professional responsibility to protect the patient's anonymity, St. Nepomuk might be acclaimed as the patron of our profession since he chose drowning in the Moldau river at the hands of a Bohemian king instead of revealing to the king his queen's confessions of her assumed infidelities.

But the strongest resistance to tape-recording comes from analysts themselves. It is not easy to expose oneself fully to the critical investigation of colleagues who all too readily infer from the interpretations given to their sources, not in the patient's material, but in the feelings and hidden motives of the analyst. In fact, it is a very sobering experience for every analyst to listen to his own voice and often less than perfect interpretations. Kubie's (1958) description reflects our own experience and the extended quote speaks for itself:

> When for the first time a student psychiatrist or an experienced analyst hears himself participate in an interview or a psychotherapeutic session, it is always a surprisingly illuminating experience. He hears himself echo the patient. Or he hears himself outshooting or outwhispering the patient, always louder or always softer. Or he hears himself playing seesaw with his patient – loud when the patient is soft, and soft when the patient is loud. Or with surprise and dismay he hears in his own voice the edge of unintended scorn or sarcasm, or impatience or hostility, or else over tender solicitude and seductive warmth. Or he hears for the first time his own unnoted tic-like noises punctuating and interrupting the patient's stream. From such data as this he and the group as a whole learn a great deal about themselves and about the process of interchange with patients and what this process evokes in them in the form of automatic and therefore indescribable patterns of vocal interplay.
>
> They learn also to watch for and to respect the subtle tricks of forgetting and false recall to which the human mind is prone. In one session a young psychiatrist reported that in a previous interview at one point his patient had asked that the recording machine be turned off while he divulged some material which was particularly painful to him. The group discussed the possible reasons for this, basing our discussion on our knowledge of the patient

> from previous seminars. Then to check the accuracy of our speculative reconstruction, the psychiatrist was asked to play to the group about five minutes of the recorded interview which had preceded the interruption, and then about five of the minutes which followed when the recording had been resumed. To the amazement of the young psychiatrist and of the group as a whole, as we listened to the recording we discovered that it had been the psychiatrist and not the patient who had suggested that the recording should be interrupted. Of his role in this, the young psychiatrist had not the slightest memory. Furthermore, as we heard the patient's halting speech, his change of pace and volume, the altered pitch and placing of his voice, it became clear to the whole group that the young psychiatrist's intuitive move had been sound: that he had correctly evaluated the patient's mounting tension and had perceived the need for this gesture of special consideration and privacy. The result was that the patient's rapport was more firmly established than before, to such an extent that the psychiatrist could now recall that it had been the patient who had suggested that the recording be resumed after a relatively brief interruption, and who then, with the machine turned on, had continued to discuss frankly and without embarrassment the material about which he had been so touchy before. The illuminating implications of this episode for the data itself and for the transference and countertransference furnished the group with material for reflection and discussion throughout the remaining course of the seminars. These could not haven been studied without the recording machine (pp. 233-234).

This study of the influence of tape-recording and transcribing on the psychoanalytic process was conducted as a doctoral thesis study by one of us (WR) under supervision (by HK and HT). We wondered if the experiences of a number of analysts over many years still justified Gill's emphatic conclusion: "We doubt that any problem will arise on the patient's part in a research analysis, which is not already known from ordinary analysis" (Gill et al. 1968, p. 236).

In designing this study we were acutely aware of the limitations imposed by the fact that we could not use a controlled design, because one cannot analyze the same patient once with and another time without a tape-recording! Moreover, we were also still under the influence of the implicit opinions of the majority of analysts against the use of tape-recording. And, to our surprise, it was only very late in our own clinical and scientific work with tape-recorded analyses that we overcame a negative bias against them. Even at the end of this investigation, when Ruberg presented the results at his formal dissertation defense, a colleague, drew our attention to a defensive quality about our undertaking. We believe that he was right and that we did indeed experience guilt-feelings and countertransference responses as part of our biases about the negative effects on the psychoanalytic process.

One source of these negative feelings lay in the high priority we attached to making precise and exact interpretations. Tape-recording and transcribing made it very easy for us to notice that we often failed to live up to our own (and other's) expectations. Nonetheless, we also gave high priority to Freud's insistence that our deepest professional obligations require us to face reality and acknowledge truth. Therefore, increasingly it seemed to us that there must inevitably be beneficial consequences for both individual patients and for the psychoanalytic community when the treating analyst looks straight in the eye what he actually communicates and does in the consulting room. We believe that if the analyst uses transcripts as an opportunity for self-examination as a means for continuous supervision either by self-reflection or by getting supervision based on transcripts, the benefits to the patient are very great indeed. We studied four psychoanalytic treatments and processes, and our own overall evaluation is a positive one: we believe that the introduction of tape-recording has no irremediable negative effects on the psychoanalytic process. On the contrary, it opens new vistas and opportunities for the analyst's work.

2. Method

1. Data

The empirical basis for this investigation rests on four long-term psychoanalytic treatments undertaken by two analysts who, later, were also part of the research team (HT and HK) About 20% of the total number of treatment sessions, 366 out of 1796, were transcribed, not for this specific study, but as part of a general data base for process studies of a variety of questions. The stratified sample covered the entire treatment ranges: out of every block of 25 sessions, 5 consecutive sessions were included (see Table 1).

Table 1

Patient/Analyst	total sessions	sample size	sample in %
A - HT	530	110	21
B - HT	517	113	22
C - HK	408	50	12*
D - HK	341	93	27
total	1796	366	mean 20

*In this treatment the analyst had considerable problems maintaining a regular tape recording plan.

There is a striking difference between the two analysts in the frequency with which sessions were in fact recorded. The junior analyst only actually recorded 12% of the sessions with his male patient compared with 20% for the senior analyst. However, technical circumstances may have contributed to this difference. The senior analyst's secretary regularly set up the tape recorder for him, while the junior analyst had to make these preparations himself. Nonetheless the difference between HK's recording rates with his male and his female patient suggests that other internal, perhaps countertransference, problems may have been present as well.

2. Variables

Since we wanted to assess the impact of tape-recording on the psychoanalytic process our first task was to select what we thought were a set of variables (ways in which the influence would be manifest) and try to operationalize them. We assumed (a) that the impact of the recording could in principle show up anywhere and any time in the material, (b) that it could assume any specific meaning for a particular patient at any given time, and (c) that it could take on different meanings at different stages of a treatment. Our basic strategy was to look at the basic rates of occurrence of these variables compared with a control set of variables that we expected to be important in all analyses.

First, we wanted to find (1) direct, manifest references to the tape-recording procedure by either the patients or the analysts. Second, because we assumed that there would also be indirect, latent or disguised allusions to the recording, we looked for three presumably related themes: (2) remarks about feeling exposed, (3) comments and feelings about being observed, and (4) references to issues of trust and confidentiality, especially in the relationship to the analyst. As control variables we looked for topics that are usually regarded as both common and significant in clinical work: (5) reactions to and feelings about payment, (6) references to the couch, and (7) the reporting of dreams.

3. Measurement - with a Computer Content Dictionary

One might imagine that the straight forward way to search for manifestations of the seven variables that we had decided upon would be to read through the entire 366 transcripts and identify each instance. But this is a big order, surpassing even the motivation of a doctoral candidate. Fortunately we were able to solve our search problem by using a technology called computer assisted content analysis (CACA) which works with the transcripts that are stored in the computer based ULM TEXTBANK (Kächele and Mergenthaler 1983; Mergenthaler 1985; Mergenthaler and Kächele, this volume). The basic method (see Stone et al. 1966) involves designing a specific computer content dictionary as the measuring instrument.

Such a dictionary consists of a set of conceptual categories representing the variables to be measured and each category is in turn defined by a list of words (nouns, adjectives and verbs) thought to exemplify manifestations or instances of the concept. Our seven variables, of course, became our seven categories:

Category No.	Category Name	Description of Word List
1	Tape	All words that refer to tape- recording.
2	Exposure	All words that refer to shame and being exposed in public. Includes positive as well as negative references.

3	Being Observed	All words that refer to the feeling of being observed, looked at, etc.
4	Trust	All words that refer to the feeling of trusting or not trusting somebody.
5	Payment	All words that relate to payment for the treatment.
6	Couch	All words that refer to lying on the couch.
7	Dreams	All words that refer to some aspect of dreams and dreaming.

We used the methods developed by Stone and his colleagues (Stone et al. 1966) to construct our dictionary. From a German thesaurus (Synonymwörterbuch von Textor 1962) – comparable to Roget's Thesaurus – and the DUDEN (a dictionary of written and spoken German) we selected all of the words that might represent or refer to each of the above seven dictionary categories. In this way we obtained a first word list of 1600 words. These words were then compared with our "Basic Vocabulary of Psychotherapeutic Language" – the part of the ULM TEXTBANK containing the vocabulary of an eight million word corpus of text – and we retained only those words that are actually used in psychotherapy sessions. We were left with 735 words distributed over the seven categories. Finally, when we first applied our newly constructed dictionary to the 366 transcripts, we were further able to reduce the list of dictionary entries to 317 because the other words did not occur in these sessions.

With this final version of the Tape-Recording Dictionary (TRD, Ruberg 1982, pp. 139-142) we analyzed the 366 sessions by using a computer text analysis package called EVA-ULM (see Mergenthaler 1985), which yields frequency scores for each of the seven categories for each of the sessions. Although it is clear that the measurement reliability of this method is perfect because the programs do not make mistakes in matching the words of the text to those of the dictionary, nonetheless a real question can be raised about their validity. The dictionary as a measure embodies a simple (if not simple-minded) linguistic hypothesis, namely that the lists of words which define the seven categories adequately capture the concepts, even while ignoring syntactic and contextual information. Nonetheless those who remain skeptical of these keyword procedures should examine some clinically compelling examples of their ability to measure some rather complex concepts (e.g. Dahl 1972, 1974, 1983).

The practical issue in this validity problem lies in the question: are the text references picked out by the computer program *really* examples of the intended meaning of a given category? To check this, one of us (WR) read all the instances, e.g. all references identified by the text analysis, 14 in the verbatim transcripts and made a commonsense judgment about whether the specific text was indeed an instance of a given category. At the same time this judge was able to identify references to the categories in the text that were not picked up by the content analysis. Table 2 summaries the false positive and false negative identifications.

Table 2 Correctness of Computer-Based Identification (in %)

category	tape 1	exposure 2	observation 3	trust 4	payment 5	couch 6	dream 7
false positive	2.6	48.0	19.8	7.0	6.3	1.0	1.5
false negative	–	3.4	5.1	2.9	2.0	1.9	0.4
total	2.6	51.4	24.9	9.9	8.3	2.9	1.9

In six out of the seven categories there were more false positives than false negatives, in other words, the program "found" instances that were in fact not instances of a category more often than it missed true instances, which is desirable for a scanning procedure. However, more than 50% of the Exposure Category references were misleadingly identified, which certainly highlights the limitations of this kind of dictionary measure.

4. Results

The misidentified or missed texts were corrected by the judge with the following results for the frequency of direct and indirect references to the tape-recording (Table 3):

Table 3 Frequency of Direct and Indirect Reactions to Tape-Recording and Frequency of Control Variables

	tape	exposure	observation	trust	payment	couch	dream
category	1	2	3	4	5	6	7
n sessions	7	169	44	48	49	36	148
% sessions	1.9	46.2	12	13.1	13.4	9.8	40.4

To our surprise only 7 of the 366 sessions contained direct references to tape-recording. Of course not all initial sessions in which the question of recording was introduced and discussed were included, but one must still consider the possibility of a sampling artifact. The rarer the events in the entire domain the less the chance that these events will appear in the sample. However to adequately study this question in more detail one needs a complete set of recordings of each treatment (see Grünzig 1985 and Grünzig, this volume).

Nonetheless, is it really surprising that analysts and patients so seldom mention the recording? The two analysts in this study had quite different backgrounds and experience. One of them (HT) was a senior analyst with more then 20 years of experience. The other analyst (HK) however, was conducting and recording his first two training analyses. Although it is reasonable to assume that they had quite different motives and reasons for participating, they at least shared enthusiasm for undertaking something as challenging and novel as tape-recording psychoanalyses. In any case, part of the answer to the question lies in the fact that neither analyst forced his patients to talk about the recording. And it is certainly a plausible hypothesis that the analysts failed to encourage their patients to talk freely about the recordings because of their own anxieties about the procedure. We will return to this matter shortly.

The main findings of the content analysis are shown in Table 4.

Table 4 Frequency of Direct and Indirect Reactions to Tape-Recording for Four Patients in % of Sessions

	tape	exposure	observation	trust	payment	couch	dream
category	1	2	3	4	5	6	7
Pat. A (N=110)	–	49.1	–	15.5	3.6	5.5	25.5
Pat. B (N=113)	2.7	35.4	18.6	3.5	22.1	19.5	60.2
Pat. C (N=50)	–	58.0	2.0	18.0	18.0	4.0	8.0
Pat. D (N=93)	4.3	49.5	23.7	19.4	11.8	6.5	51.6

One of the puzzling findings is that in this sample of the four patients only the two female patients, one from each analyst, referred to the tape-recording (Patient B, 2.7%; Patient D, 4.3%). Moreover these same female patients much more frequently talked about "being observed" than did the male patients. In fact the results indicate that patients of the same sex (A and C were male, B and D female) were more alike than patients of the same analyst (HT: A and B; HK: C and D).

5. Clinical Illustrations

Let us return now to the hypothesis that the low frequency of references to tape-recording was at least in part due to the analysts' failure to encourage the patients to talk about their responses and associations to the procedure. In an informal attempt to throw light on this question we shall provide some examples from the two treatments where we found direct references to the recording in the sample of this investigation.

Patient B

Session 101: The patient asks, after a discussion of details of her sexual problems, if the recording machine is still on. The analyst replies, "Yes." She wonders if Mrs. X, the analyst's secretary, will transcribe the session, but before the analyst answers she adds, "You need not answer. I don't care anymore." When the analyst wonders why she retreats so quickly she focuses on the fact that the secretary is female and thus might have a more truthful and stricter attitude towards sexual perversity than the analyst seems to have. Thus the topic shifts from the recording and transcribing to the patient's conflictual material.

Session 202: The patient understands one of the analyst's statements to be an explanation of his analytic technique. She highly appreciates this and wonders if there is no tape-recording during this session since the analyst seems much freer and less restricted than usual. She experiences the audio-recording as a kind of higher moral pressure under which the analyst suffers just as she suffers under the strict authority of her headmaster.

Session 352: The patient recalls that from time to time while waiting for the hour to begin she has heard funny and sometimes derogatory remarks coming from the secretary's office. She believes that these are references to typing the tapes of the patient's sessions. She has recently read an article by her analyst and had the impression that, just as the secretary must despise her, he despised the patient whom he described in the article. She is very critical of the analyst for this, feels rejected, and imagines that after the session the analyst sits down at his desk, writes an essay about her and gets excited about the session that just finished because of its scientific implications. She is reduced to a mere object of science.

Three examples were found in which the reference to the tape was not manifestly connected to the treatment. *Session 129*: The patient reports on tapes with stories from her grandmother. *Session 213*: The patient uses a tape recorder herself to conduct an opinion poll in her office. *Session 279*: The patient mentions the use of tape-recording in her own profession. Obviously all three of these incidents might be indirect references to the treatment, but the analyst did not so interpret them at the time.

In summary it appears that Patient B's reactions to the tape-recording indicated a central concern that the function of the recorder was that of a moral censor. In her third session she reported childhood memories of going to confession and compared these with the analytic situation. She said that, even today she still had trouble participating in "open confession ceremonies" as they were practiced in Catholic church services. In hour 242 (not in the sample) she told a dream in which her analysis was being conducted publicly. The analyst pointed out the connection between confession, being treated publicly and the tape-recording.

Patient D

In the introductory session this patient of the junior analyst had reacted very positively to the idea of recording, saying that her brother, who was a psychologist, could make use of the tapes himself.

Session 3: The patient talks about what the relationship with the analyst means to her. She wants to exclude any personal, emotional relations, saying, "Yeah, if one could achieve that, that would make it much easier to convey to you what comes to my mind – if I could switch you off, if I would be all on my own in this room and could talk to the tape alone." The analyst points out that this expresses her ambivalence between wishing for closeness and wishing for protective distance.

Session 4: The patient begins by asking whether the tape machine is turned off, because the dust cover is still on. She says that last night she was out and consumed quite a few glasses of wine. The analyst interjects, "So you may not want to record your present state," to which she replies with a certain irony, "No, that doesn't bother me at all. Maybe I'm concerned that you'll miss my precious utterances. But maybe the machine is running. Who knows?" The analyst suggests that perhaps the importance of the tape-recordings is what happens to them. She then reports having felt deserted over the weekend (between sessions 3 and 4) just as she had often felt during empty weekends at her school. She then reports a dream in which a girl exhibited herself in a police station to a man who got sexually aroused. In the next scene during a medical examination a physician took an x-ray and then looked only at her bare skeleton. She wanted a more satisfying examination and was disappointed. The analyst tells her that she is feeling insecure about her own attractiveness and connects this to her feelings about the tape-recording.

Session 88: The patient complains that she has nothing to talk about. She says that if she could feel that somebody likes her then she would be able to talk a lot – sometimes even too much – and "when I have the feeling that you are cool, this doesn't work at all." The analyst says that she feels an obligation to feed him. And she refers back to the previous session where she said that in every session at least one sentence from her must be useful. She feels all of these tapes are full of empty, worthless stuff. They should contain at least one precious word or else they could be thrown away. The analyst points out that she feels she has to report something special in order to be appreciated. She then recalls feeling humiliated during her initial interview with the head of the clinic; she had the feeling that she could not show him any of her positive assets and hoped that he would also listen to these tapes. Then he would learn more about her difficulties, but also have a chance to see her accomplishments, because she perceived being offered an analysis in his clinic as an act of mercy.

In summary, the tape-recording seemed to have several different but related meanings for this patient. In one instance the recordings were connected with her obligations to a powerful father figure, the chief of the clinic, to whom she felt obligated, but whom she wanted to impress. In another it represented a means of giving gifts to her client-centered therapist brother. And it confronted her with her own feelings of emptiness, unattractiveness and worthlessness, and the wish to give precious words to the analyst lest the tapes too be worthless.

6. Ethical Aspects

When a psychoanalyst asks a patient for informed consent to make audio recordings of the analysis he explicitly or implicitly informs the patient that the boundaries of the privacy of the consulting room are extended to involve other people, known or unknown to the patient. These include those who transcribe the tapes and professional colleagues who either listen to them or read and study the transcripts. Moreover, the analyst assumes the obligation to maintain the patient's confidentiality within these limits. In contrast, patients undergoing supervised analyses are rarely if ever informed of that fact and the implicit extension of the boundaries of privacy that it entails. It is curious that analysts who might be very uncomfortable with the first extension, which the patient knows about, are likely to be quite comfortable with the other extension of which the patient is typically ignorant.

We believe that the openness of the analyst's attitude, as embodied in obtaining informed consent, can contribute significantly to a therapeutic alliance based in part on the fact that both patient and analyst know that the analyst, as well as the patient, will be observed by others, that in that respect they are both "in the same boat." While it is undoubtedly true that some patients and analysts view this as an unbearable intrusion on their privacy, it is also true that others find it not only tolerable, but liberating.

We believe that an analyst not only has the negative ethical obligation to not harm his patients, but that he also has a positive ethical obligation to take any reasonable steps that promise a better and deeper understanding of his patients and thereby enhance his effectiveness as an analyst. The beneficial effects of recording may occur quite directly, as when the analyst replays all or a portion of a session during ongoing treatment, or they may occur more indirectly as a result of studying transcripts at leisure after an analysis is ended. We believe that it is healthy for an analyst to be confronted with what he *in fact* has said, with his actual interpretations, rather than be satisfied with his own fallible memory. It is healthy to relisten or reread and discover, or have one's colleagues point out that one missed some important material, just as it is healthy to note when one seems to have understood and made a useful intervention. These considerations alone would constitute sufficient reason for introducing tape-recording as a regular procedure, to say nothing of the value of the potential knowledge to be gained from systematic research.

The Ulm Textbank Management System: A Tool for Psychotherapy Research

Erhard Mergenthaler and Horst Kächele

1. Introduction

After many years of tape-recording and the production of a large collection of verbatim transcripts, we realized the need to establish a major computerized databank for psychotherapy research and education.[1] The documents stored in the ULM TEXTBANK, as it is known, are primarily a collection of open-ended text databases. The main characteristic of these databases is that they can be continuously expanded, as in, for example, a collection of transcribed brief psychotherapies. It is possible to expand such a database to include every newly undertaken brief psychotherapy without ever reaching a state of completeness or representativeness with regard to this type of text. Completeness or representativeness can only be approximated if, say, in a large set of diagnostic initial interviews, careful attention has been paid to sampling according to a variety of variables such as "sex," "age," "diagnosis," "social class," etc. Examples of closed databases are the Bible (see Parunak 1982), and Freud's collected works.

The degree of completeness exhibited by a database also influences strategies for handling the results of subsequent analyses of these texts. There are two main approaches. In the first, results of all the available analyses are actually stored with the text or in direct relation to it. In the second, texts from the database are processed as needed, according to the wishes of the researcher.

The primarily open databases make it possible to apply any new or old computational form of analysis to any of the texts at any time. Nonetheless, one of the TEXTBANK's goals has been to make available

---

[1]Supported by the German Research Foundation, Sonderforschungsbereich 129, project B2.

to many different researchers the results of previous analyses of this data, gained with such great effort. Therefore the plan is for the ULM TEXTBANK to store such results directly with the texts. Thus, the textbank management system has been designed to facilitate the following tasks:

1. The input and editing of texts selected according to many different points of view and criteria.

2. Management of an unlimited number of texts on the University of Ulm Computer Center's auxiliary storage.

3. Management of an unlimited amount of information on the texts, their authors, and the related text analyses.

4. Management of an open-ended variety of methods for editing and analyzing stored texts.

5. Providing interfaces to statistical and other user packages.

6. Providing a simple, dialogue-oriented user interface when implementing the tasks in 1 to 5 (above).

In summary, the TEXTBANK management system (TBS) is an information system, designed to administer texts and information about the texts in databases, that makes texts accessible by integrating techniques of linguistic data processing and text processing. It features a uniform user interface that assists in the input, processing, output, and analyses of texts.

2. System Architecture

According to the previous definition, the system's structure includes modules for:

(1) manipulating texts (text module)

(2) analyzing texts (analysis module)

(3) managing the databases (databank module)

The user gains access on a computer terminal via a monitor program, which also coordinates the individual functions of the system.

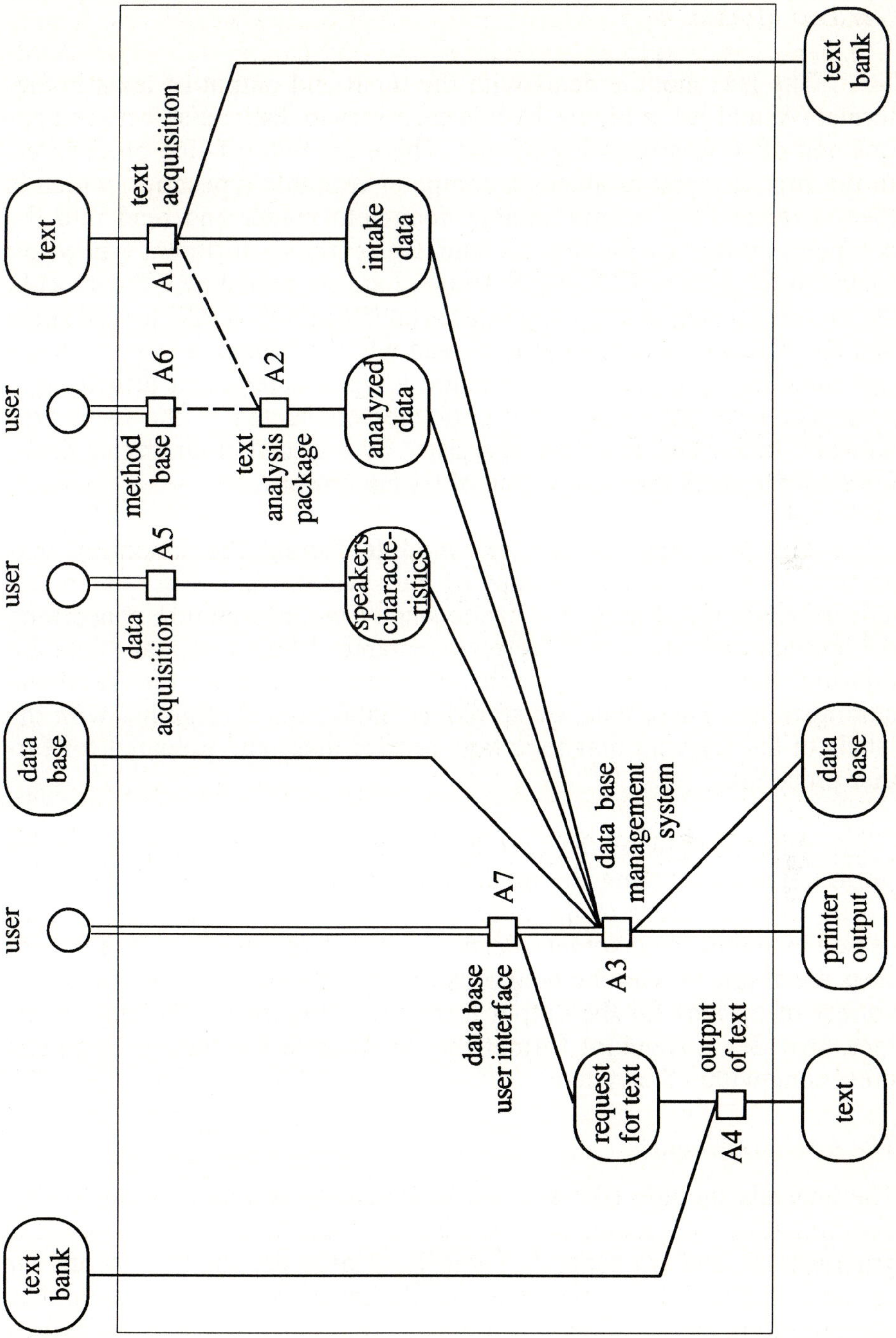
text
user
user
data base
user
text bank
text acquisition
A1
method base
A6
text analysis package
A2
data acquisition
A5
intake data
analyzed data
speakers characte-ristics
A7
data base user interface
data base management system
A3
request for text
output of text
A4
text bank
data base
printer output
text

Figure 1

The Text Module

The text module deals with the input and output of texts in any format (Al and A4 in Figure 1). It is necessary to distinguish between on-line and off-line processing of text. There are two off-line procedures. In the first, a typist produces a computer readable typescript, which is then scanned by a programmable document reader and read into the computer system by the text module. Currently six different typewriter fonts (NLQ) such as COURIER 10 or 12 are supported (see Figure 2).In the second procedure a typist produces an IBM-DOS ASCII text file on a 360 KB diskette which can also be read into the computer system by the text module. In the on-line procedure a typist enters data directly at a computer terminal or personal computer connected to the local area network. In this task the typist is assisted by a special program that deals, for example, with the recognition of typing errors.

The programs of the text module format the incoming text according to the requirements of the system and store it in the TEXTBANK (see Figure 1). At the same time information concerning the speaker and situational factors is entered. When necessary data are missing, these may be obtained and supplemented by the Textbank administrator. These data are stored as "intake data" (together with the labels of the relevant magnetic tape or hard disk) and prepared for further processing.

When output of the text is requested, the system will ask for information concerning the medium on which the requested texts are stored and the nature of the output required. This output may be processed by either the *printout interface* or the *data interface*. Printouts of texts are obtained with the help of special programs that offer the user a variety of options for the output format (see Figure 3). The data interface provides a standard format that is suitable for further linguistic processing within the system.

The Analysis Module

The analysis module (A2 and A6 in Figure 1) is a subsystem for the determination of certain characteristics of the texts: (1) formal, (2) grammatical, and (3) content (Table 1). It provides the framework for an expandable body of programs for the analysis of textual data. The module refers the standard text to these programs and stores the results of the analysis as "analyzed data" within the system until they are required for further processing (see Figure 1). Apart from the standard

```
12995503008901

T/you're late, late.

P/I know, I wouldn't 've, I should have been on time. This is all
for my face.

T/well what happened?

P/well traffic on Main street was heavy

T/uh huh

P/so I came down Irving street and went around Picadilly to the
parking lot and I sat there because the parking lot was very full
so there were three cars in front of me that had turned the
corner, you know, into Picadilly.

T/yeah

P/and they had to wait for, what happened was you had to wait for
one car to get out and then one went in, the other went out and
then one went in. (clears throat) and that was it.

T/well, so tell me, are you independent professionally? you're
still working for uh;

P/I'm not working for /

T/really;

P/they can't afford me.

T/really finished.okay.

P/I'm really finished and I'm so busy I don't know to do first.

T/why?
```

Figure 2

TEXT: 129955 EINHEIT: 0089

1 T: You're late, late.

2 P: I know. I wouldn't 've, I should have been on time. This is all for my face.

3 T: Well what happened?

4 P: Well traffic on *17 street was heavy

5 T: Uh huh

6 P: So I came down *19 street and went around *83 to the parking lot and I sat there because the parking lot was very full so there were three cars in front of me that had turned the corner, you know, into *83.

7 T: Yeah

8 P: And they had to wait for, what happened was you had to wait for one car to get out and then one went in, the other went out and then one went in. (Clears throat) and that was it.

9 T: Well, so tell me, are you independent professionally? you're still working for uh;

10 P: I'm not working for /

11 T: Really;

12 P: They can't afford me.

13 T: Really finished. Okay.

14 P: I'm really finished and I'm so busy I don't know what to do first.

Figure 3

analyses (text size, information content, redundancy, distribution of word categories, and type-token ratio), which are carried out on any text, the user can decide on additional analyses (e.g. the distribution of anxiety themes). Kächele and Mergenthaler (1983) provided an overview of text analyses carried out up to that date. Some examples of text analyses are given later in this chapter.

Table 1

characteristics	monadic	polyadic
formal	text size	speaker sequence
grammatical	verb/adjective quotient	lexical correspondence
substantive	anxiety themes	thematic continuity

The Databank Module

The databank module is a subsystem for the management of information about texts (A3 and A7 in Figure 1). It consists of programs for: (1) the definition of data, (2) data input, and (3) data analysis.

The *definition of data* clarifies the terms used in the description of texts and in the identification of relationships among these characteristics. A standard description scheme can be changed or expanded at any time, thereby controlling the consistency of the data. This program functions as a user interface in a data definition language. The *storage*, *elimination* and *modification* of information that can be described in this scheme is carried out by the programs for *data input*, which also interface with the user in a data manipulation language. During the data input phase the program checks to see if the restrictions specified in the scheme have been observed.

Queries are dealt with by programs for *data analysis*. The interface allows a user to ask questions related to the scheme in a data query language. The answer is returned to the terminal screen immediately and, if desired, forwarded within the system to the text module.

Associated Demographic data (A5 in Figure 1) are determined by a specific mask-oriented program which facilitates the protection of personal data. The structure of this and related data stored within the system is determined by the data manipulation language described above.

3. Methods and Applications

Starting from a semiotic view of language, which goes back to Peirce, the founder of semiotics, and to its further development by Morris, language is understood as a system of symbols whose structure is determined according to rules based on the relationship between form and content.

Accordingly, it is possible to distinguish between *formal*, *grammatical*, and *substantive* measurements. Each of these types of measurements can be further subdivided with regard to whether it can be applied to a speaker's text or to the entire speech activity in a conversation, i.e., to the dialogue. It is therefore possible to speak of monadic or dyadic values. It is also possible to distinguish among these types of measurements according to the kind of data they utilize. Best known are simple frequencies of occurrence, which form the basis for ratios and distributions.

It should also be noted that, according to the distinction made here, some of the approaches for formal and grammatical measurements presume substantive knowledge, either wholly or in part, for example, the denotative meaning of a word. The contrast with substantive measurements stems from the fact that the required knowledge does not come from the research field itself, namely psychoanalysis, but from the realm of methodologies, i.e., linguistics or information science.

The formal measurements can generally be determined in a simple manner. In computer-aided approaches only the capacity to segment a sequence of symbols (letters, numbers, and special symbols) into words and punctuation is necessary. The programming task is minimal; hardly any recoding is necessary. Table 2 contains a selection of such formal measurements, accompanied by indications of their applicability.

Table 2

Text size (Tokens)	Activity
Vocabulary (Types)	Diversity
Type/Token Ratio	Efficiency
Redundancy	Simplicity vs. Complexity
Distance	Variability, Flexibility
Cluster	Fixation, Focus
Filter	Continuity
Change of Speaker	Dynamic, Rigidity

The simplest and most elementary formal measurement is that of the number of words spoken by the analyst and patient. Kächele (1983) found that in a successful psychoanalytic treatment there was no correlation across 130 sessions in the number of words spoken by analyst and patient. In an unsuccessful treatment of the same analyst these word counts were significantly (+.30, N=110) correlated. O'Dell and Winder (1975) also used the text size as a measure of the therapist's activity in order to distinguish therapeutic techniques. They give 7% as the proportion of therapist's speech in analytic therapy and 31% in eclectic psychotherapy. Zimmer and Cowles (1972), in a study of one patient who visited three therapists with different orientations, also pointed out significant differences. Using the same data, Pepinsky (1979) showed that the therapist's form of activity influences the patients to act in a similar way, i.e., the speech activity of the patient conforms to that of the therapist, as if there is "a convergence of the client toward the level of talk manifested by the therapist" (Pepinsky 1979, p. 7).

The redundancy of a text is a measure adopted from information theory. Spence (1968) proposed some important ideas about psychodynamic redundancy, without testing these ideas empirically. In addition, he formulated a series of hypotheses about the course that redundancy takes in psychoanalytic treatment. Kächele and Mergenthaler (1984) confirmed one of these hypotheses, namely that the repetitiousness of a patient's speech increased in the course of treatment. The therapist's values, in contrast, remained constant.

The grammatical measures require the researcher to have linguistic knowledge about the language being studied, for example, the grammar of German. The programming and precoding tasks in the computer-aided procedures are considerable. Moreover, many kinds of questions still cannot be correctly processed automatically. An example is lemmatization, which can assign 50% to 95% of all word forms, depending on the kind of text, to the correct lemma. The psychoanalytic interview, a form of speech with the many syntactically deviant forms (such as incomplete words and sentences) that characterize spoken and spontaneous speech, falls at the lower end of this range. Accordingly, there are hardly any computer-aided studies of psychoanalytic texts using grammatical measures. Table 3 lists a selection of such measures.

The distribution by word type was used by Lorenz and Cobb (1975) to differentiate patients with different psychotic illnesses. To mention one result as an example, they determined that neurotics used more verbs but fewer conjunctions than the normal population used for comparison. At least in German, other variables have to be taken into account, as Eisenmann (1973) demonstrated for conjunctions: "The use of particular conjunctions is determined first and foremost by locality, second by sex, third by age, and lastly by language class" (Eisenmann 1973, p. 407).

The dependence of word choice on word type and semantic class was demonstrated by Busemann (1925) in investigations of children's speech. He spoke of an "active" and a "qualitative" style with regard to verbs and adjectives. He showed that these differences in style are only slightly dependent on the subject being discussed and that they belong rather to personality variables. Using a computer-aided approach to the text of a psychoanalytic interview, Mergenthaler (1985) showed that the realization of a word form within the text may definitely depend on the subject matter. However, this microanalytic view does not exclude the possibility that, viewed at a micro level, personality-dependent variables are effective as described by Busemann.

Table 3

Interjections		Noise
Word types		Cognitive Structure
	Verb Noun Adjective, Adverb Pronoun	Action, dynamic Conditions, static Features, modal Relations
Sentences	Relative clause Yes questions Questions	Complexity Support, confirm Exploration
Phrases	Nominal phrases Verbal phrases Prepositional phrases	
Passive forms	Resistance	
Tense	present past future	
Degree of description	Simple Composite	General vs. Specific
Ambiguity	pronoun syntactic lexical	
Diminution and Raising	Emotion Affect	
Ratio	Interjections/Text size Verb/Adjective Relative clause/main clause Indicative/main clause Phrases/Sentences	

The verb-adjective quotient, introduced by Boder (1940), analogous to Busemann's action quotients, was applied by Wirtz and Kächele (1983) to the first interviews of three different therapists. They concluded that this quotient is a differential measure of the therapist's speech style as well as of differences associated with sex and diagnosis.

The significance of personal pronouns for the structuring of object and self-relations in language has been taken up several times. Several studies have been undertaken on speech material from the ULM TEXTBANK (see Mergenthaler 1985, 1986).

Table 4 shows a selection of *substantive* measures. They presume, in addition to the knowledge mentioned above, detailed expert knowledge of a theory with regard to the theory's area of application. Computer-aided procedures are only able to provide approximate results and are limited to narrowly defined constructions. New approaches in information science, especially in the field of artificial intelligence, could achieve a breakthrough in such matters by establishing data bases in conjunction with a system of rules. Two approaches that strongly emphasize the rule components are Clippinger (1977) and Teller and Dahl (1981a).

Table 4

Themes	
Separation, Mutilation, Guilt, Shame	Anxiety themes
Dogmatism	Cognitive Style
Self, Other	Relationship
Positive, Negative	Affect balance
Primitive Concepts	Cognitive Structures
Speech Acts	
Clarification	Technique
Confrontation	
Exploration	
Interpretation	
Theme Association	Patterns of topics
Theme constancy (after change in speakers)	Interaction
	Synchrony

The most important kind of the quantitative method for substantive measurements has been content analysis. Gottschalk and Gleser (1969) and Gottschalk (1974) presented the scales most widely used in psychotherapy. Koch and Schöfer (1986) have edited a survey of these methods, including a section by Grünzig and Mergenthaler (1986) on computer-aided approaches. Lolas, Mergenthaler, and von Rad (1982) provide a comparison of results using a computer-aided method with those from other methods.

In a pioneering study, Dahl (1972) was able to trace the downhill course of 363 hours during a 2 1/2 year segment of an unsuccessful psychoanalysis and to convincingly categorize 25 sessions as 10 extreme "work" hours, 10 extreme "resistance" hours, and 5 directly in the middle of the range. Using single words derived from the Havard III dictionary categories he was also able to demonstrate word clusters that manifestly appear to reflect oedipal and other unconscious conflicts (Dahl 1974).

Reynes et al. (1984) used the Regressive Imagery Dictionary (RID) to compare this same patient's 10 working hours and 10 resistance hours. The working hours were characterized by increases in the dictionary categories that assessed primary process language and the resistance hours by increases in the secondary process category scores. This agrees with Freud's earlier attribution of defensive functions to the secondary processes (see Bucci, this volume).

Large continuous segments as well as selected sections of treatment transcripts may thus be examined using *computer aided text analysis* as a tool in psychoanalytic process research (Kächele and Mergenthaler 1984). Further progress requires that methods be developed even more extensively, that basic research be conducted, and that techniques from related scientific disciplines, such as information science and linguistics, be integrated. In fact, Teller (this volume) audaciously proposes artificial intelligence as a basic science for psychoanalytic research.

4. Uses and Sources of the TEXTBANK and the Text Databases

The optimal employment of a TBS in psychotherapy research requires that the text databases to be administered be able to answer the kinds of questions that are likely to be posed. The definition of individual text databases as subunits of the TEXTBANK are thus especially significant. In this regard two major areas of work have crystallized at the ULM TEXTBANK, each corresponding to a different research approach, *longitudinal* and *cross-sectional* studies.

Longitudinal studies concentrate on text from psychoanalytic treatment; their goal is the study of the change process. Because of the large number of hours of a typical psychoanalysis, it is possible to prepare transcripts for only a small number of different cases. Thus studies of variation (of many kinds) during single cases are foremost.

There are, of course, questions that go beyond variation within individual patients or therapists; these are examined using the texts of initial interviews in cross-sectional studies. Focusing on the initial interview means that many different patients with only one interview can be examined, making it possible to study the effects of variables such as sex and diagnosis, for example. Maintained separately are the text databases required for special investigations, such as those of the Balint group research, verbal exchanges during doctors' visits, and verbal interactions during family consultations.

The texts constituting the major focus of work at the ULM TEXTBANK are being systematically increased. The database of psychoanalysis texts now includes extensive excerpts from four psychoanalytic cases. Individual sessions from nine other psychoanalytic therapies are also included. The database of initial interviews includes several hundred different interviews and is referenced according to the *sex* of the patient or therapist and whether the *diagnosis* is *neurosis* or *psychosomatic disturbance*. This body of texts is being enlarged with special attention to the patient variables of *sex*, *diagnosis*, *social class*, and *age*, and the therapist variables of *experience* and *kind of* psychotherapy (de la Parra 1985).

The kind of texts included in the TBS is determined by the goals, questions, and scientific interests of the supporting and other institutions. For the Department of Psychotherapy at Ulm University this means both the establishment of an empirical basis for research in the field of psychotherapy, and for the support of teaching. The latter takes the form of demonstration materials for the education of medical students and the use of verbatim transcripts in the clinical education and supervision of resident physicians, psychologists, etc. (see Thomä and Rosenkötter 1970).

Table 5

Text type	Textbank			Audio/Video		
	P	T	S	P	T	S
1 Counseling	1	1	1			
2 Short Term Psychotherapy	4	3	14	25	8	547
3 Analytic Psychotherapy	17	11	78	8	6	782
4 Psychoanalysis	22	13	826	22	9	4557
5 Marital Psychotherapy				*2	2	17
6 Family Psychotherapy	*7	7		43		
7 Group Psychotherapy				*3	2	140
9 Group Work	*4	2		4		
11 Behavior Psychotherapy	1	1	1	3	1	9
12 Initial Interview	300	19	308	218	20	272
13 Initial Interview Report	247	12	291			
14 Psychotherapy Case Notes	5	2	23	1	1	58
15 Psychoanalysis Case Notes	2	1	59	4	1	127
18 Balint Group Work	*2		154	*5	3	150
19 Self-experiential Group	*4	2	43			
20 Dreams	36	2	55			
22 Psychological Testing	16	1	128			
23 Catamnestic Interview	24	1	24			
24 TAT (Thematic Apperception Test)	73	6	73			
25 "Narrative"	73	6	73			
26 Genetic Counseling	29	4	29			
29 Individual Reports	-	20	20			
30 Scientific Report	-	40	40			
32 Cognitive-behavioral Psychotherapy	1	1	20			
33 Supervision	6	5	16	8	5	19
34 Psychiatric Interview	8	5	8			
Total	882	16	2311	299	58	6678

P = Patient T = Therapist S = Session. * Couple, Family, Group

Two-thirds of the material in the ULM TEXTBANK has come from Ulm. The other third has been supplied as a result of scientific contacts and joint research projects with institutions outside of Ulm. In most cases these contributions were tied to the right to use the TBS services. While these donations were primarily from the narrow field of psychotherapy, the outside users were almost exclusively linguists who did not require services of the TBS other than the provision of recordings and transcripts along with word and line counts. At present there are contacts with about 30 institutes in Germany, 4 in the United States, 2 in Sweden, 2 in Switzerland and 1 in Austria. Table 5 gives an informal summary of the large variety of materials currently stored in the ULM TEXTBANK. All together, the electronically stored texts include a vocabulary of 135,000 German and 20,000 English words and a total of more than 10 million.

5. Representativeness

Questions as to the representativeness of the ULM TEXTBANK are oriented around the goals of research. However, there are general practical limits such as the large number of hours in each treatment.

In selecting the individual interviews to be stored in the TEXTBANK a number of considerations other than practical ones are important. Several of these, in order of importance, are: the numerical balance among the different therapists, diagnostic categories that are relevant to the central subject of research (anxiety), treatments lasting 300 to 500 hours, and the success of the treatment. Other criteria for selection that would be especially relevant for statistical evaluations, such as the sex distribution of patients and therapists and patients' social class, cannot be accomplished due to the small number of cases. Thus the database of psychoanalytic texts at Ulm is only representative with respect to their specific research goals.

6. Protection of Personal Data

When entering a text into the TEXTBANK, all personal names, geographic references, and other personal characteristics are coded by means of a cryptographic procedure or replaced by *pseudonyms*. While the texts which have thus been made virtually anonymous (Schlörer 1978) are processed at the University's computer center, the key data, i.e., all personal data, remain in the microcomputers used exclusively by the ULM TEXTBANK. This separate storage, as well as extensive controls on retrieval and manipulation, in large measure protect the ULM TEXTBANK against misuse. The personnel working at the TEXTBANK are subject to professional discretion and instructed as to the relevant regulations with regard to the protection of personal data. The ULM TEXTBANK is registered with the Data Protection List of Baden-Württemberg.

7. Availability and Costs

The services of the ULM TEXTBANK are available essentially free of charge to scientific institutions. Charges are made only for the costs of labor-intensive tasks, such as the transcription of tape recordings and, for university institutions, small charges for materials. In return, it is expected that the texts that are added in this way remain in the TEXTBANK, accessible to other scientists.

With regard to text material loaned by the TEXTBANK, it is expected that a copy of the report of any work using this material be supplied to the ULM TEXTBANK. In this way, in addition to the actual texts, an increasing amount of knowledge about the texts from different disciplines can be stored and made available to others. The ULM TEXTBANK is open to all who wish to store their own texts there. The opportunity for routine or individually tailored text analyses, the convenience of text management, and the variety of options for different outputs should serve as encouragement enough to use the services.

For more technical details concerning structure, data, or usage of the ULM TEXTBANK see Mergenthaler (1985).

Time-Series Analysis of Psychoanalytic Treatment Processes: Sampling Problems and First Findings in a Single Case*

Hans-Joachim Grünzig

1. Introduction

For several years our research group at Ulm University has been investigating long-term psychoanalytic treatment processes. The principal data base consists of tape-recorded treatment sessions with subsequent verbatim transcriptions (see Kächele et al. 1973; Kächele et al. 1975; Kächele et al., this volume). There are of course many different problems to be solved, only one of which is the focus of this contribution. The verbatim transcription of the tape-recorded psychotherapeutic dialogue is an extraordinarily time consuming endeavor; it takes approximately 15 to 20 hours to transcribe one 50-minute session but the transcribing permits subsequent computerized studies. For economic reasons long-term psychoanalytic treatments extending over several hundreds of sessions can therefore be investigated only by means of time sampling.

Different methods of time-series sampling may be considered e.g. random samples in different variations or a typical selection of treatment sessions in which characteristics occur which are specific for a given research question. Unfortunately, there is no sampling theory for time-series from which methods for arriving at time-series samples might be derived; the existing attempts to formulate a psychoanalytic process theory (see Thomä und Kächele 1975, 1987; Fürstenau 1977) are not yet precise enough in order to yield sampling criteria. For practical research problems we formulated a few sampling criteria which are not strictly founded in a theoretical sense:

1. The sample should cover the entire treatment process in a representative way; sessions from all important treatment phases should

*Supported by the German Research Foundation, Sonderforschungsbereich 129, project B3.

be included. However, the notion of representativity is not defined since the parameters of the distribution of the variables are not known for a single case.

2. For clinical reasons the sample should consist of blocks of several consecutive therapy sessions. Indeed, it is of special clinical interest to investigate short-term changes of variables across a number of sessions, e.g. variables such as "intervention effects," "mutative interpretation," etc.

3. Since the sampling error also is undefined and we therefore had no statistical reason for choosing any particular number of sampled sessions, we arbitrarily chose to include about 20% of the total number of sessions.

Once such criteria have led to selecting a particular sample of therapy sessions then the central question to be answered is: to what extent is there a correspondence between the view of the treatment process resulting from the investigation of the sample sessions and that which would result from an examination of the entire case? Or, to put it another way, would a different sample of different sessions arrived at by using the same criteria lead to the same process description? We have tried to answer these questions empirically by using selected variables in a single psychotherapy case. And the limitations of a single-case study should be kept in mind: the findings from this one psychotherapy can neither be necessarily generalized to other therapies, nor can the results for these particular variables be necessarily generalized to another set of variables. This report represents just a beginning exploration of the problems of time-series sampling in psychotherapy process research.

For these studies we employed the methods of computer assisted content analysis (CACA) using both the variables in the Ulm Anxiety Topic Dictionary (ATD) (see Angstthemenwörterbuch (ATW), Speidel 1979; Grünzig and Mergenthaler 1986) and a count of the number of words spoken by the patient. The ATD consists of Gottschalk and Gleser's (1969) four anxiety scales, i.e., *guilt, shame, mutilation anxiety*, and *separation anxiety*, operationalized as lists of individual words meant to represent each category. A computer program, EVA (see Grünzig et al. 1976), similar to the better known General Inquirer (Stone et al. 1966), performs the CACA by (1) comparing the transcribed text of each therapy session word by word with the ATD entries, (2) keeping track of the occurrences of text words that match the words in each of the four ATD categories, (3) summing the counts for each category,

(4) computing percentages of total text words matched in each category, and (5) counting the number of patient words spoken.

2. The First Two Samples

Several years ago the practical considerations mentioned above led to the following time sample *1a:* out of every 25 therapy sessions the first block of 5 consecutive sessions was transcribed and included in the total. Thus, after 5 consecutive sessions 20 sessions were omitted in the sample, followed by the next 5 consecutive sessions and so on; this time sample *1a* includes N = 110 sessions out of the total of 517 therapy sessions. With the exception of the end of the therapy the number of sample sessions is exactly 20% of all of the sessions and the sample blocks are evenly distributed across the entire therapy.

Another time sample, *1b,* consisted of blocks of 8 consecutive sessions interrupted by variable, random length intervals of omitted sessions. The block length of 8 sessions was chosen to allow for a reliable estimation of autocorrelations (see below) and the random intervals were chosen to compare with the 20-session fixed length omissions in sample *1a.* This time sample *1b* includes N = 112 sessions out of the total 517 therapy sessions. Although the length of the intervals between blocks was determined by random numbers (within a range), in order to minimize transcribing effort, we made minor corrections so that several sessions from the 5-session blocks that had been previously transcribed could be used for this alternative sample *1b.* Therefore these two samples were not entirely independent of each other. Table 1 shows these two samples; the correspondences in the selected sessions selected can be seen.

Our goal was to determine whether certain statistical analyses of these two time-series would lead to similar results. The theoretical basis for our analyses was the ARIMA methodology of Box and Jenkins (1976) (see also Glass et al. 1975; McCleary and Hay 1980).

For those readers who are not familiar with the ARIMA methodology, a brief summary together with a rough explanation of some technical terms is inserted. The aim of this methodology is to investigate regularities, i.e., serial dependencies within a given series of time ordered data values. A consistent increase or decrease of the time-series values over time is called a *trend* and is denoted by the letter *I* in the ARIMA abbreviation; *I* stands for *integrated* process and can adopt the values 0 (no trend; stationary time-series), 1 (for a linear trend), 2 (for a quadratic trend), etc. The value of *I* denotes the order of the integrated process.

Table 1 Schematic Presentation of the 5-Session-Block, Sample 1a and the 8-Session-Block, Sample 1b

Sample 1a 5-session-block N = 110	Sample 1b 8-session-block N = 112	Sample 1a 5-session-block	Sample 1b 8-session-block
I 1 - 5	1 - 8 I	XII 276 - 280	
II 26 - 30	25 - 32 II	XIII 300 - 304	297 - 304 X
III 51 - 55		XIV 326 - 330	
IV 76 - 80	73 - 80 III	XV 351 - 355	348 - 355 XI
V 101 - 105	98 - 105 IV	XVI 376 - 380	376 - 383 XII
	109 - 116 V		
VI 126 - 130		XVII 401 - 405	
VII 151 - 155	150 - 157 VI	XVIII 421 - 425	
VIII 176 - 180	172 - 179 VII	XIX 445 - 449	442 - 449 XIII
IX 202 - 206	202 - 209 VIII	XX 476 - 480	
X 221 - 225		XXI 502 - 506	
XI 251 - 255	249 - 256 IX	XXII 513 - 517	510 - 517 XIV

For a further description of serial dependencies, two different mathematical models are suggested: the *autoregressive* (AR) model and the *moving average* (MA) model. The *AR* model implies that the value of a variable at a given time point is dependent on the value(s) of the variable at the preceding time point(s); the number of the preceding time points determining the value of the given data point denotes the order of the AR model. For example, a 1st order AR model (AR(1) model) means that only the immediately preceding data point is determining the value at the given time point. An AR process may be thought of as a time-series having a kind of memory of the preceding data value(s).

The *MA* model implies that the value at a given time point is composed of a certain data level (which is assumed to be constant for the entire time-series) with a deviation caused by so called random shocks that occurred at the preceding time point(s); the number of the preceding time points at which those random shocks with an influence on the given data point occurred denotes the order of the MA model. For example, a 1st order MA model (MA(1) model) means that such a random shock occurred only at the immediately preceding time point. An MA process may be thought of as a homeostatic process over time, the time-series continuously trying to restore its values at the assumed constant level. Of course, all three models may be present in a given time-series.

In order to identify the presence of a serial dependency model, the autocorrelation function and the partial autocorrelation function have to be computed. Computing an *autocorrelation* means to correlate the values of the time-series with the same values being shifted for 1, 2, 3 or more time points (*lag*); at lag = 0 the autocorrelation yields a value of r = 1. The set of autocorrelations for several lags is called an autocorrelation function (*ACF*). For the computation of *partial autocorrelations*, similar to the partial correlations in classical statistics, the determining influence of the 1, 2, 3 or more preceding data points (for lag = 2, 3, 4 or more) on the given data point is eliminated and a, so to say, "uncontaminated" autocorrelation for a given lag is computed. At lag = 1, the autocorrelation is the same as the partial autocorrelation. The set of partial autocorrelations for several lags is called a partial autocorrelation function (*PACF*). The complex problem of estimating the model parameters is omitted at this place; the model parameters are further specifications of the time-series model identified.

After eliminating the identified serial dependency model from the time-series, the resulting *residual* time-series is said to be serially independent (white noise) if the ACF and the PACF of the residuals are non-significant; at the same time, this is a test of correctness for the dependency model identified.

3. Comparing the Samples *1a* and *1b*

For all 5 variables in both samples the time series are stationary without trend and with no clear periodicities. In the computation of the autocorrelation function (ACF) and the partial autocorrelation function (PACF) the "lags" between the individual session blocks are taken into consideration. Table 2 shows the ACF and the PACF up to lag 4 for the 5 variables in samples *1a* and *1b*.

For the *guilt* category there are no serial dependencies; evidently this variable consists mainly of white noise. The high values for lag 3 of *mutilation* are hints for a periodicity which, however, is not supported by values of the higher order lags; the entire ACF up to lag 50 in both samples is not significant however. The ACF and PACF of *shame* are not typical and, with their low values, do not indicate a clear dependency model; a preliminarily computed moving-average model of first order, MA(1), in both samples leads to a significant parameter and to serially independent residuals. The same is true for *separation*. A clear autoregressive dependency model of first order, AR(1), can be seen, however, in the *patient word count*. Now, we have a first answer to our central question: "Is there a correspondence between the two time samples?" In all 5 variables the values of the ACF and the PACF in the two samples correspond to a very high degree; if at all, there is a slight difference for *patient word count*.

In Table 3 the model parameters as well as the ACF and the PACF of the residuals in the two samples are shown, after the computation of a MA(1) model for *shame* and for *separation* and an AR(1) model for *patient word count*. A constant and very high correspondence between the two samples can be seen in Table 3.

Table 2 Comparison of the Autocorrelation Function (ACF) and the Partial Autocorrelation Function (PACF) in the Two Samples 1a and 1b for the 5 Variables

	ACF		PACF	
	1a	1b	1a	1b
	5-Sess. Block N = 110	8-Sess. Block N = 112	5-Sess. Block N = 110	8-Sess. Block N = 112
Shame	.208	.208	.208	.208
	-.003	.040	-.048	-.087
	.102	.036	-.076	.022
	.098	.119	-.031	.101
Mutilation	.181	.151	.181	.151
	.048	.116	.015	.096
	.243	.197	.212	.152
	.080	-.026	-.051	-.152
Guilt	.056	.048	.056	.048
	.078	.156	.075	.154
	.011	.027	-.001	.012
	-.015	-.055	-.033	-.102
Separation	.257	.241	.257	.241
	.138	.065	.077	.007
	-.009	.027	-.148	-.116
	.020	.064	-.095	.025
Patient Word Count	.368	.461	.362	.461
	.245	.372	.127	.203
	.202	.215	-.083	-.417
	.133	.198	-.353	-.963

Table 3 Comparison of the Model Parameters and the Residuals in the Two Samples 1a and 1b

	Model Parameters			Residuals ACF		Residuals PACF	
		1a	1b	1a	1b	1a	1b
Shame MA (1)	X	8.68	9.12	-.022	.004	-.022	.004
	s	2.68	2.88	-.036	-.033	-.094	-.033
	α_1	-.24*	-.25*	.116	.169	.113	-.168
				.050	.073	.047	.074
Separation MA (1)	X	10.46	10.63	.026	.004	.026	.004
	s	3.52	3.99	.101	-.03	.100	-.03
	α_1	-.24*	-.25*	-.025	-.17	-.030	-.17
				-.115	-.07	-.125	.07
Patient Word Count AR (1)	X	2937	2930	-.105	-.114	-.105	-.114
	s	910	962	.079	.142	.069	.131
	a_1	.483*	.492*	.219	.097	.238	.130
				.051	.088	.101	.098

4. Comparing Split-Half (odd-even) Samples, *2a* and *2b*

It is of course clear that a good part of this high degree of correspondence is to be accounted for by the overlapping sessions in the two samples. In order to establish two entirely independent time samples, in the sense of not having any sessions in common, sample 1b – 8-session blocks with variable intervals between – was split into two samples. Sample *2a* consisted of the therapy sessions with the even numbered blocks, and sample *2b* consisted of the therapy sessions with the odd numbered blocks. Since the initial and the final phase of a psychotherapy are typically conducted under special psychodynamic and technical conditions, the first and the last 8-session blocks were eliminated from this comparison of the two samples. Moreover these two blocks would have fallen in different samples and this could have led to unjustified differences between them.[1] Therefore these two samples *2a* and *2b* each included 6 blocks, i.e., 48 sessions. For the purpose of clarity the presentation of the findings will be restricted to the variable *patient word count* since for the *shame*, *guilt* and *separation* no clear dependency model emerged in these two samples; remarkably, *mutilation* in sample *2a* shows a clear AR(1) model although sample *1b* as well as sample *2b* are not significant in this respect.

As can be seen in Table 4 the ACF and the PACF of *patient word spoken* in sample *2a* – as was expected – indicates an AR(1) model; the parameter is significant and leads to white noise residuals. The values of the comparison sample *2b* again correspond very highly; the slightly larger differences are presumably accounted for by the smaller number of sample elements. Therefore comparing these two independent time samples again led to very similar results.

As the most conservative test of correspondence between these two samples a kind of cross-validation was performed: the autoregressive model of sample *2a* was used to predict sample *2b*. According to the AR(1) model this prediction was made as follows: the last value of the second block was taken to predict the first value of the third block; the first value of the third block was taken to predict the second value of this block, etc. Restricting the prediction to the immediately following value was necessary because a prediction over more than one time point leads to a steady increase in the error of prediction from AR(1) model. The confidence interval of the prediction therefore also steadily increases and the prediction cannot then be falsified (see methodical problems of time-series prediction: McCleary and Hay 1980).

If there really is a correspondence between the two samples the serial independence of the residuals in the "predicted" sample *2b* is to be expected. And in fact, the values of the ACF and the PACF demonstrate the serial independence of the residuals in the "predicted" sample *2b*. The mean of the predicted *patient word count* is 2787 words and the standard error of the prediction is 637; this means that the 95% confidence interval of the prediction comprises about 2500 spoken words; 15 of the 48 predicted values, that is, less than one third, are located outside of this confidence interval. In general it is true that the univariate prediction of

[1]In the previous sample comparison these two blocks could reasonably be considered because they were contained in both samples, and any irregularities would have affected both samples in a similar way.

Table 4 Comparison of the Split-Half (odd-even) Samples 2a and 2b

	Patient Word Count	
	2a even numbered blocks N = 48	2b odd numbered blocks N = 48
ACF	.348 .231 .171 .102	.377 .369 .191 .115
PACF	.384 .098 -.135 -.376	.377 .264 -.233 -.726
PARAMETER	α_1 .347*	.464*
Residuals ACF	-.066 .083 .074	-.115 .217 .012
PACF	-.066 .079 .085	-.115 .206 .059

stationary time-series without any periodicity includes substantial error variance and this error was of course present in this case. In fact when the mean of all of the values in sample *2a* was used as a constant predictor for the values in sample *2b*, only 16 values were located outside of the 95% confidence interval, just *one more* than we found by using the AR (1) model. Nonetheless these findings demonstrate the similarity between the two independent time samples and permit us to answer our central question positively. In all essential characteristics samples *2a* and *2b* have very similar corresponding values and it is therefore plausible that both represent the same actual therapy process.

5. Comparing the First with the Second Half of the Therapy

Next, consecutive samples were investigated. The 8-session block sample *1b*, covering the entire therapy process, was divided into two at the middle of the sample, omitting the first and last 8-session blocks. Again the two resulting samples were independent in the sense of not having any sessions in common. In contrast to the split-half (odd-even block) samples we could now compare the time-series analyses of the first half with those of the second half of the therapy.

On the grounds of simple clinical reasoning it is to be expected that the similarities between the first and second half samples would be smaller than those between the split-half samples, each of which covered most of the time span of the therapy. This is particularly true in the case of long-term psychoanalytic treatment (in this case 517 hours over about 4 years) in which one expects that the patient will change and that the measured variables will reflect that change. Thus it is reasonable to suppose that the serial dependencies that are detected by the autoregressive model will not remain constant over the course of the therapy. Rather it is to be expected that different treatment phases would yield different autoregressive models. We therefore examined the two halves separately.

Table 5 shows the ACF and the PACF for the two halves of the sample for the 5 variables. *Guilt* again is evidently mostly white noise (random variation), but the other 4 variables show more or less clear differences between the two samples. *Shame* follows a clear AR (1) model in the second part of the therapy whereas in the first half it does not. *Mutilation* in the first half as well as *separation* in the second half are characterized by a weak AR (1) process. *Patient word count* however appears to be quite a homogeneous process; both in the first and in the second half samples as well as in sample *1b* (covering the entire therapy time span) there is a clear first order autoregressive process which is considerably stronger in the second half (a_1 = .560) than in the first half (a_1 = .314). In both halves the residuals are serially independent.

Table 5 Comparison of Two 'Consecutive' Samples Out of the 1st and the 2nd Half of the Therapy

	A C F		P A C F	
	1st half N = 48	2nd half N = 48	1st half N = 48	2nd half N = 48
Shame	.145	.314	.145	.314
	-.277	.167	-.305	.075
	-.036	.130	.045	-.052
	.204	.036	.257	-.247
Mutilation	.230	.092	.230	.092
	.149	.178	.101	.171
	.205	.143	.111	.110
	.211	-.182	-.033	-.300
Guilt	.152	-.101	.152	-.101
	.355	.009	.340	-.001
	.121	-.042	.012	-.052
	.026	.134	-.310	-.158
Separation	.099	.229	.099	.229
	-.034	.000	-.044	-.055
	.192	-.134	.194	-.195
	.172	-.051	.137	-.019
Patient Word Count	.288	.380	.288	.380
	.270	.395	.204	.293
	.194	.208	-.011	-.240
	.215	.054	-.126	-.021

6. Discussion

Thus the results of our time-series analyses using 5 computer generated content measures have provided a reasonably clear (if nonetheless limited) answer to the important question: will different methods of sampling the sessions of an entire long-term psychoanalytic case yield similar or different results? And the answer is, *both*, depending on the kind of sample. In both samples *1a* and *1b*, each of which covered the entire span of the treatment, but which differed in the number of sequential sessions in each block and in whether a fixed or random number of sessions were skipped between each block, the 4 content variables were all stationary with no trends or periodicities while the number of *patient words spoken* followed an autoregressive dependency model. And in samples *2a* and *2b*, each derived from the odd-even blocks of *1b* (and therefore also covered the entire treatment span), the results were essentially similar to those of *1a* and *1b*. Thus, all four samples that spanned the whole treatment, though differing in other respects, were, by these measures, essentially similar.

On the other hand the last two samples each covered only half of the time span of the treatment. In these samples the results for 4 of the variables were different in the two halves, supporting the clear commonsense expectation that if the patient changes, i.e., gets better or worse, one ought to find differences between the first and second halves of the therapy if the variables used are at all appropriate, as these appear to have been.

Although the application of time-series analyses here has been limited to answering the one question about different methods of sampling, there are many other potential applications of this technology in the field of psychotherapy research, especially that of long-term psychoanalytic treatment where there will always be a great many potential data points. There is now a range of questions that are of great interest for which time-series analyses are both powerful and appropriate. In this study we used only the patient's text, but many of the most pressing questions in psychotherapy research involve the interaction between the therapist and the patient. Does the therapist suggest content to a patient who then follows with his own elaboration? Does the therapist's focus on the transference (see Hoffman and Gill, this volume) have consequences different from his not doing so? Are the referential activity levels (see Bucci, this volume) of the therapist and patient related to the therapeutic outcome? Are the different consequences of the application of techniques derived from different theories of change in psychotherapy and psychoanalysis (see Silberschatz, et al., this volume)? Indeed, Hohage and Kübler's (this volume) study of the relationship between the emotional and cognitive aspects of insight yielded the kind of data that would be suitable for rigorous time-series analyses.

Whenever one has reason to believe that two or more extended series of events occurring over time are related, as is the case with the interactions of therapist and patient, one is always interested in the *causal* nature of the interaction. Who mainly influences or follows whom? Does the patient adapt to the therapist or vice versa or neither? And so on. It is in principle within the power of appropriate time-series analyses to answer such questions, provided one wisely chooses the variables to measure. Of course such wisdom is not evenly distributed and that is an obstacle. But the larger practical obstacle at this time is the widespread ignorance among psychotherapy researchers of the techniques of time-series analyses. The reader is referred to Gottman's (1981) introduction to the subject for social scientists for nearly painless access to these important research tools.

Different Types of Suffering during a Psychoanalysis: A Single Case Study*

Lisbeth Neudert and Roderich Hohage

1. Theoretical Remarks

All psychotherapeutic schools agree that a patient's motivation to seek therapy depends decisively on the degree of suffering at the beginning of treatment. However opinions differ as to how important suffering becomes in the course of therapy. Moreover within psychoanalysis one finds contradictory views.

In "Lines of Advance in Psycho-analytic Therapy" (1919a) Freud took a strong position on this question:

> Cruel though it may sound, we must see to it that the patient's suffering, to a degree that is in some way or other effective, does not come to an end prematurely. If, owing to the symptoms having been taken apart and having lost their value, his suffering becomes mitigated, we must reinstate it elsewhere in the form of some appreciable privations; otherwise we run the danger of never achieving any improvements except quite insignificant and transitory ones (p. 163).

The technical means by which Freud tried to achieve this was the rule of abstinence in order to frustrate the patient's instinctual wishes. The energy, finding no discharge, would flow back to its infantile origins and bring their representations to consciousness, leading to the conflict being recalled instead of being acted out. From this point of view the patient must suffer in order to improve.

These considerations - anchored in Freud's theories of energies and instincts - have influenced psychoanalytic practice until today. The

*Supported by the German Research Foundation, Sonderforschungsbereich 129, project B3.

rule of abstinence, more than any other of Freud's technical recommendations, was set up as an absolute by many psychoanalysts and often has become a synonym for the psychoanalytic attitude (cf. Cremerius 1984 and Körner and Rosin 1985). "Putting the total emphasis on the attitude of abstinence in terms of a pure technique" (Cremerius 1984, p. 776) frequently created an unhealthy climate in psychoanalytic treatments so that even in 1967 Greenson warned in his popular textbook against excessive frustration of the patient because this would produce 'interminable or interrupted analyses' (p. 278). Of course many psychoanalysts soon started to justify the rule of abstinence not so much by theoretical, but by technical considerations, because they were getting more and more skeptical of the economical aspects of the libido-theory. Abstinence was no longer to maintain the suffering of the patient, but to guarantee the objectivity of the psychoanalyst - objectivity as seen from a positivistic ideal of science.

As part of the theoretical advances in psychoanalysis the perception of the principle of abstinence has also changed. Object-relation theorists, for instance, define abstinence as the ability of the psychoanalyst to not assume the role which the patient offers to him unconsciously (cf. Sandler 1976). According to this approach the patient's suffering does not represent a necessary condition for the success of the therapy. The therapeutic appropriateness of deprivation was one of the points in question as well when structural Ego disturbances came to be taken more and more into consideration. Authors such as Balint (1968), Blanck and Blanck (1974) and Kohut (1971) suggested far-reaching modifications in handling the rule of abstinence. Ego psychology also delivered a new theoretical framework for the understanding of abstinence.

There is one approach, which in our opinion deserves particular interest, namely the so-called control-mastery theory (Weiss and Sampson 1986). In this theory the patient's transference behavior is defined as an instrument of reality-testing: in the relationship with his psychoanalyst, the patient wants to test whether his unconscious pathogenic beliefs are true. These beliefs are the result not of instinctual wishes, but of a primitive theorizing originating in conflict situations of childhood. Being influenced by these theories the patient sets aside important life goals and establishes defense mechanisms, inhibitions, and symptoms. It depends on the behavior of the psychoanalyst whether these infantile theories will appear confirmed or refuted. To be abstinent in this context means to pass the patient's test, that is, to *not* fulfill his pathogenic expectations.

With regard to the patient's suffering, the control-mastery theory predicts that the psychoanalyst - by means of being abstinent according to this theoretical view - refutes the threatening beliefs and thus meets the unconscious hope that led the patient to seek help in analysis. Instead of suffering more, the patient will feel relieved and relaxed because of his psychoanalyst's passing the test. This model of the psychoanalytic process was empirically tested against the process model derived from the theory of instincts repeatedly and turned out to be superior (cf. Weiss and Sampson 1986).

Although turning away from the theory of instincts has been significant within psychoanalysis, its external image has scarcely changed. The cliché of the frustrating psychoanalyst who makes the treatment a depriving and painful experience for his patients still exists. Even well-meaning critics (such as Strupp 1978a) accuse psychoanalysis of making a virtue of suffering and of arguing for this from outdated assumptions.

We think that in these objections different sources of suffering related to the psychoanalyst get mixed up. First, it may be the expression of a patient's specific conflict. Second, he may suffer due to specific characteristics of the psychoanalyst's personality, because every negative transference reaction has a larger or smaller component that is focused on the specific personality of the psychoanalyst and how it has been shaped during his professional education, a point emphasized by Gill (1982) and Thomä (1981). And third, eventually the patient may experience suffering due to the psychoanalyst's *technique*. Only this is the context of the suffering related to abstinence.

Unfortunately neither critics nor defenders of a particular psychoanalytic view present empirical data to support their opinions. This single-case study is an attempt to offer data on this subject. We are interested in the following questions:

(1) Which part of the patient's suffering during psychoanalysis is related to his psychoanalyst? Which part has other sources? What are those?

(2) How does the suffering in regard to the psychoanalyst change in the course of treatment? Is it constantly present as one would expect according to Freud? Is it worse at the beginning, while the therapist's behavior is still unfamiliar and strange? Or is there a crisis in the course of treatment? If so, what causes it?

(3) How much suffering related to the therapist is in fact due to his abstinence?

(4) What does the therapist do when he becomes the object of the patient's suffering?

2. Methods

Here we shall be very brief since we have previously described the method (Neudert et al. 1985). We investigated a single case because only this kind of study permits an examination in detail of the variability of suffering during the psychoanalysis. It also offers the opportunity to gather complex and differentiated information, including qualitative clinical data that enable the generation of more adequate hypotheses about the psychoanalytic process. The study was carried out on verbatim transcripts of psychoanalytic sessions by means of content-analysis methods. Since none of the available content-analysis instruments for measuring painful affects (Dollard and Mowrer 1947; Dollard and Auld 1959; Mahl 1961; Gottschalk and Gleser 1969; Knapp et al. 1975, etc.) was suitable for our questions, we developed two special content-analysis manuals.

Manual I was used by independent judges to identify all sequences in the verbatim transcripts in which the patient verbalized painful or unpleasurable feelings. In a second step the judges scored the degree of suffering and the way of dealing with it as it was expressed in the pertinent sequences. This manual consists of four distinct categories and four rating scales. In this chapter we refer to only two of the rating scales:

(1) A 5-point rating scale for judging the *intensity of suffering* in every sequence of the text where suffering was expressed. The various values of intensity from one session are added up to yield a sum score of 'total suffering' (= TS) for each session.

(2) Another 5-point scale on which the independent judges mark the degree of the patient's *helplessness in dealing with his suffering* for every pertinent sequence.

After having been corrected according to the Spearman-Brown formula (cf. Lienert 1969, p. 119), Pearson's r as the coefficient of reliability between judges was .85 for both rating scales.

Manual II was used to measure what the patient suffered from or what he 'blamed' for his suffering. The coding units were the same sequences that were identified according to Manual I. The main categories are 'self' and 'environment'. The judgment is made on a 5-point scale with the poles labeled 'the suffering is exclusively related to self' and 'the suffering is exclusively related to environment'. If the environment is involved, i.e., when the judges check off one of the scale points between 2 and 5, they additionally have to choose one of the following subcategories:

(1) human environment (= h),

(2) therapist (= th),

(3) extra-human environment (= e). (This category includes weather, fortune, animals, etc.).

When the judges are not able to decide who the patient blamed, they are to choose the category 'unclear'.

The measures of agreement were also very adequate for Manual II: the rank Pearson's r (again corrected according to Spearman-Brown) for the rating scale 'relatedness of suffering' was .92 (n = 342), and the Kappa-coefficients (Cohen 1960), which we used to compute the agreement on nominal data, were .76 for the three types of environment and .75 for the category 'unclear'.

Our *sample* consisted of 7 blocks of 8 consecutive sessions each for a total of 56 sessions. We chose this type of sample in order to be able to explore thematic connections across several sessions as well as examine medium-term effects of therapeutic interventions. The 7 blocks were spread over the entire treatment at varying intervals to avoid periodically recurring effects. For a discussion of sampling problems in time-series see Grünzig (1985 and this volume).

3. The Patient

Ms X, the patient of the case-study, was in her mid-30's at the beginning of her psychoanalysis. She was suffering from hirsutism (a virile growth of hair). She lived alone and felt lonely, but had retired from social contacts because she was convinced that everybody perceived her hirsutism as a bad stigma. She was afraid to be observed and rejected, in restaurants for example, and developed a clinical erythrophobia.

Ms X still felt very close to her parents, spending weekends and vacations with them. At the same time she felt restricted by her mother's care for her. She had never had a sexual relationship with a man. In her view this was caused on the one hand by her hirsutism, which she had had since puberty, on the other by her strict religious attitude, which she blamed for her anxiety and her obsessive-compulsive symptoms. Because of these problems Ms X had developed a depressive reaction, which led her to seek psychoanalysis.

4. Results

The treatment was successfully completed after 517 sessions. Questionnaire data, the treating psychoanalyst's assessment, and a follow-up study two years later corroborated the successful outcome. Therefore we supposed that our process data would also show a successful course of treatment. The variables 'total suffering' and 'helplessness in dealing with suffering', which we considered to be appropriate indicators for improvement, were tested for monotonic trends.

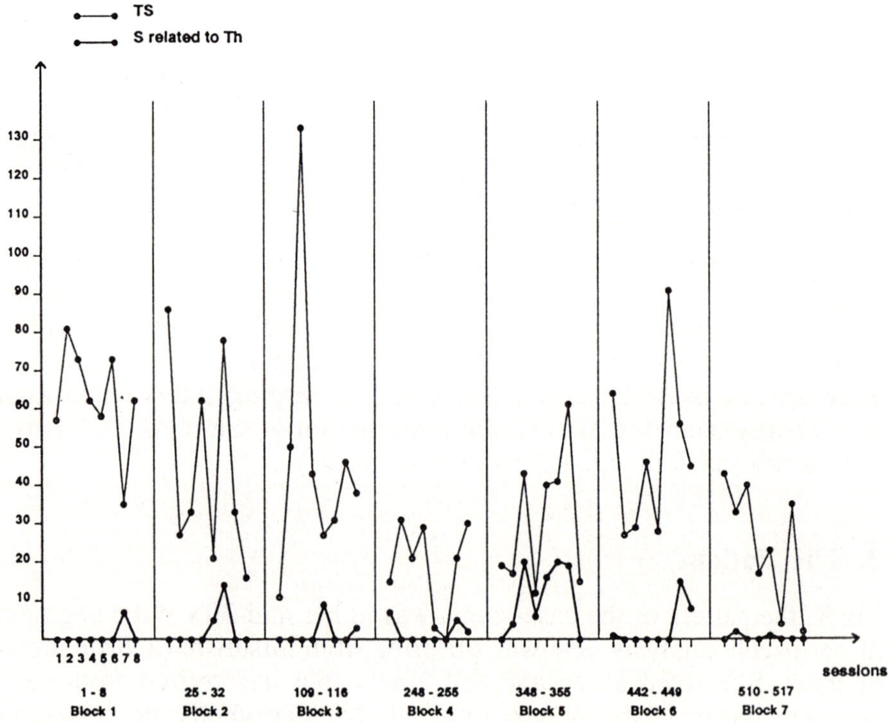

Figure 1 **Open Circles: Course of Total Suffering (= TS): Values of Intensity Summed over All of the Sequences of the Session.Solid Circles: Course of Suffering Related to the Therapist (S related to Th): Summed Values of Suffering from Sequences Which are Predominantly or Exclusively Related to the Therapist**

For this purpose we used a nonparametric trend test for dichotomous data according to Haldane and Smith (1947-1949). The course of each variable can be described as a negative monotonic trend, that is, 'total suffering' ($z = -2.14$; $p < .05$) as well as 'helplessness' ($z = -3.67$; $p < .001$) decreased significantly during treatment. Further serial dependencies according to an ARIMA-model (cf. Box and Jenkins 1976) did not exist.

To compare the proportion of the suffering related to the psychoanalyst with the total suffering, we selected all sequences in which the patient's suffering was predominantly (scale point 4) or exclusively (scale point 5) related to the therapist. Figure 1 shows the two variables over time.

It is obvious to the naked eye that the suffering related to the therapist is low in comparison to the total suffering. This is also reflected in Figure 2, which shows the average percentage of suffering related to the therapist per block.

In 6 out of 7 blocks the suffering in regard to the therapist is less than 10%, and in 3 blocks less than 5%. Only Block 5 presents a totally different result with 34.3 %. For that reason we will later explore this block in more detail from a clinical-qualitative point of view. The mean score for the whole treatment is 7.2 %.

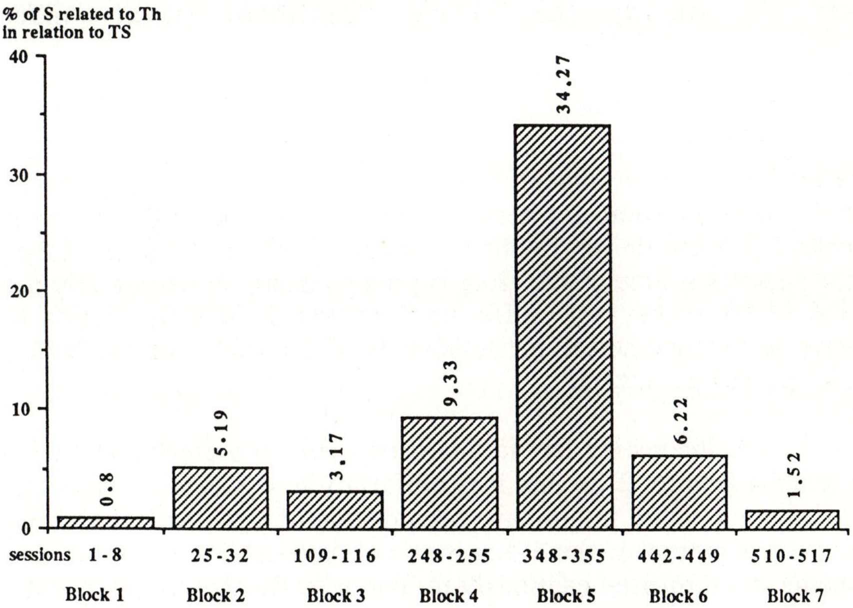

Figure 2 Mean Percentage of Suffering Related to the Therapist per Block (total suffering = 100%)

Now what are the main sources of this patient's suffering during her psychoanalysis? Figure 3 shows the percentages of the different types of suffering for the entire treatment:

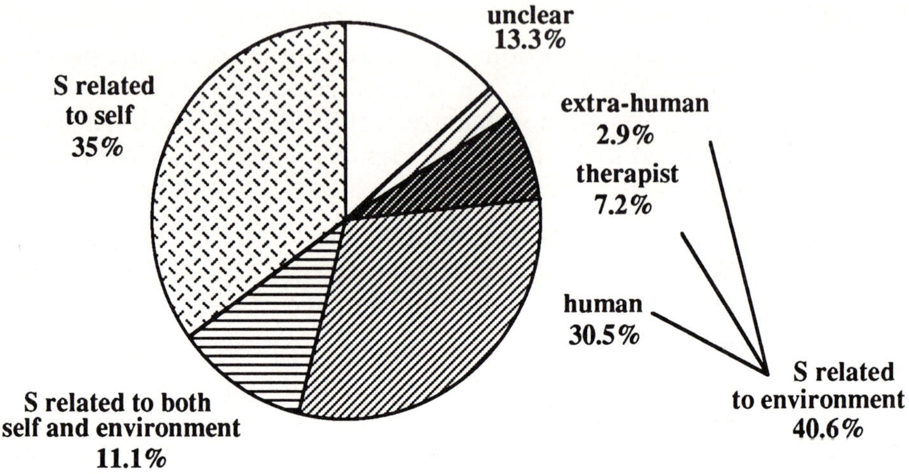

Figure 3 Percentage of the Different Types of Suffering during the Entire Treatment (total suffering = 100%)

40.6 % of the total suffering is predominantly or exclusively related to the environment. Here people outside the therapy seem most often to be the source of her suffering, 30.5% compared with the therapist's 7.2% and the 'extra-human' environment's 2.9%. 35% of the time the patient's source of suffering is predominantly or exclusively herself, and 11.1% of her total suffering is evenly divided in relation to her environment and herself (scale point 3). 13.3% of the total suffering was categorized as 'unclear'.

The interesting fact in the *distribution* of suffering related to the therapist (Figure 2) is that it is uniformly low except in Block 5. One could argue that it might have been difficult for the patient to complain about the therapist; she either may not have talked about this delicate matter at all or tried cautiously to hint at it. But not to talk about one's suffering seems incompatible with the fact that the psychoanalysis was successful. The objection that the patient might not have risked talking about it would only hold true in our opinion for the beginning of a treatment until a trusting relationship has been established. The second possibility, that the patient might have hinted at the suffering related to the psychoanalyst only very cautiously, is not supported by our data. It is likely that cautiously expressed suffering would have been reflected in an increased value of the category 'unclear'.

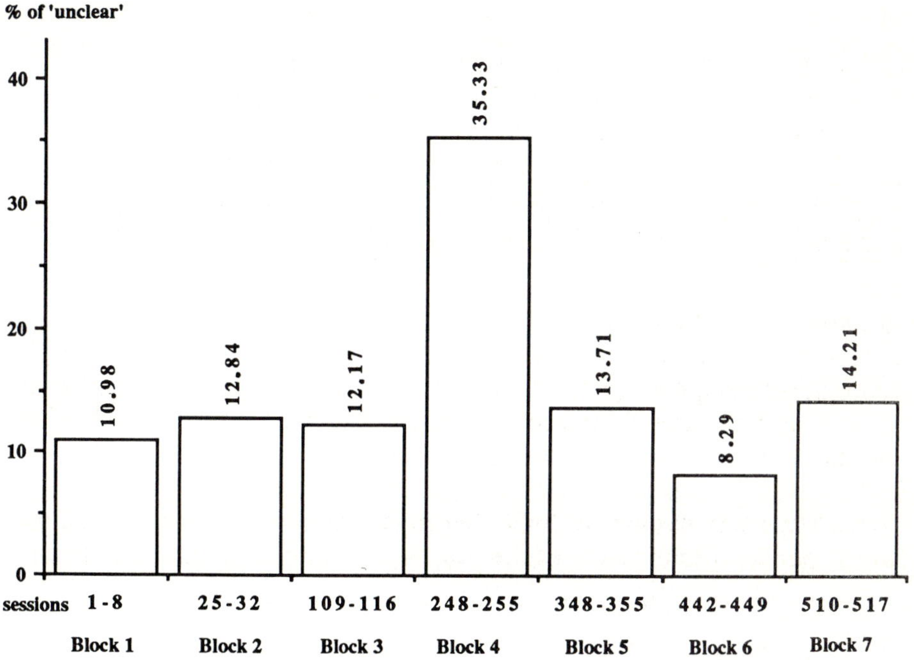

Figure 4 Mean Percentage of the Category 'unclear' for Each Block

Figure 4 represents the percentages of the category 'unclear' for the 7 blocks. The proportion of the category is not higher during the two blocks of the first 100 sessions (with 11.0% in Block 1 and 12.8% in Block 2) than it is in Block 5 (with 13.7%), where the patient obviously expressed her suffering related to the therapist in a direct manner.

So far we have considered only those sequences that received ratings of 4 and 5, i.e., suffering predominantly or exclusively related to the therapist. But the patient's cautiousness might still have found expression in reducing the degree to which her suffering was related to the therapist, thereby increasing the degree to which it was related to herself, i.e., the judges would then have chosen scale points 2 and 3 more often. It was possible to test this alternative by examining those sequences in which the patient spoke in this toned-down manner about the analyst on the one hand, and on the other hand about people who were not present and about whom she could presumably talk more easily. The data do not confirm this alternative. On the contrary, in 78% of the sequences in which any degree of suffering related to the therapist was expressed, this degree was scored as 'predominantly' or 'exclusively'. This percentage of 4's and 5's related to the therapist was even higher than the comparable 63% for sequences of suffering related to people other than the therapist.

In Block 5 suffering related to the therapist reached its peak immediately *following* Block 4 in which the *total suffering* was the *lowest* for the entire treatment (see Figure 1). What might have happened? Could it be that the sudden increase in the suffering related to the psychoanalyst was the result of the psychoanalyst having taken Freud's call for abstinence seriously? Could it be that the therapist, intending to increase the patient's level of suffering, did so by suddenly becoming more abstinent? We tried to answer this question with the help of a very simple and reliable indicator of abstinence, namely, a count of the number of words spoken by the psychoanalyst per session.

Figure 5 shows both the mean number of the psychoanalyst's words per session for each of the blocks and for comparison, the level of the patient's suffering related to the psychoanalyst for each session.

The therapist's mean number of words for the block in question is 855 which is higher than the average of 779 words for the entire treatment. The striking increase of the suffering in regard to the therapist was evidently *not* caused by the psychoanalyst's silence. In fact, if one looks at the entire course of the psychoanalysis, it was not true that the patient's suffering related to the therapist was a function of his silence. On the contrary, there is a small, not quite significant *positive* correlation ($r = .21$, $n = 56$, $p = .06$) between the number of words spoken by the psychoanalyst and the patient's suffering related to him, suggesting, if anything, that the more he talked the more the patient appeared to suffer at his hands!

What then might account for the sudden surge of suffering related to the psychoanalyst in Block 5? Our explanatory hypothesis occurred to us when we took a close look at the variation in all the types of suffering over the course of the seven blocks, as shown in Figure 6. This diagram

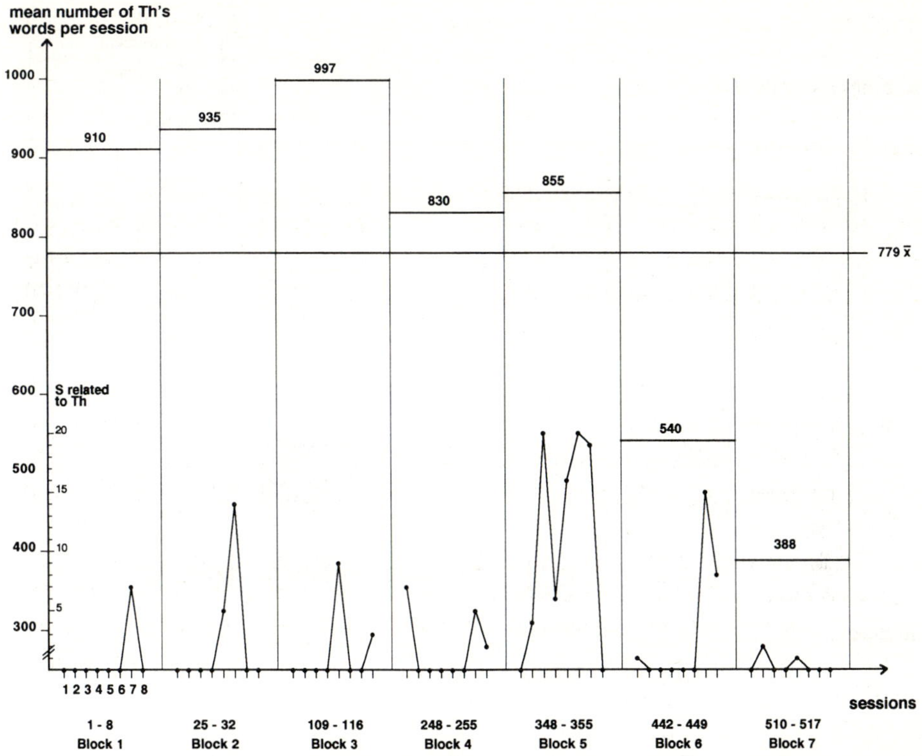

Figure 5 (a) The Psychoanalyst's Mean Number of Words per Session for Each Block and for the Entire Treatment; (b) Suffering Related to the Therapist (summed values of suffering from sequences which are predominantly or exclusively related to the therapist)

makes clear that, for the first time in Block 5, the suffering related to the environment evidently replaces the suffering in regard to herself. Until then the patient apparently had been primarily occupied with her own insufficiencies, insecurities and inhibitions. Now she began - as our data suggest - to tackle her environment, even though it was painful for her. And the psychoanalyst became the primary, and, according to the Weiss and Sampson control-mastery theory, *safe*, object for her painful conflicts. The usefulness of this hypothesis will now be examined in the light of a more detailed qualitative consideration of clinical material from Block 5.

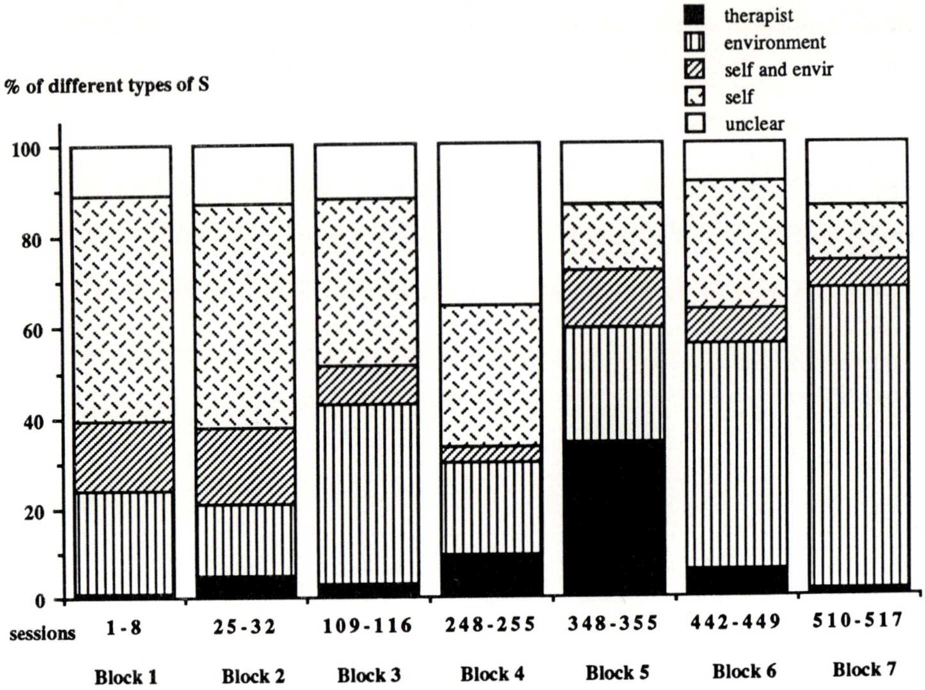

Figure 6 Mean Percentages for Each Block of the Categories: unclear, suffering related to self, suffering related to both self and environment, suffering related to environment, suffering related to therapist (subcategory)

5. Qualitative Results and Discussion

The following clinical descriptions are meant to complete the quantitative results and stick as closely as possible to the text of the verbatim transcripts. Our purpose is to make *plausible* relations among events which seem to be of importance for the psychoanalytic process. Our understanding of and reasoning about the material will proceed primarily along commonsense lines. When we use specifically psychoanalytic interpretations we shall do so explicitly.

The external situation during the sessions in question was the following: at the beginning of this period the psychoanalyst had moved his office. The consistency of the setting was disturbed; a previously unknown part of the psychoanalyst's personal life became visible to the patient.

In five out of eight sessions of this block the patient manifestly deals with topics of suffering which may be understood as paradigmatic complaints about abstinence. She complains that the psychoanalyst is silent so much, that he does not pick up on her offerings. She regards him as inaccessible and not interested in her. On the other hand there are many other sequences that contain no reference to suffering from the psychoanalyst's abstinence. The complaints in these sequences focus on a number of topics. The therapist's move has created confusion. She feels unprotected from his gaze because there are no curtains to dim the light in the new office. And here he also sits too close behind her. He expects too much from her. He asks too many questions about her holidays. And most of these complaints are based upon the patient's *assumption* about the psychoanalyst rather than on his actual behavior (e.g. he does not express any overt expectation of her, at least not verbally).

The psychoanalyst focuses on the patient's concern about both his distance (too silent, not interested, inaccessible) and his getting too close (sitting too close, seeing her too clearly, intruding on her holidays). And the patient in turn is very eager to explain why she is concerned with his getting too close. She might loose control. Her defects (especially her unwanted hair) would become too obvious. And, above all, physical closeness is forbidden: she tells of a colleague who criticized her for touching someone. In psychoanalytic terms, during this period the patient appears to be dealing with an oedipal conflict if this is defined as a conflict about gender and generational boundaries.

So far the psychoanalyst has been looked at only from the patient's perspective. What did he actually do in this block? An evaluation of his interventions shows the following:

(1) He does not intervene less than in the other treatment blocks in which suffering in regard to the therapist seldom occurs. Remember the quantitative finding that the number of the psychoanalyst's words is higher than his mean for the entire treatment.

(2) In the sessions with a high score for patient's suffering in regard to the therapist most of his interventions are focused on her critical, accusing and irritated comments about him. He explicitly encourages the patient to complain about him. When

the patient's complaints are directed toward a specific behavior he does not attempt to neutralize them, e.g. via a transference interpretation, but confirms their realistic aspects - in the manner suggested by Gill (1982). In one sequence the psychoanalyst even accepts the patient's reproach that he once used the word 'dumb' in connection with her, although this term could not be found in the verbatim transcript.

(3) A smaller group of the interventions seems to connect several of the patient's themes. For instance he links her fear of staying in the session too long with her fear of her boundaries being violated by a forbidden touch. But very few of his interventions are interpretations in a stricter sense, i.e., connections with infantile wishes or hints at (deeply) unconscious content. More often, but only in certain sequences, the psychoanalyst focuses on latent meaning.

(4) Frequently the psychoanalyst intervenes by introducing alternative ideas. For example, he suggests that silence could mean approval, not just criticism, as interpreted by the patient.

In summary one can state that during this treatment period the therapist absolutely avoided defending himself. If he had had a defensive attitude he might have glossed over the patient's criticism and suffering or have doubted their justification. And although he was not abstinent in the sense of formally complying with a rule, he handled the principle of abstinence in a functional way (according to Cremerius 1984 and Thomä and Kächele 1987), i.e., against the background of a case-specific psychodynamic understanding: to be abstinent in regard to *this* patient, during *this* phase of the psychoanalytic process means that the psychoanalyst had to avoid - even indirectly through an interpretation - personally defending himself.

Of course, the way the patient experiences the psychoanalyst's behavior is of crucial importance for the development of the therapeutic process. How then did she respond to this therapist's particular form of abstinence, that is, to his abstaining from being defensive? Fortunately we can get a clear answer to this question by examining the last hour of this block when the patient begins to talk about how she had recently been perceiving the psychoanalyst. She had repeatedly complained about the bright daylight in the new office. But suddenly, since the previous session, curtains have been put up. She realizes that the psychoanalyst must have known that this has been planned but hadn't mentioned it when she had complained about the lack of curtains. She then becomes aware that his not telling her was just what made it possible for her to clearly experience what it feels like to be subjected to someone looking at her. And she gets some insight into the benefits of the psychoanalyst's having withheld this information. She feels at ease and relieved by his calm reaction to her attacks. She describes the 'impersonal' in the therapeutic relationship as a welcome protection. And this sense of 'impersonality' becomes so strong that she suddenly can no longer remember exactly what her therapist looks like.

Finally, from a psychoanalytic point of view, one can assume that the patient perceived her psychoanalyst's calm reaction as a relief not only in regard to her aggressive attacks but also in regard to her wishes to be close, even if she still experienced these wishes predominantly as anxieties. The analyst's abstinence did not manifest itself as a rigid clinging to a rule, but was based on a correct understanding of her conflicts. Obviously he passed her test, as predicted by Weiss and Sampson's control-mastery theory, by reacting in a calm way both her criticism of him and her fear of being too close. The patient reacted according to the theory's prediction: she talked about her feelings of relief and relaxation. The 'total suffering' is very low in this session and her suffering in regard to the therapist completely disappeared.

The Emotional Insight Rating Scale*

Roderich Hohage and J. Christopher Kübler

1. Introduction

The mechanism of therapeutic change in psychoanalysis is still a matter of discussion. On the one hand the analysis of resistance and the uncovering of unconscious conflicts or of repressed memories is expected to result in changes of cognitive styles and of manifest behavior. On the other hand the patient will approach this task only in the framework of actual interactions with his analyst. Monadic and dyadic points of view are mixed up even in theories of transference and of the therapeutic relationship, as Thomä and Kächele (1987) pointed out. Self-perception and interactive behavior are related to each other in a complex way that cannot be simply reduced to dependent and independent variables.

Psychoanalytic process research too deals partly with intrapsychic changes and partly with changes of the therapeutic relationship. There are differences in research methods and designs, but not necessarily differences in the theory of therapy. It is useful to study intrapsychic changes and interactive behavior by different approaches and then to compare the results in the course of treatment (see Horowitz 1979). The CCRT-method of Luborsky (this volume) as well as the PERT-method, as provided by Hoffman and Gill (this volume) deal with relationship phenomena in the psychoanalytic process. In this presentation we report on a content analysis scale dealing with the intrapsychic aspects of emotional insight.

Insight is regarded as one of the central concepts of psychoanalytic treatment: therapeutic change should result from gaining insight and not

*Supported by the German Research Foundation, Sonderforschungsbereich 129, project B3.

from behavioral training or from suggestions of the analyst. It has been difficult, however, to define and operationalize the concept of insight for empirical studies (Roback 1974; Fisher and Greenberg 1977). The concept sometimes refers to a goal of treatment (Myerson 1965), to a prerequisite of change (Segal 1962), to a personality attribute, or even to an epiphenomenon of therapeutic change (Hobbs 1962).

Nonetheless there is some agreement among psychoanalytically oriented scientists that a kind of integrative activity of mind is a predominant feature of insight (Kris 1956; Pressman 1969; Hatcher 1973). Scharfman (see Blacker 1981) presented a very short definition: "Insight is bridging different levels of mind." The term emotional insight refers to the fact that self-knowledge is not sufficient to produce changes in patients. Emotional aspects have to be integrated with cognitive aspects of self-awareness (Reid and Finesinger 1952; Richfield 1954; Valenstein 1962).

We regard emotional insight as integration of different frameworks of self-perception. Inner experiences can either be perceived on a framework of emotional reactions or on a framework of cognitive judgments (Zajonc 1980). The patient deals with self-perceptions in an insightful manner if he is able to integrate the emotional access with a cognitive access to inner experiences. If we define insight in this way there are striking similarities between insight and the concept of tolerance of ambiguity (Frenkel-Brunswik 1949). Different frameworks of a self-perception have influence similar to the stimulus ambiguity of outer perceptions, and they may provoke certain psychic conflicts (Hohage 1985). As Kafka (1971) pointed out, tolerance of ambiguity in self-perception and in social interaction is a prerequisite of emotional growth.

2. Method: The Rating Procedure

The Emotional Insight Rating Scale is a content analysis approach using verbatim transcripts of psychotherapeutic sessions. The raters do not have to be clinically trained because the judgments are based on the language characteristics and not on clinical inferences. The rater has mainly to follow his intuitions based on his knowledge of the natural language and his common sense.

Coding units are single significant statements by the patient with a minimum length of ten lines of text. A significant statement is delimited either by the analyst's statements or by pauses of a minimum of ten seconds.

1. *Extent of Experiencing*: The coding units are rated on a 6-point scale (gwE-Scale) according to the extent of experiencing included. There are two points of view that must be taken into account. First, experiencing requires references in the patient's statements to his "inner world" (Meissner 1979), i.e., to his thoughts, feelings, fantasies, wishes, etc. If he only deals with concrete interactions or with descriptions of other people or of situations, there is no reference to experiencing. It must be possible to reformulate his statements in a meaningful way according to a statement like: "The patient is internally ... or internally does ..." Second, statements of the patient refer to experiencing only if the patient focuses his attention on this inner world. He has to deal with it consciously and to refer directly to it. The nature of insight requires that the patient recognizes internal acts. This operationalization of experiencing has important consequences: even if a patient is accusing another person in an emotional way, his statements are not rated as revealing experiencing unless he refers consciously and directly to his own feelings. If the coding unit does not refer to any experiencing, it is excluded from further ratings.

2. *Emotional Access*: The emotional access to experiencing is determined by rating on a 5-point scale to assess how much the patient is immersed in his experiences (Sub-Scale E). We choose the phrase "immersed in experiences" because it has connotations of "feelings", "lack of control", and even "overwhelmed". By analyzing portions of text that obviously showed a strong emotional access to experiencing we found three main factors indicating modes of being immersed:

1. The intensity and vividness of the experienced feelings.
2. The extent of imaginative plasticity of the experiences.
3. The extent of the spontaneity and presence of experiencing.

The first indicator refers mainly to the patient's affectivity while the second and the third indicators refer more to the primary process thinking or to the concept of regression in the service of the ego.

The following statement may illustrate how the patient is immersed in her experiencing:

> Oh, that girl, Cathy! I think sometimes I wanted to kill her! I guess she is the only person I would like to put my hands around her throat and choke – where really I must be aware not to have really bad wishes toward her; really bad, you know. She is so, so domineering and haughty, when I imagine how she walks and how she writes her name. I know about each piece of her hair and her skin and I detested her. I hated her like nobody else.

3. *Cognitive Access*: The cognitive access to experiencing is determined by rating on a 5-point scale, the degree to which the patient is at a distance from his experiences (Sub-Scale C). Again, by analyzing typical statements, we isolated three factors indicating that the patient is at some distance:

1. The extent to which the patient observes his experiencing, wonders about it, describes it ironically or expresses it in abstract terms.

2. The extent to which the patient evaluates his experiencing by classifying, by judging, by summarizing, or by confronting it with reality.

3. The extent to which the patient tries to give logical explanations or to analyze his experiences.

The cognitive access to experiencing is illustrated by the following statement:

> In a certain way I suspect that this behavior of mine is sort of tricky, and that it always plays a role. But when I reflect on this, and when I try to find my own way of living, then I am aware that it is necessary to keep on this way, and that I have to clarify my point of view, and strengthen my convictions. I think in the area of sexuality I've changed my mind in recent years,and the only problem is that I can't discuss this point of view in the right way.

4. *Rating of Ambiguity*: The raters were instructed to judge the coding units on Sub-Scale E and Sub-Scale C independently, although the scales are in some respect antagonistic. Normally opposites do not vary independently. However the independent rating procedure opens the possibility that the emotional as well as the cognitive access to experiencing is integrated and therefore present at the same time. In this case we regard the contradictions to be logical ones and integration of this contradiction is synonymous with logical ambiguity. The following statement represents this kind of logical ambiguity:

> The water in that dream, so much water! That was incredibly exciting, how this woman pulled the wagon through the water and it splashed around and she had trouble keeping the wagon on track. That was a – Oh, the water! (laughs) Now I know, oh I know what it means, the water and splashing, and before that the snake as a symbol. Oh I don't have to go on. Lately I've been very fascinated reading a report that described the origin of life, proteins, sperm, procreation, ... extraordinary and fascinating!

The combination of two sub-scales denoting opposite dimensions includes four extreme positions, as shown in Figure 1.

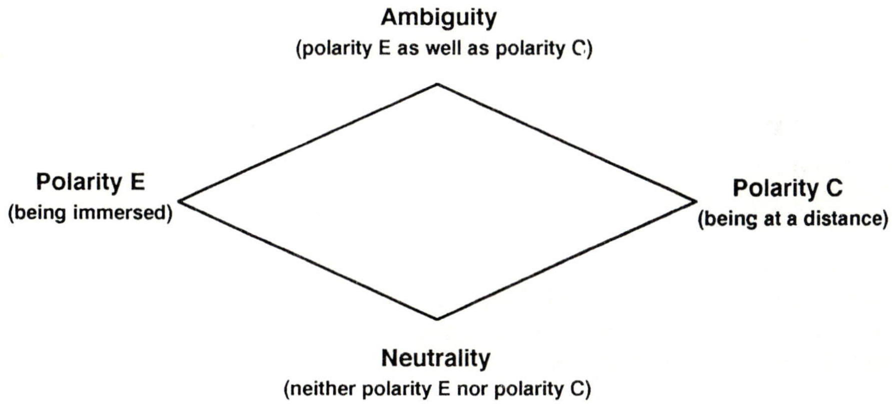

Figure 1 Extreme Positions Obtained by the Combination of Sub-Scales E and C

Polarization reflects a position in which only one access to experiencing is present. Logical ambiguity reflects a position where both kinds of access are present at the same time. If neither an emotional nor a cognitive access is present in the given text, the patient is in a neutral position. The scores of sub-scale E as well as of sub-scale C indicate some kind of active involvement of the patient. In a neutral position there is no involvement at all. We assess the total involvement of the patient by adding the scores of the sub-scales E and C (IN-Score = E/2+C/2)

In principal, ambiguity can be calculated by multiplying the scores of both sub-scales. By definition no ambiguity is observable when one sub-scale has a zero score; multiplication therefore is an adequate operation. We observed, however, that sometimes by chance there are high scores on both scales without any integration, because being immersed and being at a distance are not related to each other. To avoid such pseudo-ambiguity, the rater has to judge the extent of ambiguity on a separate 5-point rating scale (EC-Scale). He has to especially take into account the degree of tension between being immersed and being at a distance at the same time.

In summary the rater has to answer the following questions regarding the manual instructions:

1. Which are the coding units?

2. How important is the experiencing reported according to the weighting-scale?

3. How intense are the emotional access and the cognitive access to experiencing?

4. What is the extent of ambiguity?

The verbatim transcripts are judged by three raters. They obtained 5 scores from each statement: gwE-Score, E-Score, C-Score, EC-Score, and the IN-Score.

3. Empirical Investigations

We now report on changes of emotional insight in the course of a psychoanalysis. The patient in this study (Ms X, a research case; see also Grünzig, this volume, and Neudert and Hohage, this volume) is an unmarried woman, 34 years old, suffering from depression, attacks of erythrophobia, and sexual inhibitions. She has been treated by psychoanalysis for 517 sessions. The sessions were tape-recorded and samples were transcribed. We compared the initial phase of the treatment, that is the first eight sessions, to the eight sessions just before termination. This treatment was successful according to clinical judgment as well as psychodiagnostic test results. We thus expected that there would be more insight at termination than at the beginning. Therefore, all significant statements of the initial phase and of the termination phase were rated on the emotional insight scales. Table 1 shows the reliability of these ratings. Following thorough training, 3 raters showed a high degree of agreement, with reliabilities ranging between 0.85 and 0.88.

Table 1 Reliability of Statement Scores

	Cronbach Alpha Coef. (pooled for 3 judges)
E - Score	0.87
C - Score	0.87
EC - Score	0.85
IN - Score	0.88
gwE - Score	0.88
n = 216	

In comparing the initial phase of this treatment to the termination phase, we had to take into account that there are time-series dependencies among the statements during each session, so that for statistical evaluation we could not treat the single statements as independent test samples. No time-series dependency however was detected when we compared not single statements, but the mean-scores for each session.

Table 2 Average of Eight Mean Scores of the Initial Phase and of Eight Mean Scores of the Termination Phase (Pat. X)

Mean Score of Sessions	E-Score	C-Score	EC-Score	IN-Score	gwE-Score
Session 1 - 8	1.04	1.24	0.31	1.14	1.42
Session 510 - 517	1.63	1.16	0.68	1.39	1.79
n = 16	$p < 0.01$	n.s.	$p < 0.01$	$p < 0.05$	$p < 0.01$

Table 2 shows the average of 8 mean scores of the initial sessions and of 8 termination sessions. The table reveals that there is significant increase of the emotional access, of ambiguity, of involvement and of experiencing. The scores for the cognitive access show a slight decrease at the termination phase. We determined the p-value from the t-test (one-tailed). Although the number of cases is only 8 in each sample, the differences are statistically significant with the exception of the C-Scores.

The data indicate that the emotional insight increased, as we expected. The increase in the emotional access is of special clinical interest too because the patient, as described before, reacted in a self-conscious, often obsessive-compulsive manner, which is reflected in the high C-Scores in the initial phase. In this case particularly, the increase in emotional involvement appears to be an important indicator of therapeutic change.

Finally we report on a micro-analysis of three sessions (1, 2, 7) from the initial phase of this treatment. In these sessions the analyst and his patient referred directly to the "here-and-now," focusing attention on the therapeutic relationship. If we compare the scores of each statement to the manifest content obtained by systematic description, and to the statements of the analyst, we have the opportunity to study how the interaction influences the patient's access to her experiences.

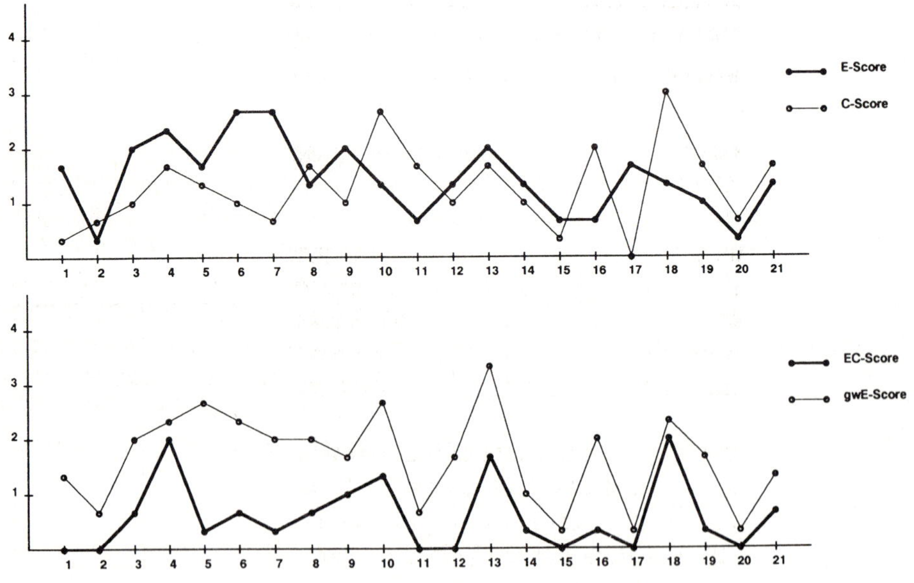

Figure 2 Course of Session No. 1 (Pat. X)

Figure 2 demonstrates the course of the first analytic session recorded.[1] The graph demonstrates high scores of emotional access that decrease slightly towards the end of the session. There are 4 peaks of manifest ambiguity at statement 4, 10, 13, 18.

If we examine the manifest content of these statements, there are two predominant themes: the patient complains that she feels lonesome (statements 5, 6, 7, 12, 13) and she criticizes herself for being too dependent (statements 5, 10, 18, 19, 20, 21). These two themes relate to each other. When describing her loneliness the patient refers to her feelings; at these statements the scores of emotional access tend to be higher than the scores of cognitive access. When the patient describes being dependent, she evaluates this experience self-critically; at these statements the scores of cognitive access exceed the E-Scores. Where both themes converge (statements 10, 13, 18) we observe peaks of insight.

The analyst in this session confines himself mainly to clarifications and encouragement. Following statement 18 however he verbalizes his observation that the patient looks at her watch. He suggests that she is afraid of staying too long and that she does not want him to close this session by himself. The patient in statement 19 agrees: she is a little bit haughty and does not want to be boring. She then says that she has problems regarding her relation to the analyst. In statements 20 and 21 the patient reinforces self-critically her dependency on other persons, especially her mother. In these statements the cognitive access to experiencing is high.

The course of this session mainly reflects a free and comfortable exchange between patient and analyst, including emotional insight and emotional involvement. This somewhat easy attitude has been described as typical for the initial phase of psychoanalytic treatment (Gitelson 1962). When the analyst confronts the patient for looking at her watch he focuses her attention on the "here-and-now." The patient's look at her watch might be a reaction to the fear of becoming dependent on the analyst. The confrontation seems to strengthen the conflictual aspects of this dependency and it is interesting that the patient reacts with agreement, but at the same time strengthens the cognitive and self-critical aspects of her feelings.

---

[1]Preceding this session there had been several initial contacts including some therapeutic interventions.

Figure 3 demonstrates the course of the second session. In the first half of this session there are high ratings of emotional access, experiencing and insight. In the second half emotionality decreases (except for the final statement, 18) and no insight is rated. The cognitive aspects of experiencing increase, however, with a peak at statement 14.

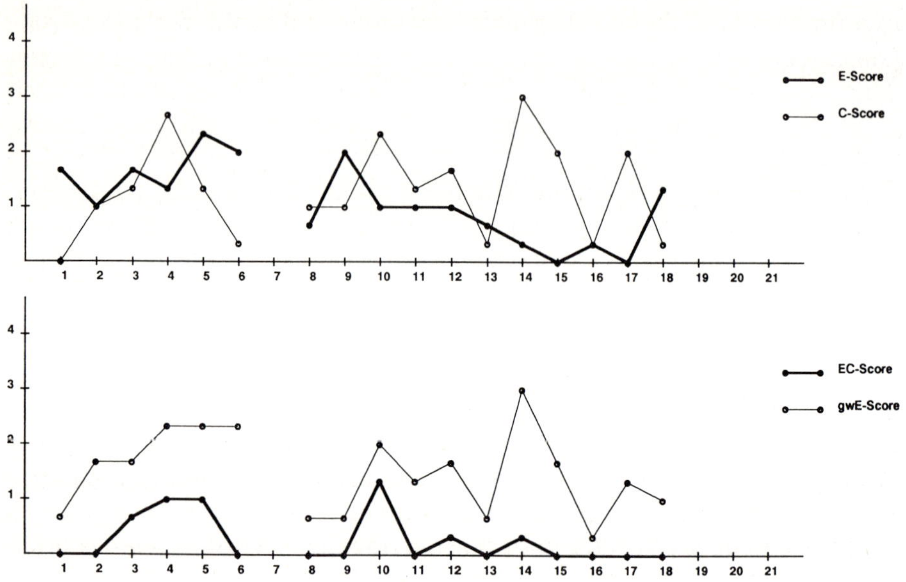

Figure 3 Course of Session No. 2 (Pat. X)

According to the manifest content of this session the patient reports that friends visited her and that she did not dare to end their visit at an appropriate time. She complains that she feels painful in such situations because she does not want to be like a bouncer and that she often is too self-conscious and anxious (statements 1 to 4). The analyst in his first interventions makes clarifications and encourages her to express her feelings. Following statements 4 and 5 he emphasizes that she had suppressed her anger at her friends. In statement 6 the patient describes her anger towards herself and her self-criticism which is in contrast to the view other people have of her. This description is plaintive and emotional. Statement 7 was not rated because the patient only describes an interaction with her chief without reference to her experiencing. She then describes herself as being inferior to her brothers, falls silent, and in statement 8 she asks the analyst for his opinion. The analyst does not answer directly, but just repeats her description.

Following this incident the patient emphasizes her tendency to feel like an underdog, doing so first more emotionally, and later on more insightfully and self-critically. The analyst asks for details and the patient offers them in statements 11, 12 and 13. During statement 13 she again looks at her watch. The analyst now gives an interpretation connecting her tendency to be concerned about somebody else with her fear of being angry. Following this interpretation the patient complains at length about her self-consciousness, her obsessive thoughts and her inhibitions. This is reflected by a peak in the cognitive ratings when she begins to wonder about the meaning of the analytic setting. She later accepts that it might be of use if the analyst does not influence her thoughts. The analyst finally connects her concern about her friends to the concern about him.

There are two important incidents in the manifest interaction of this session: (1) the question about the analyst's opinion and, (2) the renewed confrontation with her looking at her watch. The evasive answer of the analyst might have been disappointing to the patient but again – just as in the session before – she reacts with a self-critical attitude. The renewed confrontation with her looking at her watch must have been irritating too, but here again the patient is very compliant; for instance, in fantasizing about the analyst's possible reactions she does so by strengthening her self-criticism and the cognitive access to her experience. This pattern seems typical of the way the patient copes with conflicts in the therapeutic relationship.

Session 7 also reveals some important interactions referring to the here-and-now. Its course is shown in Figure 4.

According to the manifest content the patient opens this session describing business problems. In statements 5 to 7 she reports a dream that deals manifestly with a defloration scene. She wonders about this sexual content and asks repeatedly if other people have dreams like this (statements 4, 7, 8). Later on she explains that she is much afraid of being abnormal (statement 9). The analyst asks questions of his own, and makes connections to her recent experiences with sanitary tampons and finally offers an interpretation of the dream content without answering her question. In the following sequence the patient deals with problems of using tampons and thereafter with feelings of guilt about sexual excitation. In these statements (10 to 13) she strengthens the cognitive access

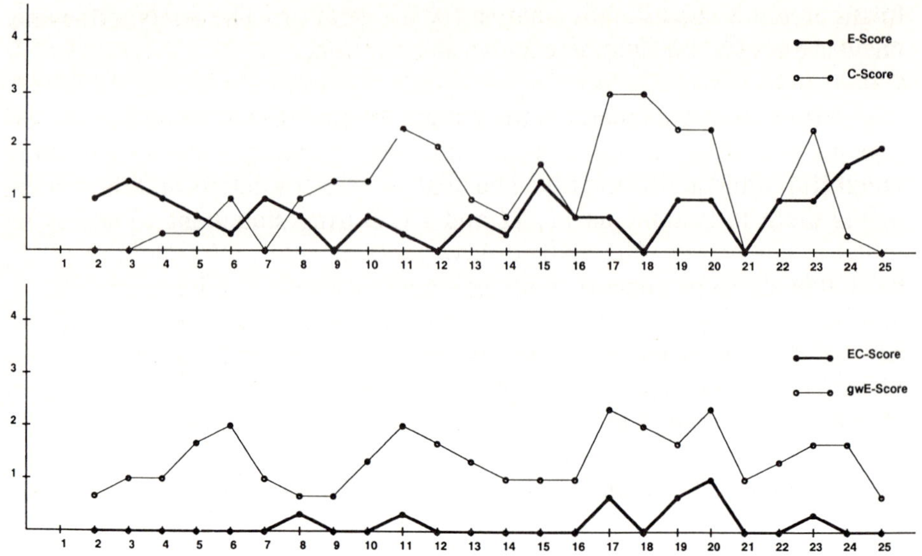

Figure 4 Course of Session No. 7 (Pat. X)

while the emotional access is low. In statement 14 the patient gives up asking questions ("I have known that you would not answer me"). She accepts the dream interpretation (statement 16), begins to ruminate about her wishes for therapeutic support, and the complains about her conscience and her dependency on other people, etc. (statements 15 to 20). This sequence is accompanied by very high scores for cognitive experiences and low scores for emotionality. Following statement 21 the patient stops talking. She resists reporting another dream that came to her mind and she argues that this dream would be depressing and indiscreet (statement 22). The analyst points out that she had momentarily tried to look at him and she replies that she feels embarrassed and surprised because he observed her impulse. In statement 23 she assures the analyst that she is accepting the treatment and then explains at greater length why she resists reporting this dream.

This session has a similar pattern to session 2: the patient asks questions and seems to be disappointed that the therapist does not answer, but she tries to be compliant and accept the dream interpretation and the analytic setting. Both analyst and patient are dealing manifestly with the here-and-now, but not directly with her disappointment and anger. Our rating scores reveal that this patient at this phase of treatment repeatedly reacts to conflicts in the therapeutic relationship by strengthening self-critical and obsessive-compulsive patterns. She withdraws from emotional experiences despite many allusions to unconscious affect. The emotional access therefore is low, and the discussion does not lead to emotional insight.

4. Discussion

We have reported on a method for assessing certain aspects of emotional insight, and we have demonstrated changes in emotional insight in the course of three early sessions taken from a psychoanalysis.

This approach consists of a quantitative assessment not only of insight itself but of the emotional and the cognitive involvement of the patient as well. Of course therapeutic change is reflected not only by different insight scores. Nonetheless it may indicate an important step if the patient begins to deal with himself and not only with other persons. In such cases an increase in the extent of experiencing is a relevant result. The patient described in this report however seems to be psychologically minded and often deals with her own thoughts and feelings. Therefore, changes in the experiencing score here are of less importance. On the other hand under the impact of psychic conflict this patient seems to strengthen her cognitive access to experiencing and it is therefore an important therapeutic change that, under the pressure of termination, she is able to remain emotionally involved. This finding is supplementary to the finding of increased insight scores.

By rating not only integration, but the emotional and the cognitive access separately as well, we differ from other content analysis approaches that quantify related phenomena, such as the Meaningfulness Scale of Isaacs and Haggard (1966), the Productivity Scale of Simon et al. (1967) and especially the Experiencing Scale, provided by Gendlin and Tomlinson (1962). The Experiencing Scale has some striking similarities to our approach, but the cognitive dimension is neglected, as criticized by Wexler (1974) and Bense (1977).

The evaluation of the rating procedure includes three different levels:

1. By comparing sequences of several hours we can examine the structural affective-cognitive patterns of the patient. If a long sequence

of hours is investigated the probability is low that the findings are based only on situational factors. So the differences between the initial phase and the termination phase of this patient are found in a total of 249 statements, most of them indicating a more insightful emotional attitude in the patient at termination. This supports the interpretation that in this respect a significant change took place.

2. Within segments of treatment we can describe and follow the mean scores for each session. In this way it is possible to study the influence of situational factors on the insight variables and to correlate insight with other variables such as anxiety level, level of suffering, etc. The results of this evaluation will be reported elsewhere.

3. If the statements within a single session are compared, as demonstrated in this paper, it is possible to study the influence of the therapist's actions and interpretations on the patient's insight. In these initial sessions the analyst confronts the patient with her looking at her watch, and he does not answer her questions. Thomä, Schrenk and Kächele (1985), referring to such clinical observations, urge a more liberal technique of answering questions to promote a good therapeutic relationship. In this case our findings seem to support their view, at least with respect to the emotional insight ratings.

One has to take into account however that this approach only determines certain aspects of insight, not insight itself. By focusing on the patient's access to experiencing, the concept of insight as an increase in self-knowledge or of insight as awareness of unconscious motives is neglected. We cannot rule out that the patient may report in an insightful way but about insignificant matters, or that she draws the wrong conclusions. The correctness of her conclusions or the significance of her thoughts can be decided only by clinical judgment, and this judgment may itself be right or wrong. On the other hand, a decrease in emotional insight as well as an increase in resistance, if observed in the course of psychoanalytic treatment, cannot simply be regarded as a step backward. The psychoanalytic process has more than one dimension and becoming more insightful is only one among many targets of the process. In the service of therapeutic progress it may be necessary that the patient develops resistances and activates conflicts. Only if it is impossible to overcome such resistances and to work through relationship problems, will the therapeutic effect be questioned. We offer the emotional insight scale to help study such developments and thereby contribute to the understanding of the therapeutic process.

Facial Indicators of Transference Processes within Psychoanalytic Treatment

Rainer Krause and Peter Lütolf

This is a report of a quasi-experiment w hose goal was to objectively define the psychophysical interactional basis of transference and countertransference reactions specific to a patient's neurosis. Two methodological paths, both leading to meaningful data, are discussed; for one of them a single case study is reported.

1. Introduction

Central to the psychoanalytic theory of neurosis is the concept of the "repetition compulsion," which can be loosely defined as the process by which patients repeatedly recreate specific fantasies, affects, and action tendencies in some, most, or all of their relevant interactions with others. Such behaviors consist of unsuccessful and unconscious attempts to correct past, but still unresolved problems (Freud 1920g; Krause 1982b). Even among European behavior therapists there is a certain agreement that disturbed behavior is more redundant and follows some sorts of plans that lead to results the patient does not want (Caspar and Grawe 1981).

Psychoanalytic therapists are trained to use their own feelings, affects, and fantasies as important information during the diagnosis and planning of treatment as well as for actual decision making during treatment. (see Argelander 1961; Brenner 1985). Despite the tremendous importance traditionally attached to such information, there have been only very rare attempts to carefully examine the claim that these feelings, affects and fantasies are a consequence of the patient's behavior and not, as critics have claimed, of the therapist's own expectations (Racker 1968).

Thus, we are confronted with a missing link in the interaction between patient and therapist. Theoretically we assume that the patient has a conscious intention or a wish as well as a set of specific behaviors that interfere with the fulfillment of that conscious wish. These are what we call "neurotic" behaviors. At the same time we assume that the therapist uses a specific decoding procedure that leads to his own feelings, which in turn are used to guide his therapeutic decision-making. This line of thinking is based partly on a multichannel model of social interaction (Scherer 1978; Krause 1982), while a related psychoanalytic version can be found in Bucci's (1985) "dual code" theory of mental representation (cf. Bucci, this volume). From a methodological point of view, investigation of the consequences of this point of view can proceed in two ways, both of which we are pursuing. We focus on one method in this paper, while mentioning the other only briefly at the end.

2. Two Possible Quasi-experimental Situations

A. Interactions Between Laymen and Mental Patients

A reasonable deduction from the concept of the repetition compulsion is that neurotic behavior should be observable in dyadic relationships in which a patient interacts with a layman who does not know that his associate is a mentally disturbed person. The laymen should, if they are not themselves disturbed, react in predictable and orderly ways, narrowing their range of feelings and behavior repertoire as compared with their interactions with healthy people. We have conducted a series of research projects to examine this prediction with schizophrenics, psychosomatic patients, and stutterers, all of whom were given the task of discussing politics with unknown laymen in a standard setting. Some of these results have been published (Hans, Krause, and Steimer 1986; Krause 1980, 1982a, 1981, 1982b; Steimer, Krause, Sänger-Alt, and Wagner 1988) and will not be further discussed here.

B. Psychotherapeutic Interactions

Dyadic psychotherapeutic interactions have some disadvantages for the investigation of transference behavior, among them the fact that the therapist is informed rather than naive and is not supposed to respond overtly to the patient's transference behavior. On the other hand we can get information that cannot be found in other settings, for example, about the interface between introspection and signaling and between verbal and nonverbal data. We can also follow the changes in transference behaviors as therapy succeeds or fails. Finally we might get valid tools for the measurement of therapeutic success. We shall now focus on a quasi-experimental use of the treatment situation.

3. Predictions

We shall report on a brief psychoanalytic psychotherapy that was completely videotaped in the above mentioned setting and lasted 12 hours. We have three videotaped catamnestic interviews up to one year after treatment as well as other outcome measures that showed constant improvement. Treatment was planned according to Malan's (1976a) Focal Therapy, which requires extensive interviewing and testing in order to be able to formulate a so-called focus that describe the patient's nuclear conflict before treatment. If our reasoning has been correct, we should expect that:

1. The nuclear conflict will show up in the transference behavior during treatment.
2. Based on our knowledge of facial activities, we should be able to predict the kind of facial behavior to be expected from the nuclear conflict.
3. If treatment is successful, this behavior will diminish and become available for conscious reflection and monitoring at least once during treatment.
4. With a fixed termination of the therapy, set in advance, transference behavior will be maximal in the middle of treatment, where we expect conscious realization in the patient of that behavior.

4. The Patient

Mr. A, a 35-year-old man, came for help at the urging of his wife because he was troubled by anxiety attacks, especially at night, during which he was afraid that he might cause a traffic accident and kill somebody during his approaching military service in which he was to drive a truck. He thought a military court would end up condemning him severely. Mr. A, on the face of it a very kind and obedient man, had lived with his younger brother and his parents up to the age of 30, when he had his first sexual relationship with his future wife. At the age of 20 his younger brother emigrated to Canada because of difficulties with his parents. The father, a very religious and controlled primary school teacher, had been in psychiatric treatment because of "problems with the other sex". He had had a lifelong obsession about the Russians invading his country and forcing him to act as an interpreter, so, to prepare himself, he learned Russian.

As a child the patient had also been in treatment because of anxiety attacks that prevented him from entering Kindergarten. He never succeeded in getting any formal certificate for his higher education, always failing the final examinations. Nevertheless he obtained a responsible job in a factory. Shortly before the emergence of his current symptoms, his former boss, whom he had secretly despised, died of cancer, and a young man with a formal certificate, whom the patient had trained, became his new boss. At the same time his wife had born him a son whom he loved very much, but he was worried that he might pass along his lifelong problems to him.

Based on the interviews as well as on independent projective testing, our team formulated his focal conflict as follows:

> The patient is warding off destructive wishes against authority figures. He is afraid that a breakthrough of his impulses will kill the weak but arrogant father figures and then, in relation, he will be punished. Despite this latent nuclear conflict he has lived most of his life without manifest symptoms. But now, in the presence of his unconscious death wishes towards his boss, three events have triggered his neurotic behavior: (1) his boss's death, (2) his former apprentice becoming his new boss and, (3) his becoming a father himself. We expect recurrent manifestations of unconscious 'destructive' behaviors as well as defensive behaviors against them. In treatment we expect that the patient will unconsciously try to defeat himself by obediently submitting to the therapist, no matter what the therapist says, especially at those very moments when he most severely doubts the therapist's skills.

5. Hypotheses about Facial Behavior

Based on Ekman and Friesen's (1975) views on facial expressions we made the following specific predictions about their occurrence during the therapy:

1. There will be a high incidence of negative affect, especially anger and/or disgust, masked by friendly social affect, especially joy and happiness in the beginning.
2. Positive affect expressions will be accompanied by indications that they are spurious.
3. Masking will diminish during treatment.
4. The therapist will smile genuinely only when the patient exhibits no facial masking.

6. Design of the Study

Based on a prediction table, which proved to be highly reliable, happiness was assumed to be present if there were innervations of action unit 6, a muscle raising the cheeks and wrinkling the eyes plus action unit 12, the zygomaticus major, which pulls up the lip corners during a smile. The indicators of anger were action unit 4, a muscle lowering the eye brows, action unit 7, the orbicularis oculi, tightening the lids, action unit 23 and 24, a ring muscle pressing or tightening the lips together. Indicators of disgust were action unit 9, a muscle wrinkling the nose or action unit 10, a muscle raising the upper lip, or action unit 15, a muscle pulling down the lip corners or action unit 17, a muscle raising up the chin boss.

In each of the 12 therapy sessions 4 samples of 40 seconds duration each – 20 seconds of speaking plus 20 seconds of listening time – were coded for both patient and therapist segments using Ekman and Friesen's (1979) FACS. The coders achieved a satisfactory reliability of .80 in Ekman and Friesen's final test. The sessions were coded in random order to prevent information about the natural progress of the treatment from biasing the coding. To assess these data the following dependent variables were constructed: (1) the percent of time during which joy was expressed along with anger and/or disgust (INCON%), (2) the percent of time during which the masking affect (joy) alone was displayed (A1%), and (3) the percent of time of the expression of the negative affects (anger or disgust) alone (A2%). This design is shown in Table 1. All three measurements are necessary because masking could drop during therapy as a result of an absolute reduction of joy, anger/disgust, or both of them together. Therefore only a diminution of masking that takes into account the absolute amount of expression of all of the affects is acceptable.

Table 1 Masking Hypotheses

Patient's face		Affect expression 1 "Joy"	
		On	Off
Affect expression 2 "Anger" and/or "Disgust"		State 1 Inconsistency visible S1 = Duration of State 1 in Sec./100 Dependent Variable: INCON% = (S1/G) (100)	State 2 Negative affect alone S 2 = Duration of State 2 in Sec./100 Dependent Variable: A2% = (S2/G) (100)
		State 3 Masking affect (joy alone) S3 = Duration of State 3 in Sec./100 Dependent Variable: A1% = (S3/G) (100) G = Total time	State 4 None of the affect visible S4 = Duration of State 4 in Sec./100 Dependent Variable: NONREL% = (S4/G) (100)

A second set of dependent measures, shown in Table 2, was created to take into account the affective expressions of the therapist as well. One of these is a measure of the simultaneous expression of the same affect in the therapist's and the patient's face while taking into consideration the absolute time of both partners' affective expression (SYNCHRON%).

Table 2 Synchronization of Smiling

Therapist's face		Affect expression "Joy" in therapist's face	
		On	Off
Patient's face	ON	State 1 Both faces smile S1 = Duration of State 1 in Sec./100 Dependent Variable: SYNCHRON% = (S1/G) (100)	State 2 Only patient smiles S 2 = Duration of State 2 in Sec./100 Dependent Variable: A2% = (S2/G) (100)
Affect expression "Joy" in "patient's" face	OFF	State 3 Only the therapist smiles S3 = Duration of State 3 in Sec./100 Dependent Variable: A1% = (S3/G) (100)	State 4 Nobody smiles S4 = Duration of State 4 in Sec./100 Dependent Variable: NONREL % = (S4/G) (100)

A third group of eight dependent measures was created to take into account the synchronization of affect in the dyad depending on the presence or absence of another negative affect. In psychological terms this means investigating whether joy in both faces depends on the presence or absence of an additional negative affect (disgust or anger) in the patient's face. The logic of this design is shown in Table 3.

Table 3 Conditional Synchronization

Patient's face		Therapist's face	
Affect expression		Affect expression 1	
2	3	On	Off
ON	ON (Factor B)	State 1 The therapist shows the investigated affect expression. Patient shows masking. S1 = Duration of State 1 in Sec./100 $SYNCHRON\%_{(p)} = (S1/G)(100) B_{(p)}$	State 2 The therapist does not show the investigated affect expression. Patient shows masking. S2 = Duration of State 2 in Sec./100 $A2\%_{(p)} = (S2/G)(100) B_{(p)}$
	OFF (FACTOR B)	State 3 The therapist shows the investigated affect expression. Patient does not show masking. S3 = Duration of State 3 in Sec./100 $SYNCHRON\%_{(A)} = (S3/G)(100) B_{(A)}$	State 4 The therapist does not show the investigated affect expression. Patient does not show masking. S4 = Duration of State 4 in Sec./100 $A2\%_{(A)} = (S4/G)(100) B_{(A)}$
OFF	ON (FACTOR B)	State 5 The therapist shows the investigated affect expression. S5 = Duration of State 5 in Sec./100 $A1\%_{(p)} = (S5/G)(100) B_{(p)}$	State 6 The therapist does not show the investigated affect expression. S6 = Duration of State 6 in Sec./100 $NONREL\%_{(p)} = (S6/G)(100) B_{(p)}$
	OFF (FACTOR B)	State 7 The therapist shows the investigated affect expression. Patient does not show an affect. S7 = Duration of State 7 in Sec./100 $A1\%_{(A)} = (S7/G)(100) B_{(A)}$	State 8 The therapist does not show the investigated affect expression. Patient does not show an affect. S8 = Duration of State 8 in Sec./100 $NONREL\%_{(A)} = (S8/G)(100) B_{(A)}$

The data were analyzed using a repeated measures multivariate analysis of variance with three factors: (1) number of the therapeutic session, (2) the segment of the hour (every quarter of an hour), and (3) speaking vs listening state.

7. Result

Figure 1 shows histograms of the first set of dependent measures across the 12 sessions: inconsistent expressions (INCON%), smiling alone (A1%), and disgust and anger (A2%).

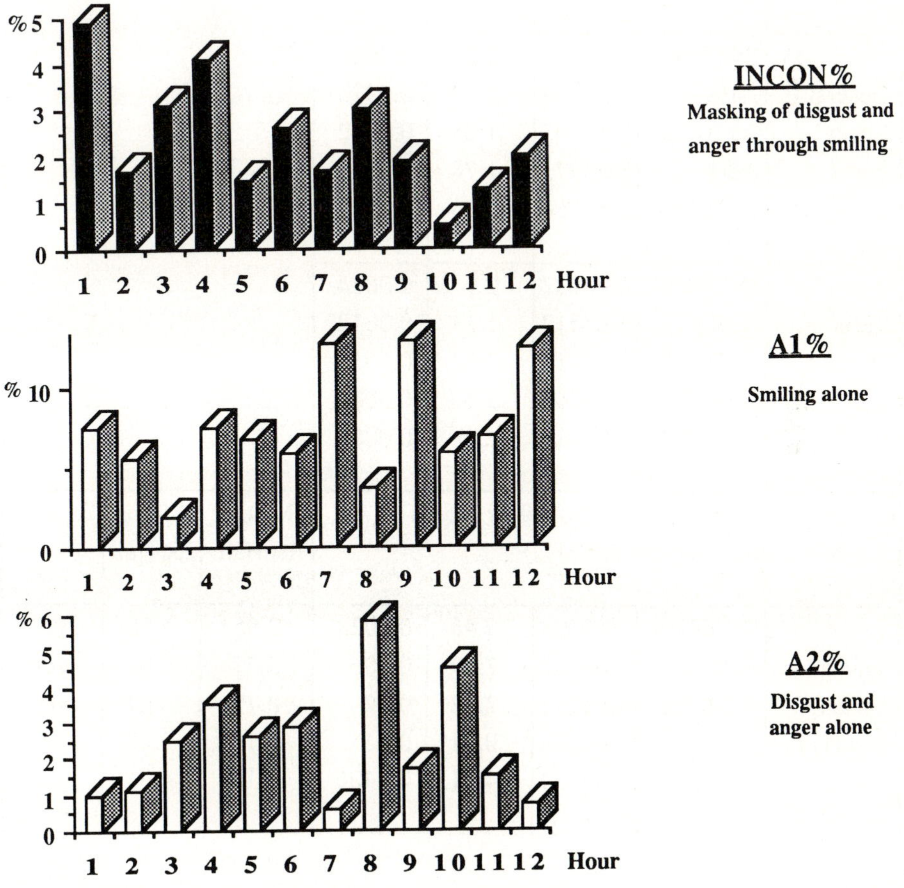

Figure 1 Changes in Patient's Masking

The analysis of variance in Table 4, indicates that there was a highly significant reduction of the masking behavior over the 12 treatment hours, taking into consideration both the covariation of the two affects and the temporal dependencies from one hour to the next. At the same time the smiling alone increased, both from the first to the last hour and from the first to the second half.

Table 4 Development of Masking: Disgust and Anger masked by Smiling

Hypotheses	Dependent Variable	Sum of Squares	F-Value	P-Value			
General Effect	INCON%	0.28751	2.22	0.0001			
	A1%	1.53514	1.39	0.0523			
	A1T0T%	1.83963	1.65	0.0072			
	A2%	0.30973	1.78	0.0025			
	A2TOT%	0.54058	2.03	0.0003			
Mean Effect	INCON%	0.03032	2.9	0.0024			
	A1%	0.23317	3.14	0.0012			
	A1TOT%	0.22717	2.82	0.0031			
	A2%	0.04746	3.66	0.0002			
	A2TOT%	0.08118	3.9	0.0001			
Contrasts of the Mean Effects and their Means					Means 1st Half	Means 2nd Half	Expected
1st Half versus 2nd Half	INCON%	0.00893	9.41	0.0028	2.95	1.58	yes
	A1%	0.05182	7.67	0.0067	5.77	9.06	yes
	A1TOT%	0.01771	2.42	0.12	8.72	10.64	yes
	A2%	0.00024	0.21	0.65	2.19	2.42	yes
	A2TOT%	0.00814	4.31	0.0406	5.15	4.01	yes

A questionnaire investigating the patient's subjective experience of disgust showed that it was highest in Hour 7 and returned to its lowest level in Hour 8.

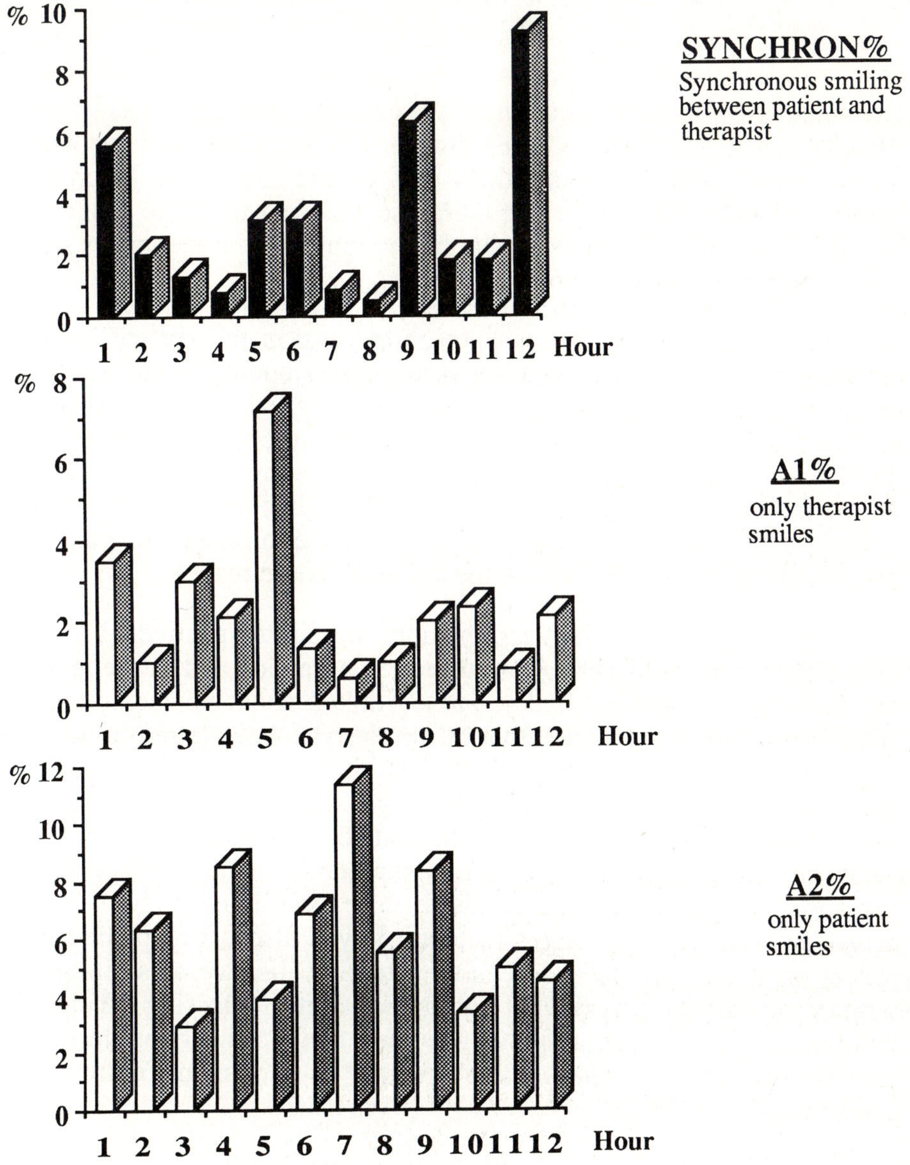

Figure 2

In the seventh hour the patient's negative transference broke through. He started the hour as follows:

> "I cannot find much anger within myself. Sure, I am angry at all these people who I think are torturing me, and angry over the boss of my apprenticeship – extremely angry. But of course I swallow it. I don't defend myself. It's funny, I find I simply can't be angry. No matter what I do, I can't."

Nonetheless he obediently continued to search for angry feelings since he thought the therapist had ordered him to. In a very intense hour with a lot of angry silences (more than half of the hour), he laughingly expressed his triumph over the therapist who had failed to make him angry. In this way he defeated what he thought was the therapist's secret master plan to cure him by making him angry.

The night before the next (eighth) session the patient became extremely anxious. Then, in Hour 8, he talked openly about what had happened in Hour 7 and his anger at the thought that the therapist would try to manipulate him into getting angry. And, although he imagined that the therapist would try to make him angry by being silent, nonetheless, during the session he had been astonished to realize that the therapist did indeed have nothing to say. (His father had once initiated a dispute with his wife in order to find out how the children would react.)

Although both patient and therapist were introspectively aware of the anger, it was minimally present in the interaction and in the motoric expressions during Hour 7. The patient talked about not being able to "find" his anger, not realizing that by doing so he actively reintroduced it into the setting. He was disgusted with the therapist, whom he saw as a looser for not being able to make him angry. Moreover, he assumed that the therapist was in turn angry with him for submissively complying. Thus, he shifted from being unable to experience his anger to both talking about it and revealing it in his facial expressions in Hour 8. This direct manifestation of anger in Hour 8 was also accompanied by a reduction in the patient's defensive affective display of smiling, for without realizing it, the patient had had a habit of showing a kind of a barely codable innervation of 12 (a *smiling trace*). This habit decreased significantly in the course of the therapy, as shown in Figure 3 and documented in Table 5.

There is an increase in synchronous smiling in the first and last hours of the treatment compared with the middle, which is not dependent on the covariate alterations of smiling by the two. The mean time therapist and patient are smiling together, is 4.61 seconds at the beginning and the end of the treatment versus 1.91 seconds in the middle of the therapy, which means the 5th, 6th and 7th hours. This difference reaches significance with a F-value of 5.95.

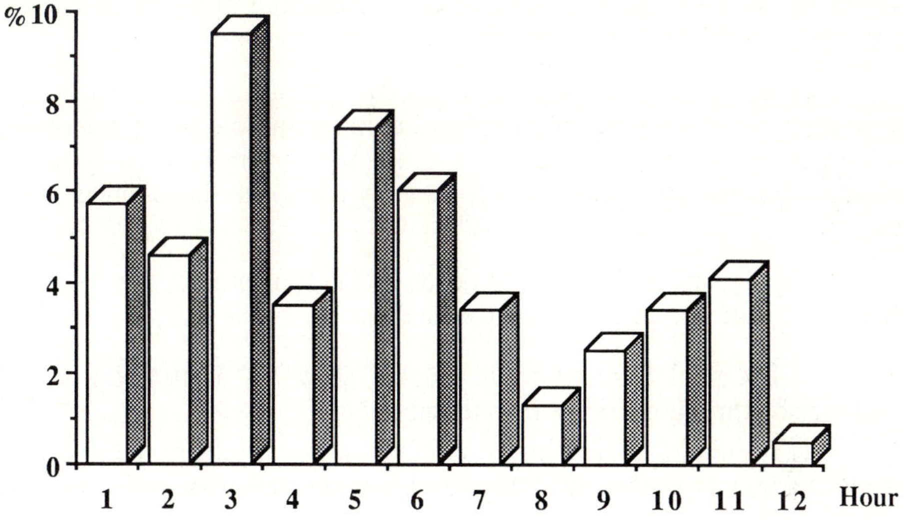

Figure 3 A1% Patient's Smiling (Trace)

Table 5 Patient's Smiling Trace

Hypotheses	Dependent Variable	Sum of Squares	F-Value	P-Value			
Effects							
General Effect	A1%	0.84101	2.38	0.0001			
Mean Effect	A1%	0.11615	3.99	0.0001			
Contrasts of the Mean Effects and the Means of them					Means 1st Half	Means 2nd Half	Expected
1st Half versus 2nd Half	A1%	0.06351	24.00	0.0001	6.16	2.52	yes

The results of the analysis of variance for conditional synchronization, revealing that the therapist smiled nearly five times more often when the patient was not masking a co-occurring negative affect expression. Again, the F-value of 16.38 is significant ($p < .0001$).

These phenomena occurred mainly without any conscious consideration by either party, although once, in the middle of treatment, the therapist mentioned the patient's tendency to smile as a defense. Nonetheless this did not seem significantly related to the changes noted above.

Finally, it is of interest that each of the four predictions we made before the study were supported by the data:

1. The nuclear conflict did indeed "show up" in the both verbal and facial expressions in the transference.

2. The facial expressions did follow rationally from the hypothesized nuclear conflicts: the masking of anger and disgust by smiling diminished over the treatment; smiling alone increased; and anger and disgust were correlated with the transference manifestations.

3. The outcome measures supported the conclusion that the treatment was successful; *and* during hours 7 and 8 the patient did consciously reflect on his intense anger and assumption of arrogance in his therapist.

4. The manifest expression of the nuclear conflict was indeed maximal during the 7th and 8th hours (middle of treatment) of the 12 hour treatment.

5. Subjective experience of the affect was not correlated to the expressive system within the 7th Hour during which the negative transference and the resistance against it broke through. The patient felt a lot of negative affects, but did not show it. In the consecutive 8th Hour during which a working through of that episode happened, the patient showed a lot of negative affects, but he did not feel negative affects anymore, at least not in relation to the therapist.

However, it must be acknowledged that one of the most interesting findings, namely that the therapist smiled nearly five times more often when the patient was not masking his anger and disgust, was *not* predicted.

8. Discussion

Nonspecific effects play a great role within psychotherapy, suggesting that in important domains we do not know explicitly how to account for our everyday successes (or failures) in treatment. Our treatment manuals do not cover all of the curative factors, especially representations of actions, that appear to function in psychodynamic psychotherapies. It may well be that implicit learning processesallow us to perceive and process peripheral details of the inter*actions* between patient and therapist. Krause (1985) has suggested that part of the curative factors in psychoanalytic psychotherapies can be explained within the theoretical framework of conditioning procedures and vice versa.

If, for example, a therapist only smiles genuinely when the patient does not show ambivalent feelings, we might expect this to have certain effects on the course of the therapy. However, it is likely that the specific affective stimuli are processed not consciously but preconsciously, using the information in the facial expression, and that it is in this information that one may find the manifest expressions of unconscious wishes, fears, and defenses. One of the reasons why it is so extremely difficult to obtain explicit knowledge of these inter*actions* is probably related to the fact that the relationship between (1) the multiple communication channels that humans use and (2) the traditional classification of intentions according to their degrees of consciousness is highly dependent both on the type of neurosis and on numerous idiosyncratic factors.

9. Future Studies

In future studies of short term psychotherapy we plan to explore the relations between linguistic variables and motoric affective expressions in the dyadic situation. We end with some preliminary observations of a particular patient that have served as a kind of pilot study to guide us in designing new ways to study the role of affect in the psychotherapy setting.

A 45-year-old lady with severe psychosomatic disturbances and severely disturbed relations with men, which had indeed turned her into the spinster she had always feared she would become, showed, during the first hour of brief psychotherapy, a specific kind of facial expression consisting of a mixture of contempt and disgust. With the exception of a false smile, only this expression occurred. It was coordinated with her speaking, occurring only when she paused and took a breath.

Although the therapist did not explicitly code this as an affective expression, he nevertheless found it very hard to tolerate, and oscillated among countertransference responses of rage, helplessness and disgust.

In this hour the patient talked about presents she used to get from men, which in retrospect she did not consider very flattering, since they were never quite what she wanted. While talking about a piece of land her father had given her when she was a girl, she said she didn't like it at all because he did it to get a tax deduction. The therapist interrupted her stream of complaints by saying to her, "This must have something to do with what your father thought about you." At that point the patient made the contempt-disgust face and replied, "I do not know what my father thought about me."

What is of particular interest, given the assumed importance of facial affective expressions, is the relation of this woman's idiosyncratic facial expression (and its ability to arouse strong countertransference responses) to a number of hypotheses about how to understand her reply. Four of these are:

1. She is consciously lying, and she knows what her father thought about her.

2. She did not know what her father thought about her, but unconsciously she knows that he despised her. Her facial expression reflected an identification with her father's attitude toward her. It can be understood as a kind of identification with the aggressor.

3. She did not consciously know what her father thought about her and she did not know what she thought about him. Nevertheless her face reflected her attitude toward him.

4. All this has nothing to do with her attitude, conscious or not, toward her father, but is an indicator of (a) her reaction to the intervention, or (b) to the therapist, from who she expected inappropriate gifts, or (c) it was a commentary on the therapist as a male or as a representative of all males.

Of course these hypotheses are not mutually exclusive and it is possible that all of these hypotheses might be correct. Nonetheless we need to do more studies in which we examine the intricate interrelationships among the linguistic and the motoric affective expressions of both patient and therapist. This should lead to a better understanding of defensive processes, especially those mechanisms that directly alter the "hardware" of social interaction. Although most of the defense mechanisms described in psychoanalysis refer to alterations of mental processes, today we know that a whole group of *defenses against affect* are manifested directly by the body. In the long run it might even lead to knowledge that would enable us to improve therapists' skills in dealing with these often very-short-duration expressions of patients' feelings.

What Makes Psychoanalysts Tick? A Model and the Method of Audio-Recorded Retroreports*

Adolf-Ernst Meyer*

1. Introduction

Among the unsurpassed virtues of audiorecordings are their incorruptibility and their completeness. Word for word, laughters or sighs, stutters or stammers, irritated or soothing tone of voice, the duration of silences, all is faithfully and completely stored, to be studied and restudied at will. Although in use for over 50 years, audiorecordings of psychoanalyses or psychotherapies are not generally accepted by the analytic community. A recent exchange of arguments may be found in Frick (1985) and in Gill's (1985) response to it (for a more recent review see Kächele et al., this volume).

Nonetheless, such audiorecordings present at least two problems for the researcher:

The Problem of Dual Self-Selection

Dual means that both analysts and patients who agree to record are not representative of the population of analysts and patients. The only analysts who volunteer are those willing to reveal themselves unguardedly with all their uncertainties, hesitancies, clumsy formulations and blunders to their colleagues' perhaps not always benevolent scrutiny. Moreover only those analysts truly committed to rigorous empirical study of the analytic process are likely to even seek their patients' consent

*A collaborative study of Sonderforschungsbereich 115, Hamburg, project B 20, and Sonderforschungsbereich 129, Ulm, project B 2. Thanks for grants are due to the German Research Foundation (Deutsche Forschungsgemeinschaft)

*The present evaluation was made possible by a senior scientist grant from the Breuninger Foundation to the author, which is gratefully acknowledged.

to recording. In addition patients whose anonymity might be compromised have to be omitted.

The Gap in Audio-Recordings

A significant problem with audiorecordings of therapeutic sessions is that they include only what the therapist actually said, thus omitting the very processes that led him to formulate his interventions. Heimann (1969, 1977) has described that an analyst, listening to a patient, conducts an inner, silent "running commentary," searching for hidden meanings, constructing "working models" of the patient, etc. The nature of this inner running commentary is hardly known and rarely studied systematically. The central goals of this study were (1) to propose a method for studying these cognitive and affective processes in the analyst and (2) to offer a preliminary model of what makes the analyst tick.

Although we did the empirical study first and then constructed the model, here I will describe the model first in order to make it easier for the reader to assimilate a very unfamiliar kind of clinical material.

2. The Schematic Model

Figure 1 is a schematic model of the psychoanalytic interaction as seen from the analyst's point of view.

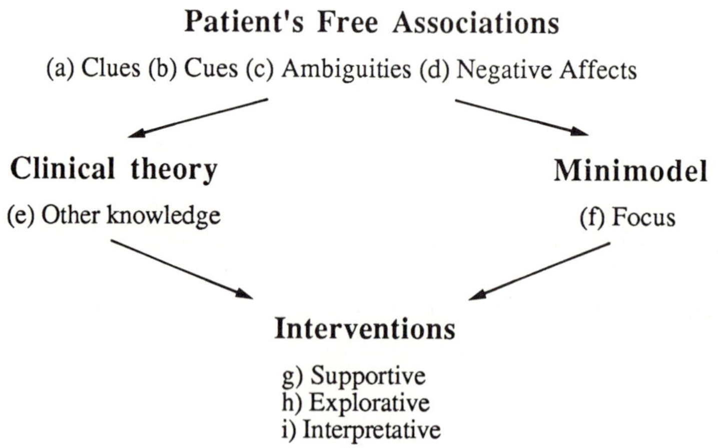

Figure 1 A Flow Chart of the Interaction in the Analytic Process

Classification of the Information from the Patient's Free Associations (a, b, c, d)

The model stipulates that the analyst classifies the free associations into four broad categories: (a) clues, (b) cues, (c) ambiguities and (d) negative affects. Clues are patient statements that the analyst classifies provisionally as an example of certain clinical concepts, which function as prototypical minimodels, e.g. "The patient has a distorted cognition that there are only rulers and slaves," might be classified as sado-masochism. Cues are statements that the analyst classifies as new instances of the same minimodel, e.g. "Making the strong leader even stronger by overlooking his weakness." Ambiguities are statements that the analyst has not yet clearly categorized, e.g. B 3.6: "... I could not make very much of this dream, therefore I ... asked her to associate to this and that detail... ." Negative affects include such feelings as anxiety, discomfort, helplessness, feeling rejected, sadness and worry, which are clear examples of Dahl's (1978) negative ME emotions, whose function is feed-back information about the status of the patient's important wishes.

Clinical Theories and other Knowledge (e)

Ramzy (1974) has argued that a psychoanalyst follows "general principles of reasoning" and hence is "a therapeutic logician or a logical physician." Our data point to the contrary: psychoanalysts employ a highly special set of conceptualizations, quite different from Ramzy's "general principles of reasoning." Their competence seems to lie both in their special theories about the nature of human conflict and in their detailed knowledge about specific patients. It is in this domain of clinical theory where most of the battles among schools of analysts originate.

Minimodels and Focus (f)

"Minimodels" is a substitute expression for Greenson's (1960) "working model" of the patient. However, in agreement with Bowlby (1969) and Peterfreund (1975) the use of the plural is deliberate and meant to convey that an analyst does not employ a single conceptualization, but rather a set of different models to organize his understanding at any given moment. "Mini" indicates that the models actually identified in our retroreports are rather small and circumscribed.

If and when the analyst believes that a certain minimodel has therapeutic potential it becomes a "focus" (see Fig. 1). Such a focus is then given preference for cognition and intervention. Once a focus has been formed the analyst scans the patient's report for "cues" for his focus (see Fig. 1). Hence there is an implicit strong tendency in this model for the analyst, once he has constructed any focus, to perceive what were formerly clues as cues, thus reinforcing his prior theories. To a lesser degree this applies equally to a minimodel and tends to lead to making interpretations based on that particular minimodel (Bowlby 1979).

Interventions (g, h, i)

Three types of interventions are stipulated in the model: (g) supportive, (h) explorative, (i) interpretative. The implicit theory claims that: (1) negative affects tend to evoke supportive interventions, (2) ambiguous statements give raise to exploratory activity such as asking for clarification and (3) successful classification of clues and cues into minimodels or foci leads to interpretations to expand the patient's knowledge.

3. The Empirical Study - Method

Because we wanted to find out what the analyst was thinking during the sessions that was not reflected in his interventions, we asked analysts to dictate a two-part *retroreport* immediately after each session at the end of the same tape that recorded the hour. Both of these were transcribed.

Free Part: In this portion the analyst was asked to free associate, with the hope that his wishes, frustrations, therapeutic plans, personal problems aroused by the patient's remarks, etc., would show up .

Structured Part: In the second part, called the *"explanation of the intervention,"* the analyst's task was to identify three interventions (among all those that he made during the hour) which he thought were most important. "Important" was loosely operationalized as "inducing change," in the topic or affect or leading to fresh material. For each of these he was asked to state: (1) the source, (2) the aim and (3) the actual time during the session when it occurred. By "source" we meant a wide range of the analyst's knowledge including theory and his own and the patient's past and present associations. By "aim" we meant what he wanted to accomplish with the intervention at that very moment.

Our sample of psychoanalysts was derived from twenty German analysts, all known for their research interests, who were asked to participate. Only three agreed to do so. In Table 1 the total number of sessions recorded, the number of hours retroreported, the number of retroreports missed (for various reasons), and the numbers of the recorded sessions are listed.

Table 1

Analyst	No of sessions	Hours reported	Hours skipped	Hour Nos.
A	21	14	7	436 - 457
B	630	620	10	1 - 630
C	12	10	2	1 - 12

For obvious reasons the initial twelve sessions of one patient cannot be compared with sessions 430 to 460 of another. Our study was designed to compare separately the first ten retroreports of analyst B and C with each other and sessions 430 to 460 of A with the same numbered sessions of B; and within B to compare early versus late hours. However, here I will only report some selected comparisons of the first ten hours of analysts B and C.

4. Data Analysis

The first step in the data analysis consisted of marking homogenous topics[1] in the retroreports and grouping them into similar topic categories. This yielded nine topics which, though not exhaustive, included the intuitively satisfying categories shown in Table 2.

[1]Each topic was numbered according to session number and its sequence in the session; for example, B10.9 designates analyst B, hour 10 and the 9th topic within the retroreport of this hour.

Table 2 Topic Categories in the Retroreports of Analysts B and C

Impact of the study situation
Minimodels
Sources for interventions
Aims of interventions
Transference
Registering changes in the patient
Counterreactions
General descriptions of the session
Reflections on technique

The raw number of these topics reported by analysts B and C is shown in Table 3. The obvious differences in the frequency of the topics is a likely result of the difference in the length of their retroreports. B's retroreports were 3 to 6 pages long, while C's were only one page on the average. Time and space do not allow a complete presentation. In order to illustrate the method and the usefulness of the information gained by means of our retroreports I will only present the results of the first four categories of Table 2.

Impact of the Study Situation

The conditions imposed by our study design obviously had their impact on the participating analysts. However, the two analysts, B and C, differed markedly in the way they reacted to and fulfilled the instructions. B indicated the many ways in which the experimental procedure was stressful for him, while C' s reports did not offer a single clue about how he was influenced by the situation. In contrast, B's actual interventions in the session were well-formed prose, while C's were often ungrammatical and filled with false starts, etc.

Table 3 Number of "Topics" Discussed in each of B's and C's first available 10 Retroreports

	Main topics		Sub-topics	
	B	C	B	C
Session				
1	4	rm	1	rm
2	11	3	0	0
3	9	7	1	0
4	12	4	2	1
5	7	4	4	1
6	8	rm	4	rm
7	10	3	0	4
8	11	6	2	0
9	6	5	2	0
10	11	5	5	1
11	na	11	na	0
12	na	5	na	0
Sum	89	53	21	7

Key: A sub-topic is a topic embedded in another topic
rm = recorder malfunctioned; na = not analyzed

Minimodels

Analyst B, in his first two retroreports, made three psychodynamic formulations, which he classified as an hysterical wish for acceptance:

> ***B 1.4*** She intends to make herself smaller than she is; . . . It's important for her that the analyst likes her and she believes that the analyst expects more from her than she can offer.
>
> ***B 2.4*** We are in the middle of a hysterical need to be accepted, and only at its surface . . . In the intervals I pondered about . . . Hoffmann's . . . guidelines of the hysterical character. This frenetic, "I want to be loved – if I am not loved, I am nothing." Or "because I am nothing, I must be loved to prove to me and the world that precisely I am not nothing." Some formula of this sort that I cannot get together.
> ***B 2.11*** You believed you had lost your mother's love.

A new minimodel, sadomasochism, began to emerge in session 4:

> ***B 4.5*** The patient has a distorted idea that there are only rulers and slaves.
>
> ***B 4.9*** I suddenly have the feeling the patient is saying something like: "There are only masters and slaves, and there are brutal rulers and mild rulers. I (patient) am a mild ruler so that others can not rule brutally over me."
>
> ***B 4.12*** To cajole men is dangerous. They may start manipulating you.
>
> ***B 5.6*** Because there are only rulers and subjects, there is a constant struggle for power . . . The focus is not right; it leaves out that the patient enjoys being raped in daydreams.
>
> ***B 6.6*** Initially you make yourself helpless and ask for guidance; only later this irritates you and you rebel.
>
> ***B 6.7*** "Making the strong leader even stronger by overlooking his weakness."
>
> ***B 7.1*** So there are two Lisa's, one who wants to be led and for this makes herself weak; another Lisa says: "My ideal is the opposite. I myself want to be leading."
>
> ***B 8.9*** The patient believed her father unswervingly, that an adult's life consists only of trouble and punishment, and this blind faith has to do with master and slave and being led.

Looking at the repetitions of these two minimodels reported for the first 8 sessions we observe a shift from a mini-hysterical model to a mini-sadomasochistic model. In B's retroreports he did not explain how he explained the shift to himself (cf. with the CCRTs in Luborsky, this volume). However there is circumstantial evidence: B retroreported in 3.7 ". . . this is an intervention which somehow pulls in the known problem structure of the patient . . . masochistic fantasies and also the sexual defense . . .". And in 4.12 B reported, "Thus I have combined the need for acceptance of the patient with the fear of men who might rape her." Since there were no sadomasochistic cues in the first two sessions B must have known about these from his intake interviews, which, very probably, made him formulate a sadomaochistic model. However in the first two sessions acceptance needs predominated. Accordingly B formulated such a minimodel. In session 3 (and more strongly in session 4) sadomasochistic clues appeared, and could soon be combined (in B 4.12) with the acceptance model.

Two other minimodels were referred to in the material; the first pertained to a completely different kind of concept, namely, the patient's resistance because she did not want to tell a dream (B 9.5). The other, ambivalence, could as well be classified as an example of sado-masochism, as in the following two examples:

B 7.6 and ***B 10.5*** The analyst assumes an ambivalence minimodel for the phobic anxiety of the patient, that her husband could have had an accident. She wants to be rid of him to be free to develop, but she is afraid she is too weak to succeed without his protection. Even this could be seen as: the slave wants to dethrone her master and be independent, but is afraid she will be lost without a patron.

Analyst C's minimodels appear far more diverse with much less repetition than B's, as illustrated in the following sequences:

C 2.2 The patient's defense against needs for exhibition and being liked.

C 3.3 The patient's wholesale confession to his wife of his own adultery served two purposes, (a) to relieve himself, and (b) to pressure his wife.

C 3.4 An aggression inhibition and its reversal into passive submissive-ness.

C 4.1 The patient's not asserting himself, so as to make himself liked, stems from his childhood experiences as a refugee.

C 5.2 My fee regulation is perceived by the patient as anally castrative and the patient's body schema is an expression of castration anxiety: nose = penis.

C 5.3 The patient has to intensify this to remain a victim.

C 5.4 A very impressive connection between symptom formation and unconscious fantasies, which are related to activity of the right arm and the anxiety that others perceive this and despise him.

Retroreport C 5.4 is highly condensed. The transcript showed that patient C reported two dreams of automobile accidents where he was severely wounded. The analyst then recalled that the patient reported earlier of feeling physically deficient. The patient described at some length the alleged malformation of his nose and then complained of pains in his right arm which usually preceded a torticollis attack.

C 7.3 Analyst C speaks of the masochism of the patient, neither going to a doctor nor taking a pill to alleviate his backache.

C 9.4 An ongoing oscillation between masochism and rebellion.

C 8.5 As he is very superego determined (see his remarks concerning belief and his religious attitude) I am afraid that after such an outburst he would have to suffer additionally under the pressure of his self reproaches.

C 8.6 The patient could not stand separation (informal or legal) from his wife.

We may raise the question of whether it is possible to construct a more encompassing and coherent model from the given elements? Indeed I think any experienced analyst could, e.g. castration inferiority engenders submission (one form of masochism) and inhibition of exhibition (because of anxieties to be found out being deficient). Both are reinforced as a reaction formation against aggressivity by the social fact of being a refugee. Submission is secondarily ideologized (more precisely christianized) as the victim being morally superior to the aggressor. All this is embodied in a strong superego.

However, there is no evidence from C's retroreports that he consciously formulated such a coherent integration (or another) of these minimodels, which then would be an example of a Greenson "working model."

Another minimodel seems to be an example of Mitscherlich's "two phasic defense operation":

C 11.6 There is a remarkable resurfacing of blushing anxiety, which had for the time being completely disappeared after the development of torticollis.

B's and C's reported psychodynamic patterns were of uniformly low complexity. Neither analyst spelled out a larger working model (gestalt) in a single coherent formulation. Frankly, it surprised me that minimodels appear to be all that these analysts reported under the conditions of this experiment.

The question then is, since we know - as shown above - that analysts do indeed construct larger models, when and under what conditions is this done? I presume that such more encompassing working models of a patient remain preconscious until in what Heimann (1977) called a third "ego configuration," such as a candidate reporting to his supervisor, the supervisor instructing his candidate, an analyst preparing a paper or presenting it to a case conference, or filing a health insurance claim.

In the preceding paragraph I used the term "preconscious." Indeed it is highly plausible that composite larger models like <hysteric-phobic-acceptance needs with a sadomasochistic pattern> or <reaction formation against castration inferiority with symptom formation and an inhibition of exhibitionistic wishes>, are part and parcel of analysts' everyday thinking. Although such composites may well have influenced our two analysts, remarkably, they were not consciously verbalized. I surmise that minimodels are both necessary and sufficient in the here-and-now situation of therapy - and more would potentially be harmful - because all encompassing conceptualizations would risk overtaxing the patient.

Sources of and Aims for Interventions

Sources and aims will be discussed together because they relate to the same intervention, thus allowing a more integrated and parsimonious description. Both analysts were rather lax in respect to the "explanation part" of their retroreports, as illustrated by B's comment:

> ***B 5.5*** Yes – oh no – . . . I have not read . . . the instruction for the homework . . . Thought I had them in my head . . . And today I read them through . . . I should also explain my interventions, not only label them . . . Yesterday I did do it in a way. Today I will try to make amends.

In contrast to B, C, in his brief reports, did not clearly distinguish between the two tasks.

Analyst B's comments about sources reflected an impressive variety:

B 4.2 Another patient who had this mechanism
B 4.5 The image of the raging and terrorizing father
B 4.8 The patient's description of how she controls men
B 5.7 The transference concept
B 6.7 The patient described overlooking her strong girl friend's weaknesses.
B 9.2 The resistance concept
B 10.6 Learning theory
B 10.7 Pornography

A similar variety seemed to exist for aims:

B 4.11 Counteracting the negative transference
B 8.10 Show her that sex is a topic
B 10.7 To make her feel better and support her
B 10.8 To reduce anxieties

Let us now examine B's retroreports about sources and aims in detail through the ten sessions. In the first two sessions B was clearly anxious that his patient might flee, as she had several times before.

> ***B 1.1*** Although, I must say, I said more than I usually would say in a first hour, simply not to let the patient wait too long for a response. I must say that in other cases I would allow a bit more frustration.

> ***B 2.2*** . . . I made . . . perhaps half a dozen supportive interventions. But much less than in the first session, where I had the feeling that I had to carry her along.

These examples suggest both an aim and a source. Manifestly his aim was to support, comfort and protect her so that she would stay in treatment. We might speculate that the source of these anxieties were related to B's investment in the patient as a research case.[2]

In session 3 the patient reported a dream in which three dangers appeared: (1) F. J. Strauß,[3] (2) men from the local red light district, and (3) a spider. B then reported:

> ***B 3.6*** Beyond this I could not make very much of this dream, therefore I asked a lot of questions and asked her to associate to this and that detail.

When B asked for the patient's impression of Strauß he referred to him as "Landesvater (father of the country) Strauß," which prompted the patient to reminisce about her own father. To the spider the patient associated to her brother. B then made an interpretation and retroreported:

> ***B 3.7*** "Then all the dangers in the dream seem to be men." This is the most important intervention, not because the patient reacted to it or that I was quite sure of the meaning. But I believe this is an intervention which somehow pulls in the known problem structure of the patient. The feeling and these – yes – masochistic fantasies and also the sexual defense against the husband and all these things. She needs two men. Her husband must not look at another woman and all these (inaudible) and masochistic things. Yes, this thus would be the most important intervention.

In this passage it seems clear that B used a minimodel, <hysteric sadomasochism>, that he arrived at during the intake interviews; the aim was to help her see that all her fears were of men.

---

[2]As a matter of fact, patients (i) with a classical neurosis, (ii) with marked impairment, (iii) a reasonable prognosis for psychoanalysis, and (iv) no previous psychotherapy, who were also willing to consent to tape-recording and research were few and far between.

[3]The well-known Bavarian prime minister.

In the fourth session B, perhaps reflecting his uncertainty about the meaning of the dream in 3.7, recalled the fact that the patient associated to her own father after the analyst had referred to Strauß as the Landesvater and then reported:

> ***B 4.5*** I thought of the patient's father as the archetypical beer-drinking Bavarian. I think I have produced a bit of a Rosenthal effect.

Later the following exchange took place:

B: The brutal tyranny, that you fear from men, you react to by becoming the victim.
P: I am not a victim; instead I am pretty aggressive.
B: So, you meet force with force.
P: (14 s pause) Hmm. (12 s pause).
B: So men do not rape you. You rape men.
P: (14 s pause) Mmhmm, but not sexually.

As a source for this B mentioned :

> ***B 4.8*** The patient's description of how she controls men.

Then he described his third important intervention and gave the source for it:

> ***B 4.12*** "The dangerous men have to be cajoled, so that they become kind and approving." Thus I have combined the need for acceptance of the patient with the fear of men who might rape her. I then continued, "This procedure has its drawbacks. If one cajoles men, they might easily get the idea that one is a victim, inviting manipulation or domination." This is also an interpretation, I would say, which stems from clinical experience. There was another patient I once had with her relentless begging for love, who was often understood sexually or abused sexually, when she only wanted to be cuddled and rocked. I believe she was a kind of model, or played a role, for this interpretation.

The following exchange took place in session 5:

P: (Daydreams that one of her girl friends is raped and she catches this man and beats him until he gives up.) It must be pretty hard for me, since I dislike and am so afraid of men, to have any kind relationship with them. (2 minute, 24 second pause punctuated by several sighs)
B: Right now it seems that you're also having trouble with me.
P: I, no, I don't know, I don't think so . . . One – some men one sees only as professional colleagues or so. And I certainly do not see you as a man right now, but as a doctor or –

In his retroreport of this exchange B stated:

> *B 5.7* With this I wanted to point out to her that I too am a man. It struck me that she was silent today much more than usual. Or was she hiding something? . . . The interpretation did not bear fruit. In effect she said: "For me you are only a doctor and not a man." Still I believe it will have a sort of educational effect that I point out to her to that thoughts about me – or everything which happens – has to be seen on the basis of her relationship to me.

It seems clear that this is an example of the patient's resistance to the experience of the relationship with the therapist (see Hoffmann and Gill, this volume).

The minimodel, <negative father transference>, continues to evolve in each of the following sessions:

> *B 6.7* I told her, "You believe that anybody who dominates you has to be strong. And if you don't find someone, you simply make her stronger." This occurred to me (6 minutes earlier) when she denied the weaknesses of her strong girl friend.

And in session 7:

> **P**: I still blame my mother that my father turned out like he did.
> **B**: Yes, you think your mother is the real villain.

As a source for this B reported:

> *B 7.7* Said this mainly from theoretical considerations.

> *B 8.7* Came to my mind, "You look for a mild form of slavery" but this seemed too negative, so 1-2 minutes later I put it positively, "You are looking for a better father who doesn't drink and is not so domineering."

In the ninth session B retroreported:

> *B 9.2* Already in my mind: Is there something she consciously keeps secret? So when she said, "Don't you believe me?" (that her mind is blank), I was silent for awhile, let her fret and said: "A part of you must know something, otherwise you would not be so anxious. You think that what you don't know won't hurt you." Then she admitted that she had had a dream.

B continued to work with the PERT minimodel: <resistance to the experience of the relationship with the therapist> and he tentatively confronted the patient – and succeeded.

In the 10th session the patient reported that for the first time in her marriage of 8 years that she, instead of her husband, went out to buy breakfast rolls. B intervened: "It almost looks as if this was a result of yesterday's session that you got the rolls today." The patient acquiesced and suggested that freedom probably begins with little things. B made her repeat this and then emphatically said, "Exactly."

> ***B 10.6*** Here I am obviously somewhat infected by learning theory when I find this to be the most important intervention.

It may come as a surprise that in the midst of a resistance situation as portrayed by the quotations and retroreports of the previous sessions, the analyst was "infected" with a well-known hobby horse of his. Whatever the merit of his <learning> minimodel for the understanding of this situation is, it underscores the patient's concept that this is a process of many small steps.

In contrast to B, analyst C's brevity in reporting is illustrated by his complete retroreports of session 2:

> ***C 2.1*** My interventions had two aims. For one I tried to help the patient familiarize himself with the analytic situation. This aim was served by my initial encouraging remarks.

> ***C 2.2*** It was above all about focusing on his defense against his need for recognition and exhibition. The patient acknowledged these interpretations positively. I believe that his repeated confirmations were correct – correct – altogether emotionally authentic and I see in it the relevant interpretations of this second hour.

> ***C 2.3*** The later questions served to orient me about his work situation and furthermore they also naturally had the aim of pointing out to the patient that I am also interested in this area. End of the retroreport.

C mentioned four aims, but no sources. Nonetheless when I examined the transcript it was easy to find plausible candidates for sources. However I will abstain from speculation. From the retroreport of session 3 I quote only those passages that related to sources or aims.

> ***C 3.2*** In the beginning of the hour I focused on the working alliance.

> ***C 3.3*** Theoretically the topic of his general confession to his wife was probably the most important. From this I deduced that the patient couldn't stand it any more and therefore unburdened himself on his wife, evidently quite permanently, even though the relationship had eased in between.

However, if we look at the actual interventions, C took a different line:

> **C**: Uhm, you had also connected your somewhat specific confession with your general confession that, uhm you – that this is, uhm, will give up the other relationship – that you –
> **P**: Yes, uhm.
> **C**: With this, uhm, through the with the, confession, uhm, you wanted to control yourself in this way.
> **P**: Correct.
> **C**: Is it?
> **P**: Yes, yes, yes, yes.
> **C**: So that no one else will attract you.

Thus C actually interpreted that P informed his wife in order to erect a barrier against his own adultery. The discrepancy between transcript and retroreport lies in the fact that the actual intervention stressed the patient's need to control himself with the confession, whereas the retroreport emphasized the unburdening and aggressive function of the confession.

This is one of several examples found in the present investigation that a psychoanalyst's dictated report - even immediately after a session - may be prone to serious distortion. There is ample evidence that this is unfortunately equally valid for reports made during the session (see Meyer 1981).

Later in the same session, as the following sequence of paraphrases of C's interventions shows, the sources and aims of a new topic emerged:

> C – Repeats selectively that the patient feels entitled to ask for a raise because of costs of his illness. Then explores the reasons for and amounts of these costs. Subsequently points out that it is easier for the patient to beg for support than to demand reward for work, and reminds him of concrete examples of his extra efforts at work. Then explores the amount the patient wants, how much it is relative to his basic salary and what the chances are of getting it; learns that the raise is very small and there is a very good chance of getting it. Finally C said, "Thus, what I mean is that it is easier for you – yes, perhaps I exaggerate a bit – to act like a beggar than to, uhm, fight for something you've earned, isn't it, with, uhm, uh or uhm?"

And C concluded that this problem had existed before, but that the illness made it worse. He then retroreported:

C 3.5 His inhibition of aggression and the reversal into passive submissivity became distinct in connection with his inability to argue for a wage increase for his extra work. He has an idea that he can argue with his superiors using his illness and what it costs him. My references in the middle of the hour were addressed to this.

The sources seemed to lie in the clinical material itself and the minimodel of <passive aggression> is everywhere. C's aim was to try to help the patient understand this.

After session 4 he reported:

C 4.1 The theme of the hour culminates at the end in P's insight that his trying to make himself generally popular has its roots in his experiences as a refugee child. My interpretations led to this development, which I had intended. In the middle there was the topic of making oneself popular, not being able to be direct because this is too closely associated with being aggressive. Right at the beginning of the hour I made some references to this which I repeated during the hour.

C 4.2 Also it was important to me to make him aware that – for his own relief – he has to become forceful, because when he feels under pressure he relieves it by getting angry.

Up to this point C's strategy seems to have been to actively analyze the patient's conflicts based on the here-and-now transference manifestations and his prior clinical theory. But in the next report there was another aim:

C 4.4 Also important to me was – and my questions were aimed at this – to collect genetic material, because as of now I still know very little of the patient's history and his – and the vicissitudes of some of his typical behaviors.

In session 5 the topic of money entered into the transference in C's retroreport:

C 5.1 Especially important are those transference interpretations, which I made, of a small detail, namely the patient's concerns about the fee. The fact that he has to pay his own money for the treatment was quite certainly experienced as anally castrative by the patient. Another topic was also important in the hour – especially his disturbances of his body schema as an expression of his castration anxiety: nose = penis. I felt it was important to make an interpretation about this equation. In addition, these feelings are so strong for the reason that he could not argue with me and had to remain a victim.

C 5.2 These interpretations naturally had the aim of mobilizing his aggression.

From the last two retroreports I now offer a reconstruction of what made C tick. He took his patient's reaction to having to pay the fee himself as an example of the minimodel <anal assault>. In the transcript there are many other instances of a variant of this model. These refer to hypochondrical preoccupations with the size of his nose and his penis, classifiable into a minimodel of <castration anxiety>. The aim of C's interpretations was to point out to P the defensive strategy of remaining a victim, e.g. <if I submit, he won't attack>.

Editors' Coda:

It seems to us that this reconstruction is an excellent example of the fact that Meyer's model has captured the pervasive tendency in the analysts' mental processes to represent free associations as *cues* rather than *clues*. It thus highlights Bowlby's (1979) claim that the task of the clinician lies in maximizing the value of positive evidence, whereas the task of the researcher lies in maximizing the value of negative evidence.

Author's Coda:

I am deeply obliged to the three contributing psychoanalysts for their courage in submitting to the novel conditions of this investigation – conditions not generally accepted in the psychoanalytic community – and for their dedication in spending additional time and effort for research. I can only hope that they will feel that the findings constitute a reasonable, or even a good result. Equal thanks are due to the patients for their willingness to share their intimate secrets with unknown observers in the name of science. Even if they could not foresee the full extent of their commitment when they consented, none of them withdrew as they became aware of it.

I am also grateful to two of the editors, Dahl and Kächele, who shortened and condensed my elaborate and bulky treatise to a third of its original lenght. Through this it has gained in argumentative force and readability – although, of course, I do miss many of the examples that were omitted. And finally I especially thank Ruth Limpinsel for her patient and painstaking dedication in typing many versions of the manuscript.

From Calvin to Freud: Using an Artificial Intelligence Model to Investigate Cognitive Changes during Psychoanalysis*

Marianne Leuzinger-Bohleber and Horst Kächele*

"There is the old joke about not really understanding something until you have taught it to somebody else. The new version now says you don't really understand it until you've programmed it into a computer." (Randall Davis)

1. Introduction

Can you imagine a greater difference than the one existing between a computer and a patient?

> *"You know for some reason I just thought about the bill and about payment again. (You shoudn't give me a bill.) <Uh->I was thinking that I (shoudn't be given a bill) of asking you whether it wouldn't be all right for you not to give me a bill. That is, I usually by (the end of the month know the amount of the bill), well, I immediately thought of the objections to this, but my idea was that I would simply count up the number of hours and give you a check at the end of the month."* (Clippinger 1977, p. 146)

Perhaps you will find it hard to believe that this text was not taken from a verbatim transcript of a psychoanalytic session, but was produced by a computer program called ERMA, written by J. Clippinger (1977). Indeed, the text produced by his computer program is nearly the same as the actual discourse in the transcript of a real psychoanalytic session that Clippinger originally used to conceptualize the possible cognitive pro-

*To Ulrich Moser for his 60th birthday

*Supported by the German Research Foundation, Sonderforschungsbereich 129, project B6.

cesses of the patient, processes that may indeed have "run" inside her "black box" and led to this verbalization.

The program's production of this text may serve as evidence that the cognitive theory upon which the computer program was based is an adequate model of most of the cognitive processes involved. This technique of computer simulation to test theories (psychological in this case) is one application of the rapidly developing field of Artificial Intelligence (AI) (cf. Teller, this volume).

In our opinion this approach to testing complex psychological theories can also be fruitful for psychoanalysis. The models derived from AI theories, partly because of being tested by computer simulation, have a high degree of precision, consistency and clarity in the terminology used. Moreover they take into account, much more than psychoanalytic concepts do, modern knowledge from other scientific disciplines such as neurophysiology, brain research and research on memory structures. These advantages are one reason why we have used a theory of cognitive processes based on computer simulation models in our study of changes in these processes in psychoanalytic patients. Borrowing an AI model in an empirical study of psychoanalytic processes also helps to avoid the dangers of circularity, i.e., using a psychoanalytic model to justify itself.

Clippinger's theory of cognitive processes was convincing to us because it embodies the conception of conflicting processes taking place inside a black box, just as the structural theory in psychoanalysis does. That is, it conceptualizes cognitive processes as being determined by the interaction of separate cognitive modules. The processes (programs) running in one module can complete, modify or inhibit and interrupt those running in other modules. Among other things, this leads to characteristic structures in the interaction of the different modules and specific ways of perceiving and processing information.

In this study we used Clippinger's model in a modified form by defining the six modules shown in Figure 1. These modules perform the following tasks:

MOZART selects what is attended to.
CALVIN represents the superego and the patient's values, and acts as censor.
MACHIAVELLI develops problem-solving strategies.
CICERO translates cognition into verbalizations.
MARX perceives and tests reality.
FREUD introspects and performs specific ego functions.

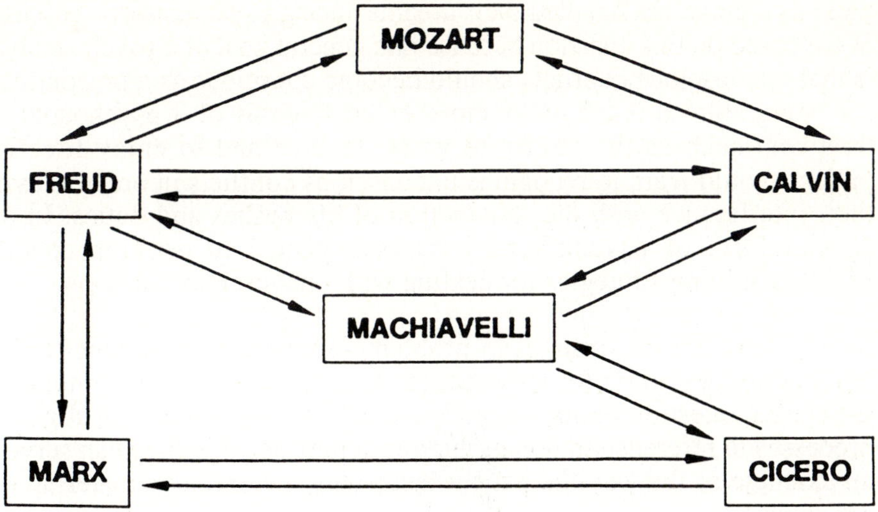

Arrows indicate paths of communication among the cognitive modules.

Figure 1 Interaction of Cognitive Modules

The psychoanalytic notion of the Id as a source of unconscious motivation is not explicitly represented in this model. Clippinger includes the concept of motivation in his sequential representation of cognitive processes, but its exposition here would take us too far afield. For a detailed understanding of the operation of the model the reader is referred to Clippinger (1977). Nonetheless it is obvious that unconscious motivations ultimately reveal themselves in cognitive processes, and it is the manifestation of these in the transcripts of what patients verbalize on the couch that we study.

2. Overview of the Study

In our empirical study we aimed at describing and analyzing changes in the problem-solving cognitive processes of five patients during their long-term psychoanalyses. We studied modifications of the way the patients themselves handled their dreams during psychoanalytic sessions. We focused on this question because one general goal of a psychoanalysis is that unconscious conflicts should become conscious as a precondition for being able to reach other more external goals of a psychoanalytic treatment such as the ability to work, to love and to enjoy life. The patient should learn to recognize unconscious conflicts in order to avoid their interference with the satisfaction of his wishes and duties. In this special form of psychotherapy he is expected to develop specific problem-solving strategies for dealing with unconscious conflicts.

Therefore the changes in problem-solving cognitive processes as one important criteria for the success of a psychoanalytic treatment was the central question in our research project. We analyzed such cognitive processes in reference to dream interpretations because they can serve as an example of the way the patient deals with unconscious material, e.g. his dreams.

Here we shall give a highly condensed overview of a few of the results of our project. In the first phase of our study we generated hypotheses from a single case study by exploring dream associations as recorded in a transvestite patient's (Leuzinger-Bohleber 1987) diary during the first and last hundred hours of his psychoanalysis. In the second phase we tested our hypotheses by using four additional psychoanalytic cases from the Ulm Textbank. Using two kinds of theory-directed content analyses, we compared each patient's dream reports taken from the first hundred with those from the last hundred psychoanalytic sessions.

In all that follows it should be understood that we use a very broad definition of "cognitive processes" as inner processes of perceiving and processing information that are always connected with physiological and emotional processes and cannot be studied separately (Pfeifer and Leuzinger-Bohleber 1986)

3. Methods: Theory-Directed Content Analysis by Complex Ratings and Computer-Aided Content Analyses

Our tools for testing the hypotheses derived from the Clippinger model consisted of (1) computer-aided content-analyses and (2) ratings by trained judges of transcribed sessions and written dream reports. We used two "naive" raters and two "expert" (psychoanalyst) raters in this study. The judges were intensively trained to understand our model of cognitive processes. In several pretests they were acquainted with the kind of material to be rated. The training was very time-consuming, but we finally achieved reasonable interrater reliabilities. The raters judged randomly ordered sessions taken from early and late in the treatment in which there were dreams and dream associations, including the patients' own interpretations of their dreams.

The following examples of diary reports from our first patient are taken from one early and one late session:

Session 19

> Let me first tell you a dream: There is a church, large, modern architecture, triangular walls with large windows. Daniela (a girlfriend) and me, probably also her relatives went with us into the church. While entering I already felt anxious that those relatives wouldn't sit nearby an exit door. To me it was clear in a war one would safeguard the possibility of rapid evacuation. In the church there was a staircase leading upward to a second story. Some people moved up there. To my satisfaction, we placed ourselves where I wanted to be seated. The pulpit was like a wooden cage. It was swinging on ropes fixed on the ceiling. Suddenly I heard the noise of aircraft; I hurried and left the church and hid myself behind a wall. I knew there was no absolute protection, but at least some shelter. Then I saw the airplanes dropping bombs, very clearly, especially the bombs. I felt like being in a nightmare so strong was my anxiety.
>
> Associations: The church, its triangular shape reminds me of Lionel Feininger, the architect; maybe it's also influenced by the famous chapel of Ronchamps by Le Corbusier. As I myself am interested in architecture and do some drawings too from time to time, this church has attracted me very much. On specific questioning by my analyst, what interests me most are the curbs, the roof and the shadows, the uneven walls and the non-rectangular shapes.
>
> I once went with Daniela into the church. Because she was used to going to church every Sunday, I thought that I would want to justify my prejudices. But it was no prejudice; I felt my judgment confirmed, especially with regard to the Catholic church.
>
> The bombs: I used to construct many models as a boy, airplanes and tanks. The airplanes had bombs as well, and I did it with special perfection. About eight years ago I used to be very interested in war materials. I was especially excited by their technical perfection. I was caught up by that in a way that I didn't realize how much human misery and suffering the technical world spreads in such ways. In the war movies I've seen, the technical aspects were exaggerated and the human aspects neglected. When I realize today

the way I felt then, it makes me shiver. I realize the way I used to be; that interest in technical aspects is basically there but still I have discovered these inconsistencies and now am trying (with some success) to mold this interest in more human concerns. The fear that I may be forced in the long run to earn my money in a technical job still remains. I also still feel anxious that I may relapse into this ideological thinking – I doubt it, but it is still there. Another aspect of this apprehension is combined with my sophistication for technical innovations; it might well be that I would invent something really new with a lot of controversial consequences. When I was nine years old I used to construct rockets, which really intrigued me.

How would I have developed if I had become an engineer in the war industry, terrible thought, isn't it? The interest in this stuff was not directly influenced by my parents; it seems to have developed out of my search for something elementary, out of my problems and circumstances surrounding me.

There is another event I remember: as a child I went Christmas shopping with my parents. I saw a tank and wanted to have it. My father said, "Look, what an ugly (maybe dangerous, but not inhuman) toy." With my construction kit I couldn't build a tank; it was late in school when I was able to build my first tank, which I was very proud of.

No, I haven't really worked it through. Whenever I daydream that I would stay alone in a house and a burglar would try to break in, I place such a little tank in front of him and would then be able to really shoot and hurt him. It looks as if I am preoccupied with defending myself, even in fantasy, against an invisible intruder and being invisible myself. All this is related directly or indirectly to the bombs, which I had a clear picture of in the dream.

Session 617

I had a dream: a shop, I stand in front of the shelf with stockings, but I cannot find the right ones. I leave the shop. I have about three quarters of an hour before my analytic session begins. Change of scenery. I wake up and find out that I have missed the analytic session. I should call my analyst and tell her, or else she might be worried. Something keeps me from doing it, but having missed the first session I should take care that I don't miss a second. This session will take place in X; taking a bike I should be able to make it just in time. While riding there I suddenly am confronted with a mountainous road, hard to follow and very difficult. The situation frightens me. In a small hut there is a young man with long hair; he's got to do something about the bad road. Time runs very short and though I see X on the horizon I am not able to make it in time. I am very anxious, feel stiff; I look at the freaky young man working and I think I should try to retrieve my bike which had been lost somewhere in the mountain.

> Associations: It's not only my (female) analyst, but I can't reach any woman; I cannot open myself; I pretend to come to X. I am wondering, did I betray her? Could it be that the analysis has not been as successful? In the dream I have missed two session whereas in reality I never skipped one. Has it to do with the fear of not being loved any longer? The issue around men: do I want to observe them and imitate them; what could it be? It was yesterday that I realized what my analyst had in mind when she said there was a wish to imitate another man, but this is very hard. Most men I know have their difficulties so that there is very little to identify with, anyway at least with regard to my technical abilities. I always was a very efficient observer and looked carefully at how things work. However there are areas where I am not able to observe so keenly. What does X stand for? Well it looks as if I am on the verge of establishing a new part of my identity; recently I talked to my boss about a chance to share a social worker's position with someone else. I had this idea a few days ago. I had even disputed it with a friend of mine; however, I think this does not belong to the dream anymore.

Now, what hypotheses were being rated?

From CALVIN to FREUD - An Example

One of the central concepts in Clippinger's model is that cognitive processes are determined by the interaction of programs running both in and between cognitive modules. Accordingly, our first hypothesis was that in the diary notes (or verbatim protocols) from the early part of the psychoanalysis the programs of the CALVIN module would especially dominate those of the FREUD module. In other words, the introspective associations of the patient would be inhibited by interventions of a rigid forbidding superego structure. In contrast, we postulated that we would find the FREUD module dominating in the sessions at the end of psychoanalysis, corresponding to the possibility of "freer" associations as one result of psychoanalysis.

The raters were asked to judge whether, after having read the material of a session dealing with dream associations (as in the examples above), they had the impression that the cognitive processes operating in each of the different modules: (1) were controlled by those of other modules (1, on the scale); (2) could have "run" without being inhibited by those of other modules (2, on the scale); or (3) controlled the cognitive processes of other modules (3, on the scale).

3. Results

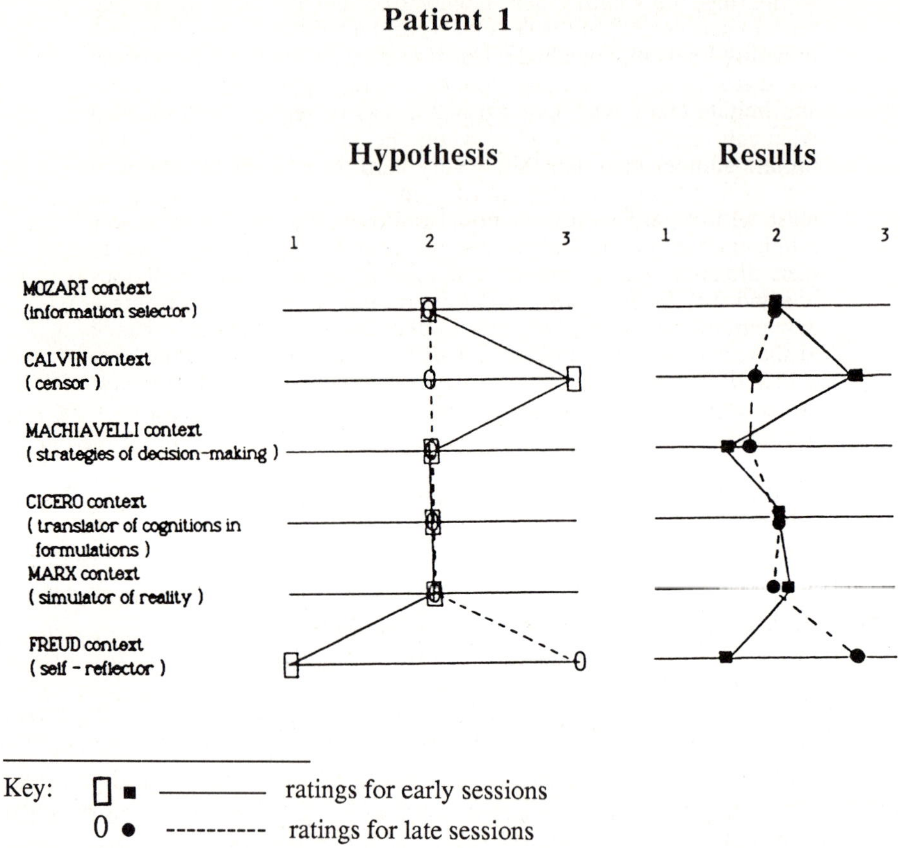

Figure 2 Hypotheses and Results: Rating of the Interactions of Cognitive Modules

The results, shown in Figure 2, supported our hypothesis. We were surprised at how easily the different clinical outcomes of the five psychoanalyses were distinguished by this pattern. Patients 1 and 5 supported our hypothesis in the most impressive way; patients 2 and 4 also supported it, but less strongly, and Patient 3 did not show the expected changes. The outcomes were assessed by: (1) global clinical impressions of the analysts of the patients, (2) the judgments of two independent analysts, and (3) the results of our theory-guided computer-aided content analyses. The outcomes of Patients 1 and 5 were judged to be "very successful," Patients 2 and 4 were judged "moderately successful," and Patient 3 was judged "unsuccessful," although this treatment had not yet been concluded at the time of our study. Indeed, the global clinical impressions were sharpened, modified and corrected in some dimensions by our empirical study.

Other hypotheses focused more on changes of the content of the programs running inside the different modules. Figure 3 shows a few examples from the CICERO module for Patient 1.

1. How do you feel about the way the analysand expresses himself?

   Is his personal language

not striking, normal	......x.........o........	striking, special
simple	......x.........o........	complicated
idiosyncratic original	.....................ox..	socially adapted
plain, simple	........x.........o......	sophisticated
hard to read	.................o....x.	easy to read
unpleasant	.................o......x	pleasant
egocentric	..........o............x..	communicative

2. How do you judge the range of the dream interpretation?

narrow	...o......................x	broad

3. Are there taboos in the themes in the sequences of dream-interpretation?

hardly observable	....x................o....	clearly observable

4. Do you find indications in the text that the patient takes into account to whom his notes are directed (normally his analyst)?

hardly observable	...o...........x........	clearly observable

5. How "psychoanalytic" do you feel the expressions of the patient are?

   psychoanalytic in a "technical" sense?

minimal	....o......x...............	clearly

   psychoanalytic in an "integrated" sense?

minimal	......o..................x ..	clearly

Key: o = rating of early sessions
x = rating of late sessions

Figure 3 Questions for the Raters Concerning the CICERO Module

Please note that the different questions are not independent of each other. The aim of this part of our study was to generate hypotheses. The questions focus on the real or fictitious effect of the diary notes on the real or fictitious reader – the instrumental aspect of language as Bühler (1934) called it – which is part of the function of the CICERO module in our model.

We interpret the many different results as indications that the expression of language in the second part of the diary came closer to the purpose of such a diary, i.e., the language was simpler, plainer, and less exaggerated. The language also more closely served the function of communication with a real or imagined partner, one reason why the notes were judged to be more readable and desirable by the raters. We also think that we have found indications that several aspects of the language performance and the knowledge of social relationship of the patient were expanded by psychoanalysis, i.e., broader range of themes, fewer taboos in the notes, greater range of performance and of psychoanalytic knowledge, and taking into account the effect on the possible partner in communication.

Two examples will illustrate how the results of these ratings were supported by our computer-aided content analyses. First, the judgment of fewer taboos late in the analysis was supported by the fact that the late diary entries contained more direct sexual terms than early ones. Second, the impression of the raters that the patient took the reaction of a possible reader of the diary more into account at the end of the psychoanalysis was supported by the fact that interventions of the analyst were mentioned in only 5 percent of the early entries, whereas in the late ones 16 percent contained reflections on the analyst's statements. Furthermore, only 2 percent of the early references were to the analyst's interpretations, but this increased later to 10 percent; and the early references tended to be the analyst's questions, confrontations and clarifications, compared with later reflections on his interpretations.

Summary of all Five Patients

I. Changes in Problem-solving Cognitive Processes: Interactions among Cognitive Modules

The problem-solving cognitive processes of the two successful patients at the end of their psychoanalyses can be characterized by a high degree of flexibility, by an enlarged cognitive range, an associative and "gestaltlike" way of thinking, and by a capacity for a functional and realistic style of problem-solving. Different information could be perceived and worked on at the same time and led to a process of generating and testing hypotheses that could compete with, modify, or contradict each other. Cognitive dissonances were recognized, reflected, and influenced, among other things, the decision-making process.

Unpleasant affects had an important function as signals indicating cognitive processes to be taken into account in the problem-solving process. In terms of our model, we found: (1) increased cognitive and affective knowledge used in a functional way in different modules, (2) interrupt programs that functioned well and corresponded better to reality, and (3) an uninhibited interaction of cognitive processes in the different modules. The two moderately successful patients showed results tending in the same direction, but not as impressive as the two very successful patients. Up to this point in the treatment, the unsuccessful patient had not yet changed his cognitive processes in the ways described.

Changes Within the Cognitive Modules

*1. **MOZART**: Changes in What was Attended To*

In the sessions at the end of the psychoanalyses of the successful patients the following changes were observable, according to our raters:

- More of the text of the dreams was attended to and worked over cognitively.
- The context of the dreams was taken into account.
- The analyst's interventions were part of the patient's dream associations.
- The patients pursued hypotheses about their dreams more systematically.
- The process of generating hypotheses took place easily, without much hesitation.
- The patients considered more than one hypothesis about the meaning of a dream.

In a separate assessment we observed the following systematic changes in three dimensions of the manifest dream content, based on the model by Moser et al. (1980): *Expressed relationships, dream atmo-*

sphere and problem solving. In the late dreams of the successful patients we observed:

Expressed Relationships:
-The dreamer expressed better relationships with both his objects and himself.
-The range of interactions in these relationships was increased e.g. in the late dreams he was more often alone, as well as interacting with one or more partners.
-Although the relationships were more often tender and friendly than in early dreams, to our surprise, they were also seldom neutral, and included conflictual relations – an indication, to us, that the range had been increased.

Dream Atmosphere:
-The variety and intensity of affects in the manifest dream content was increased.
-The atmosphere was more positive with less anxiety, but aggressive, sad and frightened moods were also expressed. This contradicted our original hypothesis that a single positive mood would prevail.

Problem solving:
-More problem-solving strategies were recognizable.
-Problem solving was more successful than not and the dreamer was more active in doing it, and seldom avoided it.
-The range of problem solving was greater than in early dreams.

In the content analyses we found less concern with the major psychopathological symptoms in the successful patients. In the late dreams the content was more personal, with a greater variety of expressed activities. Moreover, the patients' dream interpretations were more "dialogue oriented," more convincing and more directed at understanding the unconscious meanings of the dream. The associations were more constricted early and more varied in the late sessions. These are hints that the range of attention of the successful patients was enlarged.

*2. **CALVIN:** Changes in the Superego and Internal Values*

The raters observed significant changes in the internal values of the successful patients. Their criticisms and judgments grew more mature, milder, more flexible, more adequate, and more encouraging, but remained consistent with inner ethical values already present at the beginning of their treatments. This included how patients judged themselves as well as how other relevant other persons judged them. The content analyses supported the raters' findings.

3. *MACHIAVELLI: Changes in Problem-Solving Strategies for Dreams*

The raters judged that the successful patients increased their ability to interpret their dreams. In late sessions they displayed more strategies for interpreting their dreams, such as working with dream symbols, integrating different themes in the dream and associations, and dealing with contradictory information.

Since free associations are an essential part of dream interpretation, we defined five dimensions for assessing the strategies employed: *quantity* (the amount of free association), *variability* (the range of strategies employed), *quality* (the usefulness of the associations), *introspection* (the ability to reflect on the interpretations), and *incapacity* (helplessness in the face of the task). All five dimensions discriminated the very successful from the moderately successful and from the unsuccessful patients.

4. *CICERO: Changes in Language Expression*

We found a variety of changes in both the ratings and the content analyses of the patients' language. Three of these changes were: (1) the language became more socially communicative rather than egocentric; (2) affects were more integrated into expressions rather than remaining isolated; and (3) the vocabulary became more varied in later sessions.

5. *MARX: Changes in Reality Perception and Reality Testing*

We observed fewer changes in these functions than we had expected. We had significant results only in changes in the patient's *self-descriptions*. The four "very" and "moderately" successful patients all described themselves more realistically and less conflictually in the late sessions. And by the end the two very successful patients became more "empathic" in their self-descriptions.

6. *FREUD: Changes in the Capacity for Introspection*

Here the differences in clinical outcome were clearly observable. The raters found that the very successful patients showed the most increase from the beginning to the end in their ability to introspect. Moreover, their introspections were "productive" (complex, profound, more intensely experienced) rather than "intellectualized" or "rationalized," and led to new insights and thorough working-through of conflicts. The raters also found more "good" late analytic sessions in the successful patients. There were also some instances in which the successful patients reflected on their own dream interpretation strategies. Finally, although raters could not find support for our hypothesis that these capacities would be based on demonstrable identifications with the analyst, the analysts and patients were emotionally "closer" to each other at the end. Thus we concluded that the introspective capacities of the successful patients were less inhibited and analytically more fruitful.

7. Changes in Patients' Motivation to Understand Dreams

The raters found an increase in the motivation to understand dreams in one of the very successful patients (P1) and the two moderately successful patients (P2 and P4). Patient 5, the other very successful patient, was already highly motivated to understand his dreams at the beginning of analysis and continued so. The unsuccessful patient showed no increase in this motivation.

4. Summary

We have presented a brief and sketchy overview of a study designed both to generate and to empirically test hypotheses about changes in problem-solving cognitive processes of five patients during their psychoanalyses. In Phase 1 the hypotheses were generated and empirically supported in a project in which we analyzed a diary kept by a transvestite patient on his dreams while in psychoanalysis. In Phase 2 the hypotheses were further tested using verbatim transcripts of four other psychoanalyses stored in the Ulm Textbank (see also Leuzinger-Bohleber in preparation).

The five psychoanalyses were independently and reliably assessed by each of the treating analysts and by two independent analysts, resulting in three outcome categories: "very successful" (Patients 1 and 5), "moderately successful" (Patients 2 and 4), and "unsuccessful" (Patient 3). The most striking result of the study was that the ratings of four judges of a substantial number of theory-derived variables, as well as our computer-aided content analyses, discriminated among the three outcome categories. Of course even our five combined single-case studies are still a small empirical base, but the many results differentiating the three outcomes can serve as specific predictors of success to be tested in future studies of other cases.

Finally, methodologically, our use of an Artificial Intelligence model as a guide for our theory-centered ratings and our computer-aided content analyses has proved quite fruitful. The variety and face validity of many of our results should lead to a better understanding of changes in cognitive processes during psychoanalysis. We believe that this innovative trial of the model was worthwhile and provided us with more consistent, precise, differentiated and practical foci for further empirical studies than existing psychoanalytic theories. We do not go as far as Teller (this volume) when she suggests that Artificial Intelligence can be a basic science for psychoanalysis, but we believe these approaches can be quite useful.

References

Abelson RP (1981) Psychological status of the script concept. American Psychologist 36:715–729

Argelander H (1961) Das Erstinterview in der Psychotherapie. Wissenschaftliche Buchgemeinschaft, Darmstadt

Arlow J (1969a) Unconscious fantasy and disturbances of conscious experience. Psychoanal Q 38:1–27

Arlow J (1969b) Fantasy, memory, and reality testing. Psychoanal Q 38:28–51

Arlow J (1980) The revenge motive in the primal scene. J Am Psychoanal Assoc 28:519–541

Baguet J, Gerin P, Sali M, Marie-Cardine M (1984) Evolution des themes transferentiels individuals dans une psychotherapie de groupe (Application de la méthode du relationnel central) (Evolution of individual transference themes in a group psychotherapy: Application of the core relationship method). Psychotherapies 1-2:43–49

Balint M (1968) The basic fault: therapeutic aspects of regression. Tavistock, London.

Bartlett FC (1932) Remembering. Cambridge Univ Press, Cambridge

Bellak L, Smith MB (1956) An experimental exploration of the psychoanalytic process. Psychoanal Q 25:385–414

Benjamin LS (1974) Structural analysis of social behavior. Psychol Rev 81:392–425

Benjamin LS, Giat L, Estroff S (1981) Manual for coding social interactions in terms of Structural Analysis of Social Behavior (SASB). Unpublished manuscript. Department of Psychiatry, University of Wisconsin School of Medicine, Madison, WI

Bense A (1977) Das Erleben in der Gesprächspsychotherapie. Beltz, Weinheim

Bergin AE, Lambert MH (1978) The evaluation of therapeutic outcomes. In: Garfield SL, Bergin AE (eds) Handbook of psychotherapy and behavior change: an empirical analysis, 2nd ed. Wiley, New York, pp 139–190

Bibring E (1954) Psychoanalysis and the dynamic psychotherapies. J Am Psychoanal Assoc 2:745–770

Blacker KH (1981) Insight. Clinical conceptualizations. J Am Psychoanal Assoc 29:659–671

Blanck G, Blanck R (1974) Ego psychology. Columbia Univ Press, New York

Boder DP (940) The adjective-verb-quotient: a contribution to the psychology of language. Psychological Record 3:310–343

Bollas C (1983) Expressive uses of the countertransference. Contemp Psychoanal 19:1–34

Bowlby J (1969) Attachment and loss, vol I, Attachment. Basic Books, New York

Bowlby J (1979) Psychoanalysis as art and science. Int Rev Psychoanal 6:3–14

Box GEP, Jenkins GM (1976) Time-series analysis: forecasting and control. Holden Day, San Francisco

Brenner C (1985) Countertransference as compromise formation. Psychoanal Q 54:155–163

Bruner JS (1967) On cognitive growth. In: Bruner JS, Olver RR, Greenfield PM et al (eds) Studies in cognitive growth. Wiley, New York, pp 1–67

Bucci W (1984) Linking words and things: basic processes and individual variation. Cognition 17:137–153

Bucci W (1985) Dual coding: a cognitive model for psychoanalytic research. J Am Psychoanal Assoc 33:571–607

Bucci W, Freedman N (1978) Language and hand: the dimension of referential competence. J Pers 46:594–622

Bühler K (1934) Sprachtheorie. Jena

Busemann A (1925) Die Sprache der Jugend als Ausdruck der Entwicklungsrhythmik. Jena

Bush M, Gassner S (1986) The immediate effect of the analyst's termination interventions on the patient's resistance to termination. In: Weiss J, Sampson H, and the Mount Zion Psychotherapy Research Group, The psychoanalytic process: theory, clinical observation, and empirical research. Guilford, New York, pp 299–322

Cartwright R (1966) A comparison of the response to psychoanalytic and client-centered psychotherapy. In: Gottschalk LA, Auerbach AH (eds) Methods of research in psychotherapy. Appleton-Century-Crofts, New York, pp 517–529

Caspar FM, Grawe K (1981) Widerstand in der Verhaltenstherapie. In: Petzold H (eds) Der Widerstand. Ein strittiges Konzept in der Psychotherapie. Junfermann, Paderborn, pp 349–383

Caston J (1986) The reliability of the diagnosis of the patient's unconscious plan. In: Weiss J, Sampson H, and the Mount Zion Psychotherapy Research Group, The psychoanalytic process: theory, clinical observation, and empirical research. Guilford, New York, pp 241–255

Clairborn, CD (1982) Interpretation and change in counseling. J Counseling Psychol 29:439–453

Clippinger J (1977) Meaning and discourse: a computer model of psychoanalytic speech and cognition. Johns Hopkins Univ Press, Baltimore

Cohen J (1960) A coefficient of agreement for nominal scales. Educ Psychol Measurement 20:37–46

Cohen J, Cohen P (1975) Applied multiple regression/correlation analysis for the behavioral sciences. Wiley, New York

Colby K (1981) Modeling a paranoid mind. Brain and Behav Sci 4:515–534

Collins AM, Quillian MR (1972) Experiments on semantic memory and language comprehension. In: Gregg LW (ed) Cognition in learning and memory. Wiley, New York, pp 117–137

Cremerius J (1984) Die psychoanalytische Abstinenzregel. Psyche 38:769–800

Crits-Christoph P (1986) Assessing conscious and unconscious aspects of relationship themes through self-report and naturalistic protocols. Paper presented at the MacArthur Foundation Program on Conscious and Unconscious Mental Processes, Palo Alto, California

Crits-Christoph P, Mintz J, Luborsky L (1987) The size of therapist effects and the problem of non-independence in psychotherapy research. Paper presented to Society for Psychotherapy Research, June 1987

Curtis JT, Silberschatz G (1986) Clinical implications of research on brief dynamic psychotherapy. I. Formulating the patient's problem and goals. Psychoanal Psychol 3:13–25

Curtis JT, Silberschatz G, Sampson H, Weiss J, Rosenberg SE (1988) Developing reliable psychodynamic case formulations: an illustration of the plan diagnosis method. Psychother 25:256-265

Dahl H (1972) A quantitative study of a psychoanalysis. In: Holt RR, Peterfreund E (eds) Psychoanalysis and contemporary science. Macmillan, New York, pp 237–257

Dahl H (1974) The measurement of meaning in psychoanalysis by computer analysis of verbal context. J Am Psychoanal Assoc 22:37–57

Dahl H (1978) A new psychoanalytic model of motivation: emotions as appetites and messages. Psychoanal Contemp Thought 1:373–408

Dahl H (1979a) Word frequencies of spoken American English. Verbatim, Essex

Dahl H (1979b) The appetite hypothesis of emotions: a new psychoanalytic model of motivation. In: Izard CE (ed) Emotions in personality and psychopathology. Plenum Press, New York, pp 199–225

Dahl H (1983) On the definition and measurement of wishes. In: Masling J (ed) Empirical studies of psychoanalytical theories, vol 1. Lawrence Erlbaum Associates, Hillsdale NJ, pp 39–67

Dahl H, Bucci W (in preparation) Characteristics and identification of frames. In: Miller N, Docherty J, Luborsky L (eds) Psychodynamic treatment research. Basic Books, New York

Dahl H, Stengel B (1978) A classification of emotion words: a modification and partial test of de Rivera's decision theory of emotions. Psychoanal Contemp Thought 1:269–312

Davies J (1988) The development of interpersonal and emotional structures in three-year-old children. Doctoral dissertation, Adelphi University, Garden City NY

De la Parra G (1985) Differentielle Textmaße. Auswertungen an einem psychoanalytischen Erstinterviewkorpus. PSZ Verlag, Ulm

Dollard J, Auld F (1959) Scoring human motives: a manual. Yale Univ Press, New Haven

Dollard J, Mowrer OH (1947) A method of measuring tension in written documents. J Abnorm Soc Psychol 42:3–32

Edelson M (1977) Psychoanalysis as science: its boundary problems, special status, relations to other sciences, and formalization. J Nerv Ment Dis 165:1–28

Edelson M (1985) The hermeneutic turn and the single case study in pychoanalysis. Psychoanal Contemp Thought 8:567–614

Ehrenberg DB (1982) Psychoanalytic engagement. Contemp Psychoanal 18:535–555

Eisenmann, F (1973) Die Satzkonjunktionen in gesprochener Sprache. Niemeyer, Tübingen

Ekman P, Friesen WV(1975) Unmasking the face. Prentice-Hall, Englewood-Cliffs

Ekman P, Friesen WV (1979) Manual for the facial action coding system. Consulting Psychologists Press, Palo Alto

Elliot R (1983) Fitting process research to the practicing psychotherapist. Psychother Theory Res Pract 20:47–55

Elliot R (1984) A discovery-oriented approach to significant change events in psychotherapy: interpersonal process recall and comprehensive process analysis. In: Rice L, Greenberg LS (eds) Pattern of change. Guilford, New York, pp 249–286

Ellis A (1970) The essence of rational psychotherapy: a comprehensive approach to treatment. Institute for Rational Living, New York

Finn RH (1970) A note on estimating the reliability of categorical data. Educ Psychol Measurement 30:71–76

Fisher S, Greenberg RP (1977) The scientific credibility of Freud's theories and therapy. Basic Books, New York

Fiske DW (1977) Methodological issues in research on the psychotherapist. In: Gurman AS, Razin AM (eds) Effective psychotherapy: a handbook of research. Pergammon, New York, pp 23–46
Frank J (1982) Persuasion and healing: a comparative study of psychotherapy, 2nd ed. The Johns Hopkins Press, Baltimore
Frenkel-Brunswick E (1949) Intolerance of ambiguity as emotional and perceptual personality variable. J Pers 18:108–143
Fretter PB (1984) The immediate effects of transference interpretations on patient's progress in brief, psychodynamic psychotherapy. Dissertation Abstracts International 46 (6)
Freud S (1897) Letter 69 (to Fliess). SE vol I, pp 259–260
Freud S (1900a) The interpretation of dreams. SE vol IV/V, pp 1–625
Freud S (1905e) Fragment of an analysis of a case of hysteria. SE vol VII, pp 1–122
Freud S (1912b) The dynamics of transference. SE vol XII, pp 97–108
Freud S (1916/17) Introductory lectures on psycho-analysis. SE vol XV/XVI, p 18
Freud S (1918b) From the history of an infantile neurosis. SE vol XVII, pp 1–122
Freud S (1919a) Lines of advance in psycho-analytic therapy. SE vol XVII, pp 157–168
Freud S (1920g) Beyond the pleasure principle. SE vol XVIII, pp 1–64
Freud S (1937d) Constructions in analysis. SE vol XXIII, pp 255–269
Freud S (1940a) An outline of psycho-analysis. SE vol XXIII, pp 139–207
Frick EM (1985) Latent and manifest effects of audiorecording in psychoanalytic psychotherapy. In: Langs R (ed) Yearbook Psychoanalytic Psychotherapy, pp 151–175
Fürstenau P (1977) Praxeologische Grundlagen der Psychoanalyse. In: Pongratz LJ (ed) Handbuch der Psychologie, vol 8 (Klinische Psychologie, 1. Halbband), Hogrefe, Göttingen, pp 847–888
Gardner H (1983) Frames of mind: the theory of multiple intelligences. Basic Books, New York
Gardner H (1985) The mind's new science. Basic Books, New York
Garduk EL, Haggard EA (1972) Immediate effects on patients of psychoanalytic interpretations. Psychological Issues 7, Monograph 28:1–85. Int Univ Press, New York
Garfield SL (1978) Research on client variables in psychotherapy. In: Garfield SL, Bergin AE (eds) Handbook of psychotherapy and behavior change, 2nd ed. Wiley, New York, pp 191–232
Gassner S, Sampson H, Weiss J, Brumer S (1982) The emergence of warded-off contents. Psychoanal Contemp Thought 5:55–75
Gedo J (1979) Theories of object relations: a metapsychological assessment. J Am Psychoanal Assoc 27:361–373
Gendlin ET (1986) What comes after traditional psychotherapy research? Am Psychol 41:131–136
Gendlin ET, Tomlinson TM (1962) The experiencing scale. Mimeographed paper. Wisconsin Psychiatric Institute, Univ of Wisc
Gergen KJ (1985) The social constructionist movement in modern psychology. Am Psychol 40:266–275
Gill MM (1979) The analysis of the transference. J Am Psychoanal Assoc 27 Supplement:263–288
Gill MM (1982) Analysis of transference I: theory and technique. Int Univ Press, New York
Gill MM (1984) Transference: a change in conception or only in emphasis? Psychoanal Inquiry 4:489–523
Gill MM (1985) Discussion - a critique of Robert Langs' conception of transference, evidence by indirection, and the role of frame. In: Langs R (ed) Yearbook Psychoanalytic Psychotherapy 1:177-187

Gill MM, Hoffman IZ (1982a) Analysis of transference II: studies of nine audio-recorded psychoanalytic sessions. Int Univ Press, New York
Gill MM, Hoffman IZ (1982b) A method for studying the analysis of aspects of the patient's experience of the relationship in psychoanalysis and psychotherapy. J Am Psychoanal Assoc 30:137–168
Gill MM, Simon J, Fink G, Endicott NA, Paul IH (1968) Studies in audio-recorded psychoanalysis. I. General considerations. J Am Psychoanal Assoc 16:230–244
Gitelson M (1962) The first phase of psycho-analysis. Int J Psychoanal 43:194–205
Glass G, Willson V, Gottman JM (1975) Design and analysis of time-series experiments. Colorado Assoc Univ Press, Boulder
Glover E (1955) The technique of psychoanalysis. Baillière, Tindall & Cox, London
Gomes-Schwartz B (1978) Effective ingredients in psychotherapy: prediction of outcome from process variables. J Consult Clin Psychol 46:1023–1035
Gottman JM (1981) Time-series analysis: a comprehensive introduction for social scientists. Cambridge Univ Press, Cambridge
Gottman JM, Markman HJ (1978) Experimental designs in psychotherapy research. In: Garfield SL, Bergin AE (eds) Handbook of psychotherapy and behavior change, 2nd ed. Wiley, New York, pp 23–62
Gottschalk LA (1974) The psychoanalytic study of hand-mouth approximations. Psychoanal Contemp Sci 3:269–291
Gottschalk LA, Gleser GC (1969) The measurement of psychological states through the content-analysis of verbal behavior. Calif Univ Press, Berkeley
Greenberg LS (1982) Psychotherapy process research. In: Walker E (ed) Handbook of clinical psychology. Dorsey Press, Homewood IL, pp 164–204
Greenberg LS (1986) Change process research. J Consult Clin Psychol 54:4–9
Greenson RR (1960) Empathy and its vicissitudes. Int J Psychoanal 41:418–424
Greenson RR (1967) The technique and practice of psychoanalysis. Int Univ Press, New York
Grünbaum A (1984) The foundations of psychoanalysis: a philosophical critique. The University of California Press, Berkeley
Grünzig HJ (1985) Zeitreihenanalyse psychoanalytischer Behandlungsverläufe: Stichprobenprobleme und erste Ergebnisse bei einem Einzelfall. In: Czogalik D, Ehlers W, Teufel R (eds) Perspektiven der Psychotherapieforschung: Einzelfall - Gruppe - Institution. Hochschulverlag, Freiburg, pp 566–581
Grünzig HJ, Holzscheck K, Kächele H (1976) EVA - Ein Programmsystem zur maschinellen Inhaltsanalyse von Psychotherapieprotokollen. Med Psychol 2:208–217
Grünzig HJ, Mergenthaler E (1986) Computerunterstützte Ansätze. Empirische Untersuchungen am Beispiel der Angstthemen. In: Koch U, Schöfer G (eds) Sprachinhaltsanalyse in der psychosomatischen und psychiatrischen Forschung. Psychologie Verlags Union, Weinheim München, pp 203–212
Haldane JBS, Smith CAB (1947-49) A simple exact test for birth-order effect. Ann Eugenics 14:117–124
Hans G, Krause R, Steimer E (1986) Interaktionsprozesse bei Schizophrenen. In: Nordman E, Cierpka M (eds) Familienforschung in Psychiatrie und Psychotherapie. Springer, Berlin Heidelberg New York Tokyo, pp 30–51
Harway NI, Dittman AT, Raush HL et al (1955) The measurement of depth of interpretation. J Consult Clin Psychol 19:247–253
Hatcher RL (1973) Insight and self-observation: the development of the concept of insight in psychoanalysis. J Am Psychoanal Assoc 21:377–398
Hayes-Roth F, Waterman D, Lenat D (1978) Principles of pattern-directed inference systems. In: Waterman F, Hayes-Roth F (eds) Pattern-directed inference systems. Academic Press, New York, pp 577–601
Heimann P (1969) Gedanken zum Erkenntnisprozeß des Analytikers. Psyche 23:2–24

Heimann P (1977) Further observations on the analyst's cognitive process. J Am Psychoanal 25:313–333
Hobbs N (1962) Sources of gain in psychotherapy. Am Psychol 17:741–747
Hoffman IZ (1983) The patient as interpreter of the analyst's experience. Contemp Psychoanal 19:389–422
Hoffman IZ (1985) Merton M. Gill: A study in theory development in psychoanalysis. In: Reppen J (ed) Beyond Freud: A study of modern psychoanalytic theorists. Analytic Press, New York, pp 135–174
Hohage R (1985) Das Selbst zwischen Ambivalenz und Ambiguität. Zur Theorie des unbewußten Konfliktes. Forum Psychoanal 1:189–200
Holt RR (1978) Methods in clinical research,vol II: prediction and research. Plenum Press, New York
Horowitz L (1977) Two classes of concomitant change in a psychotherapy. In: Freedman N, Grand S (eds) Communicative structures and psychic structures. Plenum, New York pp 419–440
Horowitz L, Sampson H, Siegelman EY, Wolfson AQ, Weiss J (1975) On the identification of warded-off mental contents. J Abnorm Psychol 84:545–558
Horowitz L, Weckler D, Doren R (1983) Interpersonal problems and symptoms: a cognitive approach. In: Kendall PC (ed) Advances in cognitive-behavioral research and therapy, vol 2:82–127, Academic Press, New York
Horowitz MJ (1979) States of mind: analysis of change in psychotherapy. Plenum, New York London
Horowitz MJ, Marmar C, Krupnick J, Wilner N, Kaltreider N, Wallerstein R (1984) Personality styles and brief psychotherapy. Basic Books, New York, pp 51–67
Hoyt MD, Marmar CR, Horowitz MJ, Alvarex WF (1981) The therapist action scale and the patient action scale: instruments for the assessment of activities during dynamic psychotherapy. Psychotherapy: Theory, Research and Practice 18:109–116
Isaacs K, Haggard EA (1966) Some methods used in the study of affect in psychotherapy. In: Gottschalk LA, Auerbach AH (eds) Methods of research in psychotherapy. Appleton-Century-Crofts, New York, pp 226–239
Jones E, Windholz M (submitted for publication) The psychoanalytic case study: toward a method for systematic inquiry. Paper presented to the George Klein Research Forum at the American Psychoanalytic Assoc., Dec. 1987
Kächele H (1983) Verbal activity level of therapists in initial interviews and long-term psychoanalysis. In: Minsel WR, Herff W (eds) Methodology in psychotherapy research. Lang, Frankfurt, pp 125–129
Kächele H. Mergenthaler E (1983) Computer-aided analysis of psychotherapeutic discourse. In: Minsel WR, Herff W (eds) Methodology in psychotherapy research. Lang, Frankfurt , pp 116–161
Kächele H, Mergenthaler E (1984) Auf dem Wege zur computerunterstützten Textanalyse in der psychotherapeutischen Prozeßforschung. In: Baumann U (ed) Psychotherapie: Makro-/Mikroperspektive. Verlag für Psychologie Dr. CJ Hogrefe, Göttingen, pp 223–239
Kächele H, Schaumburg C, Thomä H (1973) Verbatimprotokolle als Mittel in der psychotherapeutischen Verlaufsforschung. Psyche 27:902–927
Kächele H, Thomä H, Schaumburg C (1975) Veränderungen des Sprachinhaltes in einem psychoanalytischen Prozeß. Schweizer Archiv für Neurologie, Neurochirurgie und Psychiatrie 116:197–228
Kafka JS (1971) Ambiguity for individuation. Arch Gen Psychiatry 25:232–239
Kernberg OF (1975) Borderline conditions and pathological narcissism. Aronson, New York

Kernberg OF (1982) Supportive psychotherapy with borderline conditions. In: Cavener JO, Brodie HK (eds) Critical problems in psychiatry. Lippincott, Philadelphia

Kernberg OF (1984) From the Menninger Project to a research strategy for long-term psychotherapy of borderline personality disorder. In: Williams JBW, Spitzer RL (eds) Psychotherapy research: where are we and where should we go? Guilford Press, New York

Kernberg OF, Burstein E, Coyne L, Appelbaum A, Horowitz L, Voth H (1972) Psychotherapy and psychoanalysis. Bull Menn Clin 36:1–178

Kiesler DJ (1966) Some myths of psychotherapy research and the search for a paradigm. Psychol Bull 65:110–136

Klein MH, Mathieu PL, Gendlin ET, Kiesler DJ (1970) The experiencing scale: a research training manual. Madison, WI, Univ of Wisconsin

Klerman GL, Weissman MM, Rounsaville BJ, Chevron ES (1984) Interpersonal psychotherapy of depression. Basic Books, New York

Knapp PH, Greenberg RP, Pearlman CH, Cohen M, Kantrowitz J, Sashin J (1975) Clinical measurement in psychoanalysis: an approach. Psychoanal Q 44:404–430

Koch U, Schöfer G (1986) Sprachinhaltsanalyse in der psychosomatischen und psychiatrischen Forschung. Psychologie Verlagsunion, Weinheim München

Koenigsberg HW, Kernberg OF, Haas G (1985) Development of a scale for measuring techniques in the psychotherapy of borderline patients. J Nerv Ment Dis 173:424–431

Kohut H (1971) The analysis of the self: a systematic approach to the psychoanalytic treatment of narcissistic personality disorders. Int Univ Press, New York

Körner J, Rosin U (1985) Das Problem der Abstinenz in der Psychoanalyse. Forum Psychoanal 1:25–47

Krause R (1980) Stuttering and nonverbal communication: investigations about affect inhibition and stuttering. In: Giles H, Robinson WP, Smith PM (eds) First international conference on social psychology and language. Pergamon Press, Oxford, pp 261–266

Krause R (1981) Sprache und Affekt. Untersuchungen über das Stottern. Kohlhammer, Stuttgart

Krause R (1982a) A social psychological approach to the study of stuttering. In: Fraser C, Scherer KR (eds) Advances in the social psychology of language. Cambridge Univ Press, Cambridge, pp 77–122

Krause R (1982b) Kernbereiche psychoanalytischen Handelns. Nervenarzt 53:504–512

Krause R (1985) Psychotherapie. In: Lantermann ED, Herrmann T (eds) Persönlichkeitspsychologie. Ein Handbuch in Schlüsselbegriffen. Urban & Schwarzenberg, München, pp 147–154

Kris E (1956) On some vicissitudes of insight in psychoanalysis. Int J Psychoanal 37:445–455

Kubie LS (1958) Research into the process of supervision in psychoanalysis. Psychoanal Q 27:226–236

Lacan J (1968) The language of the self. Johns Hopkins Press, Baltimore

Langs, R (1978) Technique in transition. Jason Aronson, New York

Lawlis GF, Lu E (1972) Judgment of counseling process: reliability, agreement, and error. Psychol Bull 78:17–20

Leary T (1957) Interpersonal diagnosis of personality. Ronald Press, New York

Leeds J (1986) A reliable method for the detection of repetitive structures in a transcript of an analytic session. Paper presented at annual meeting of Society for Psychotherapy Research, Boston, Mass.

Leeds J (1988) Repetition, science and psychoanalysis: theoretical considerations and an empirical study. Doctoral Dissertation, Adelphi University, Garden City NY

Leuzinger M (1984) Psychotherapeutische Denkprozesse. Kognitive Prozesse bei der Indikation psychotherapeutischer Verfahren. PSZ-Verlag, Ulm

Leuzinger-Bohleber M (1987) Veränderung kognitiver Prozesse in Psychoanalysen, vol I Eine hypothesengenerierende Einzelfallstudie. Springer, Berlin Heidelberg New York Tokyo

Leuzinger-Bohleber M (in preparation) Veränderung kognitiver Prozesse in Psychoanalysen, vol II Fünf aggregierte Einzelfallstudien.

Levenson E (1983) The ambiguity of change. Basic Books, New York

Levine FJ, Luborsky L (1981) The core conflictual relationship theme method: a demonstration of reliable clinical inferences by the method of mismatched cases. In: Tuttman S, Kay C, Zimmerman M (eds) Object and self: a developmental approach. Int Univ Press, New York, pp 501–526

Lienert GA (1969) Testaufbau und Testanalyse. Beltz, Weinheim

Loewald H (1960) On the therapeutic action of psychoanalysis. Int J Psychoanal 41:16–33

Loewald H (1971) The transference neurosis: comments on the concept and the phenomenon. J Am Psychoanal Assoc 19:54–66

Lolas F, Mergenthaler E, Rad von M (1982) Content analysis of verbal behavior in psychotherapy research: a comparison between two methods. Br J Med Psychol 55:327–333

Lorenz M, Cobb S (1975) Language and a woman's place. Harper & Row, New York

Luborsky L (1967) Momentary forgetting during psychotherapy and psychoanalysis: a theory and research method. In: Holt RR (ed) Motives and thought: psychoanalytic essays in honor of David Rapaport. Int Univ Press, New York, pp 177–217

Luborsky L (1970) New directions in research on neurotic and psychosomatic symptoms. American Scientist 58:661–668

Luborsky L (1975) Clinicians' judgments of mental health: specimen case descriptions and forms for the Health-Sickness Rating Scale. Bull Menn Clin 35:448–480

Luborsky L (1976) Helping alliance in psychotherapy: the groundwork for a study of their relationship to its outcome. In: Claghorn JL (ed) Successful psychotherapy. Brunner/Mazel, New York, pp 92–116

Luborsky L (1977) Measuring a pervasive psychic structure in psychotherapy: the core conflictual relationship theme. In: Freedman N, Grand S (eds) Communicative structures and psychic structures. Plenum Press, New York, pp 367–395

Luborsky L (1984) Principles of psychoanalytic psychotherapy: a manual for supportive-expressive psychotherapy. Basic Books, New York

Luborsky L (latest ed 1986) The core conflictual relationship theme (CCRT) method: a guide to scoring and rationale. (unpublished, available upon request)

Luborsky L, Auerbach AH (1969) The symptom-context method. J Am Psychoanal Assoc 17:68–99

Luborsky L, Strupp H (1962) Research problems in psychotherapy: a three-year-follow-up. In: Strupp HH, Luborsky L (eds) Research in psychotherapy, vol II. American Psychological Association, Washington DC, p 308–329

Luborsky L, Bachrach H, Graff H, Pulver S, Christoph P (1979) Preconditions and consequences of transference interpretations: a clinical-quantitative investigation. J Nerv Ment Dis 167:391–401

Luborsky L, Chandler M, Auerbach AH, Cohen J, Bachrach HM (1971) Factors influencing the outcome of psychotherapy: a review of quantitative research. Psychol Bull 75:145–185

Luborsky L, Crits-Christoph P, Alexander L, Margolis M, Cohen M (1983) Two helping alliance methods for predicting outcomes of psychotherapy: a counting signs versus a global rating method. J Nerv Ment Dis 171:480–492

Luborsky L, Crits-Christoph P, Mellon J (1986) The advent of objective measures of the transference concept. J Consult Clin Psychol 54:39–47
Luborsky L, Graff H, Pulver S, Curtis H (1973) A clinical-quantitative examination of consensus on the concept of transference. Arch Gen Psychiatry 29:69–75
Luborsky L, Kächele H (1988) (eds) Der zentrale Beziehungskonflikt. Ein Arbeitsbuch. PSZ-Verlag, Ulm
Luborsky L, Mellon J, Alexander K, Van Ravenswaay P, Childress A, Levine F, Cohen KD, Hole AV, Ming S (1985) A verification of Freud's grandest clinical hypothesis: the transference. Clin Psychol Rev 5:231–246
Luborsky L, Mintz J, Auerbach A, Christoph P, Bachrach H (1980) Predicting the outcomes of psychotherapy: findings of the Penn Psychotherapy Project. Arch Gen Psychiatry 37:471–481
Luborsky L, Singer B, Hartke J, Crits-Christoph P, Cohen M (1984) Shifts in depressive state during psychotherapy: which concepts of depression fit the context of Mr. Q's shifts? In: Rice L, Greenberg LS (eds) Patterns of change. Guilford Press, New York, pp 157–193
Macalpine I (1950) The development of the transference. Psychoanal Q 19:501–539
Mahl GF (1961) Measures of two expressive aspects of a patient's speech in two psychotherapeutic interviews. In: Gottschalk LA (ed) Comparative psycholinguistic analysis of two psychotherapeutic interviews. Int Univ Press, New York, pp 91–114
Mahrer AR (1985) Psychotherapeutic change: an alternative approach to meaning and measurement. Norton, New York
Malan DH (1963) A study of brief psychotherapy. Tavistock, London
Malan DH (1976 a) The frontiers of brief psychotherapy: an example of the convergence of research and clinical practice. Plenum Press, New York
Malan DH (1976 b) Toward the validation of dynamic psychotherapy. Plenum Press, New York
Mandler G (1984) Mind and body. Norton, New York
Mann J (1973) Time-limited psychotherapy. Harvard Univ Press, Cambridge
Marziali EA (1984) Prediction of outcome of brief psychotherapy from therapist interpretive interventions. Arch Gen Psychiatry 41:301–304
Marziali EA, Sullivan J (1980) Methodological issues in the content analysis of brief psychotherapy. Br J Med Psychol 53:19–27
Masterson JF (1976) Psychotherapy of the borderline adult: a developmental perspective. Brunner/Mazel, New York
McCleary R, Hay RA jr (1980) Applied time series analysis for the social sciences. Sage, London
McNair DM, Lorr M (1964) An analysis of professed psychotherapeutic techniques. J Consult Clin Psychol 28:265–271
Meichenbaum D, Gilmore JB (1984) The nature of unconscious processes: a cognitive-behavioral perspective. In: Bowers K, Meichenbaum D (eds) The unconscious reconsidered. Wiley, New York, pp 273–298
Meissner WW (1979) Internalisation and object relations. J Am Psychoanal Assoc 27:345–360
Mergenthaler E (1985) Textbank systems: computer science applied in the field of psychoanalysis. Springer, Berlin Heidelberg New York Tokyo
Mergenthaler E (1986) Die Ulmer Textbank - Entwurf und Realisierung eines Textbankverwaltungssystems als Beitrag der Angewandten Informatik zur Forschung in der Psychoanalyse. Springer, Berlin Heidelberg New York Tokyo
Meyer AE (1981) Psychoanalytische Prozeßforschung zwischen Skylla der "Verkürzung" und der Charybdis der "systematischen akustischen Lücke". Z Psychosom Med Psychoanal 27:103–116

Minsky M (1975) A framework for representing knowledge. In: Winston PH (ed) The psychology of computer vision. McGraw-Hill, New York, pp 211–277
Mintz J, Luborsky L (1971) Segments versus whole sessions: which is the better unit for psychotherapy process research? J Abnorm Psychol 78:180–191
Mintz J, Luborsky L, Auerbach AH (1971) Dimensions of psychotherapy: a factor-analytic study of ratings of psychotherapy sessions. J Consult Clin Psychol 36:106–120
Mitchell KM, Berenson BG (1970) Differential use of confrontation by high and low facilitative therapists. J Nerv Ment Dis 151:303–309
Mitchell KM, Bozarth JD, Krauft CC (1977) A reappraisal of the therapeutic effectiveness of accurate empathy, non-possessive warmth, and genuineness. In: Gurman AS, Razin AM (eds) Effective psychotherapy: a handbook of research. Pergamon Press, New York, pp 482–502
Morgan R, Luborsky L, Crits-Christoph P, Curtis H, Solomon J (1982) Predicting the outcomes of psychotherapy by the Penn Helping Alliance method. Arch Gen Psychology 39:397–402
Moser U, Pfeifer R, Schneider W, Zeppelin I von (1980) Computersimulation von Schlaftraumprozessen. Berichte aus der Interdisziplinären Konfliktforschungsstelle der Universität Zürich, Nr. 6
Myerson PG (1965) Modes of insight. J Am Psychoanal Assoc 13:771–792
Neisser U (1976) Cognition and reality. Freeman, San Francisco
Neudert L, Kübler JC, Schors R (1985) Die inhaltsanalytische Erfassung von Leiden im psychotherapeutischen Prozeß. In: Czogalik D, Ehlers W, Teufel R (eds) Perspektiven der Psychotherapieforschung: Einzelfall - Gruppe - Institution. Hochschulverlag, Freiburg, pp 120–135
O'Dell J, Winder P (1975) Evaluation of a content-analysis system for therapeutic interview. J Clinic Psychol 31:737–744
Ogden T (1982) Projective identification and psychotherapeutic technique. Jason Aronson, New York
O'Malley SS, Suh CS, Strupp HH (1983) The Vanderbilt Psychotherapy Process Scale. J Consult Clin Psychol 51:581–586
Orlinsky DE, Howard KI (1978) The relation of process to outcome in psychotherapy. In: Garfield SL, Bergin AE (eds) Handbook of psychotherapy and behavior change: an empirical analysis, 2nd ed. Wiley, New York, pp 283–329
Paivio A (1971) Imagery and verbal processes. Holt, Rinehart & Winston, New York
Paivio A (1978) The relationship between verbal and perceptual codes. In: Carterette EC, Friedman MP (eds) Handbook of perception: perceptual coding 8. Academic Press, New York, pp 375–397
Parloff MB, Rubinstein EA (1962) Research problems in psychotherapy. In: Rubinstein EA, Parloff MB (eds) Research in psychotherapy, vol I. American Psychological Association, Washington DC, p 276–292
Parloff MB, Waskow IE, Wolfe BE (1978) Research on therapist variables in relation to process and outcome. In: Garfield SL, Bergin AE (eds) Handbook of psychotherapy and behavior change: an empirical analysis, 2nd ed. Wiley, New York, pp 233–282
Parunak DV (1982) Data base design for biblical texts. In: Bailey RW (ed) Computing in the humanities. North-Holland, pp 149–161.
Pepinsky HB (1979) A computer-assisted language analysis system (CALAS) and its applications. ERIC Document Reproduction Service, Arlington
Peterfreund E (1975) How does the analyst listen: on models and strategies in the analytic process. Psychoanal Contemp Sci 4:59–101
Pfeifer R, Leuzinger-Bohleber M (1986) Applications of cognitive science methods to psychoanalysis: a case study and some theory. Int Rev Psychoanal 13:221–240
Piaget J (1952) The origins of intelligence in children. Int Univ Press, New York

Pressman MD (1969) The cognitive function of the ego in psychoanalysis. I. The search for insight. Int J Psychoanal 50:187–196

Protter B (1985) Toward an emergent psychoanalytic epistemology. Contemp Psychoanal 21:208–227

Racker H (1968) Transference and countertransference. Int Univ Press, New York

Ramzy I (1974) How the mind of the psychoanalyst works: an essay on psychoanalytic inference. Int J Psychoanal 55:543–550

Raskin NJ (1949) An analysis of six parallel studies of the therapeutic process. J Consult Clin Psychol 13:206–221

Reid JR, Finesinger JE (1952) The role of insight in psychotherapy. Am J Psychiatry 108:726–734

Reynes R, Martindale C, Dahl H (1984) Lexical differences between working and resistance sessions in psychoanalysis. J Clin Psychol 40:733–737

Rice L, Greenberg LS (1984) The new research paradigm. In: Rice L, Greenberg LS (eds) Pattern of change. Guilford Press, New York, pp 7–26

Rich E (1983) Artificial intelligence. McGraw-Hill, New York

Richfield J (1954) An analysis of the concept of insight. Psychoanal Q 23:390–408

Roback HB (1974) Insight: a bridging of the theoretical and research literatures. Can J Psychol 15:61–88

Rogers C (1957) The necessary and sufficient conditions of therapeutic personality change. J Consult Psychol 21:95–103

Rosch E (1978) Principles of categorization. In: Rosch E, Lloyd B (eds) Cognition and categorization. Erlbaum, Hillsdale, pp 27–48

Rosen VH (1974) The nature of verbal interventions in psychoanalysis. Psychoanal Contemp Sci 3:189–209

Rosenbaum M, Friedlander J, Kaplan S (1956) Evaluation of results of psychotherapy. Psychosom Med 18:113–132

Rosenberg S, Silberschatz G, Curtis J, Sampson H, Weiss J (1986) A method for establishing reliability of statements from psychodynamic case formulations. Am J Psychiatry 143:1454–1456

Rounsaville BJ, Chevron ES, Weissman MM (1984) Specification of techniques in interpersonal psychotherapy. In: Williams JBW, Spitzer RL (eds) Psychotherapy research: Where are we and where should we go? Guilford Press, New York

Ruberg W (1982) Untersuchung sprachlicher Reaktionen von Patienten auf Tonbandaufnahmen. Doctoral Dissertation, University of Ulm

Rubinstein B (1978) Psychoanalytic hypotheses and the problem of their confirmation. In: Irani K, Horowitz L, Myers G (eds) Pathology and consciousness. Haven, New York pp 35–50

Sachs JS (1983) Negative factors in brief psychotherapy: an empirical assessment. J Consult Clin Psychol 51:557–564

Sampson H, Weiss J (1986) Testing hypotheses: the approach of the Mount Zion Psychotherapy Research Group. In: Greenberg LS, Pinsof W (eds) The psychotherapeutic process: a research handbook. Guilford Press, New York, pp 591–613

Sandler J (1976) Countertransference and role-responsiveness. Int Rev Psychoanal 3:43–48

Sargent, HD, Horowitz L, Wallerstein RS, Appelbaum A (1968) Prediction in psychotherapy research. Psychological Issues 6

Schacht TE, Henry WP (1983) Vanderbilt interpersonal locus of control scale (VILCS). Unpublished instrument. Department of Psychology, Vanderbilt University, Nashville, TN

Schacht TE, Binder JL, Strupp HH (1984) The dynamic focus. In: Strupp HH, Binder JL Psychotherapy in a new key: a guide to time-limited dynamic psychotherapy. Basic Books, New York, pp 65–109

Schacht TE, Strupp HH, Henry WP (1984) On integrating psychotherapy research: the principle of P-T-O congruence (unpublished manuscript)
Schafer R (1980) Action and narration in psychoanalysis. New Lit Hist 12:6185
Schaffer ND (1982) Multidimensional measures of therapist behavior as predictors of outcome. Psychol Bull 92:670–681
Schank RC, Abelson RP (1977) Scripts, plans, goals, and understanding: an inquiry into human knowledge structures. Erlbaum, Hillsdale
Scherer KR (1978) Personality inference from voice quality: the loud voice of extroversion. Eur J Soc Psychol 8:467–487
Schlörer J (1978) Probleme des Datenschutzes und der Datensicherung bei "anonymen" Daten. Med. Welt 29:777–781
Segal H (1962) The curative factors in psycho-analysis. Int J Psychoanal 43:212–217
Silberschatz G (1978) Effects of the analyst's neutrality on the patient's feelings and behavior in the psychoanalytic situation. Doctoral Dissertation, New York University
Silberschatz G (1984) Effect size and the unit of measurement in psychodynamic psychotherapy research. Paper presented at the National Institute of Mental Health conference on methodologic challenges in psychodynamic research, Washington, D. C.
Silberschatz G (1986) Testing pathogenic beliefs. In: Weiss J, Sampson H, and the Mount Zion Psychotherapy Research Group, The psychoanalytic process: theory, clinical observation, and empirical research. Guilford Press, New York, pp 256–266
Silberschatz G, Curtis JT (1986) Clinical implications of research on brief dynamic psychotherapy. II. How the therapist helps or hinders therapeutic progress. Psychoanal Psychol 3:27–37
Silberschatz G, Fretter PB, Curtis JT (1986a) How do interpretations influence the process of psychotherapy? J Consult Clinic Psychol 54:646–652
Silberschatz G, Sampson H, Weiss J (1986b) Testing pathogenic beliefs versus seeking transference gratifications. In: Weiss J, Sampson H, and the Mount Zion Psychotherapy Research Group, The psychoanalytic process: theory, clinical observation, and empirical research. Guilford Press, New York, pp 267–276
Simon HA (1981) The sciences of the artificial, 2nd ed. MIT Press, Cambridge
Simon HA, Newell A (1970) Human problem solving. Am Psychologist 25:48–59
Simon J, Fink G, Endicott NA (1967) A study of silence. J Hillside Hospital 16:224-233
Singer JL (1984) Transference and the human condition: a cognitive-affective perspective. Paper presented at the meeting of the American Psychological Association, Toronto
Slap J (1986) Some problems with the structural model and a remedy. Psychoanalytic Psychology 3:47–58
Slap J, Slaykin A (1983) The schema: basic concept in a nonmetapsychological model of the mind. Psychoanal Contemp Thought 6:305–325
Sloane RB, Staples FR, Cristol AH, Yorkston NJ, Whipple K (1975) Psychotherapy versus behavior therapy. Harvard University Press, Cambridge MA
Smith EE (1985) Cognitive psychology (correspondent's report). Artificial Intelligence 25:247–253
Smith ML, Glass G, Miller T (1980) The benefits of psychotherapy. Johns Hopkins University Press, Baltimore
Speidel H (1979) Entwicklung und Validierung eines Wörterbuches zur maschinell-inhaltsanalytischen Erfassung psychoanalytischer Angstthemen. Psychol. Dipl.-Arbeit, Konstanz und Ulm
Spence DP (1968) The processing of meaning in psychotherapy: some links with psycholinguistics and information theory. Behav Sci 13:349–361

Spence DP (1982) Narrative truth and historical truth: meaning and interpretation in psychoanalysis. Norton, New York

Steimer E, Krause R, Sänger-Alt C, Wagner G (1988) Mimisches Verhalten von Schizophrenen und ihren Gesprächspartnern. Z Klin Psychol 2:132–147

Stern DP (1985) Some controversies regarding constructionism and psychoanalysis. Contemp Psychoanal 21:201–208

Stiles WB, Shapiro DA, Elliott R (1986) Are all psychotherapies equivalent? Am Psychologist 41:165–180

Stone L (1967) The psychoanalytic situation and transference: postscript to an earlier communication. J Am Psychoanal Assoc 15:3–58

Stone PJ, Dunphy DC, Smith MS, Ogilvie M (1966) The general inquirer: a computer approach to content analysis. The MIT-Press, London

Strunk W jr, White EB (1972) The elements of style. MacMillan, New York

Strupp HH (1957) A multidimensional system for analyzing psychotherapy techniques. Psychiatry 20:293–306

Strupp HH (1978a) Suffering and psychotherapy. Contemp Psychoanal 14:73–97

Strupp HH (1978b) Psychotherapy research and practice: an overview. In: Garfield SL, Bergin AE (eds) Handbook of psychotherapy and behavior change: an empirical analysis, 2nd ed. Wiley, New York, pp 3–22

Strupp HH (1980a) Success and failure in time-limited psychotherapy: a systematic comparison of two cases (Comparison 1). Arch Gen Psychiatry 37:595–603

Strupp HH (1980b) Success and failure in time-limited psychotherapy: a systematic comparison of two cases (Comparison 2). Arch Gen Psychiatry 37:708–716

Strupp HH (1980d) Success and failure in time-limited psychotherapy: further evidence (Comparison 4). Arch Gen Psychiatry 37:947–954

Strupp HH (1986) Psychotherapy: research, practice and, public policy (How to avoid dead ends). Am Psychol 41:120–130

Strupp HH, Binder JL (1984) Psychotherapy in a new key: A guide to time-limited dynamic psychotherapy. Basic Books, New York

Strupp HH, Hadley SW (1979) Specific versus nonspecific factors in psychotherapy: a controlled study of outcome. Arch Gen Psychiatry 36:1125–1136

Strupp HH, Chassan JB, Ewing JA (1966) Toward the longitudinal study of the psychotherapeutic process. In: Gottschalk LA, Auerbach AH (eds) Methods of research in psychotherapy. Appleton-Century-Crofts, New York, pp 361–400

Teller V, Dahl H (1981a) The framework for a model of psychoanalytic inference. Proceedings of the Seventh International Joint Conference on Artificial Intelligence 1:394–400

Teller V, Dahl H (1981b) Clinical artificial intelligence - a commentary on Colby (1981). Behav and Brain Sci 4:549–550

Teller V, Dahl H (1984) Recurrent structures in psychoanalytic discourse: candidates for pattern-directed inference. Technical Report CS-TR 84-01, Computer Science Dep, Hunter College CUNY

Teller V, Dahl H (1986) The microstructure of free association. J Am Psychoanal Assoc 34:763–798

Textor AM (1962) Sag es treffender, 4th edn. Essen

Thomä H (1981) Schriften zur Praxis der Psychoanalyse: Vom spiegelnden zum aktiven Psychoanalytiker. Suhrkamp, Frankfurt am Main

Thomä H, Kächele H (1975) Problems of metascience and methodology in clinical psychoanalytic research. Annu Psychoanal, vol III. Int Univ Press, New York, pp 49–119

Thomä H, Kächele H (1985) Lehrbuch der psychoanalytischen Therapie, vol 1 Grundlagen. Springer, Berlin Heidelberg New York Tokyo

Thomä H, Kächele H (1987) Psychoanalytic practice, vol I Principles. Springer, Berlin Heidelberg New York Tokyo

Thomä H, Rosenkötter L (1970) Über die Verwendung audiovisueller Hilfsmittel in der psychotherapeutischen Ausbildung. Didacta Medica 4:108–112
Thomä H, Schrenk H, Kächele H (1985) Der psychoanalytische Dialog und die Gegenfrageregel. Forum Psychoanal 1:4–24
Tinsley HE, Weiss DJ (1975) Interrater reliability and agreement of subjective judgments. J Counsel Psychol 22:358–376
Tomkins SS (1979) Script theory: Differential magnification of affects. In: Howe HE, Diensbier RA (eds) Nebraska symposium on motivation. University of Nebraska Press, Lincoln, vol 26, pp 201–236
Truax CB (1963) Effective ingredients in psychotherapy. J Counsel Psychol 10:256–263
Truax CB, Mitchell KM (1971) Research on certain therapist interpersonal skills in relation to process and outcome. In: Bergin AE, Garfield SL (eds) Handbook of psychotherapy and behavior change: an empirical analysis. Wiley, New York, pp 299–344
Valenstein AF (1962) The psycho-analytic situation: affects, emotional reliving, and insight in the psychoanalytic process. Int J Psychoanal 43:315–324
Wachtel PL (1982) Vicious circles: The self and the rhetoric of emerging and unfolding. Contemp Psychoanal 18:259–273
Wallerstein RS, Sampson H (1971) Issues in research in the psychoanalytic process. Int J Psychoanal 52:11–50
Waterman D, Hayes-Roth F (eds) (1978) Pattern-directed inference systems. Academic Press, New York
Weiss J (1986) Theory and clinical observations. In: Weiss J, Sampson H, and the Mount Zion Psychotherapy Research Group, The psychoanalytic process: theory, clinical observation, and empirical research. Guilford Press, New York, pp 3–138
Weiss J, Sampson H, and the Mount Zion Psychotherapy Research Group (1986), The psychoanalytic process: theory, clinical observation, and empirical research. Guilford Press, New York
Weizenbaum J (1966) ELIZA - a computer program for the study of natural language communication between man and machine. Communications of the ACM 9:36–45
Wexler DA (1974) A cognitive theory of experiencing, self actualisation and therapeutic process. In: Wexler DA, Rice L (eds) Innovations in client-centered therapy. Wiley, New York, pp 49–116
Winston PH (1984) Artificial intelligence. Addison-Wesley, Reading
Wirtz EM, Kächele H (1983) Emotive aspects of therapeutic language: a pilot study on verb-adjective-ratio. In: Minsel WR, Herff W (eds) Methodology in pychotherapy research. Lang, Frankfurt, pp 130–135
Yeaton W, Sechrest L (1981) Critical dimensions in the choice and maintenance of successful treatments, strength, and effectiveness. J Consult Clinic Psychol 49:156–157
Zajonc RB (1980) Feeling and thinking: preferences need no inferences. Am Psychol 35:151–175
Zetzel ER (1971) A developmental approach to the borderline patient. Am J Psychiatry 127:867–871
Zimmer JM, Cowles KH (1972) Content analysis using FORTRAN. J Counsel Psychol 19:161-166
Zolik ES, Hollon TW (1960) Factors characteristic of patients responsive to brief psychotherapy. Am Psychol 15:387

Name Index

E

F

G

H

I

J

K

L

M

N

O

U

V

W

Y

Z

Subject Index

A

B

C

D

E

F

N

O

P

T